PocketRadiologist™
Head and Neck
100 Top Diagnoses

PocketRadiologist™
Head and Neck
100 Top Diagnoses

H Ric Harnsberger MD

Professor of Radiology
R C Willey Chair in Neuroradiology
University of Utah School of Medicine
Salt Lake City, Utah

Patricia A Hudgins MD

Professor of Radiology/Neuroradiology
Head and Neck Imaging
Emory University Hospital
Atlanta, Georgia

Richard H Wiggins III MD

Assistant Professor of Radiology
Head and Neck Imaging
University of Utah School of Medicine
Salt Lake City, Utah

H Christian Davidson MD

Chief of Radiology, VA Medical Center
Salt Lake City, Utah

Assistant Professor of Radiology
University of Utah School of Medicine
Salt Lake City, Utah

With contributions by: *Anne G Osborn*
                           Karen L Salzman

With 200 drawings and radiographic images

Drawings: *Lane R Bennion MS*
                 James A Cooper MD
Image Editing: *Ming Q Huang MD*
                 Melissa Petersen

AMIRSYS

W. B. SAUNDERS COMPANY
An Elsevier Science Company

ii

AMIRSYS
A medical reference publishing company

First Edition

Text – Copyright H Ric Harnsberger 2002

Drawings – Copyright Amirsys Inc 2002

Compilation – Copyright Amirsys Inc 2002

First Printing: November 2001
Second Printing: April 2002

Composition by Amirsys Inc, Salt Lake City, Utah

Printed by K/P Corporation, Salt Lake City, Utah

ISBN: 0-7216-9697-X

Preface

The **PocketRadiologist**™ series is an innovative, quick reference designed to deliver succinct, up-to-date information to practicing professionals "at the point of service." As close as your pocket, each title in the series is written by world-renowned authors, specialists in their area. These experts have designated the "top 100" diagnoses in every major body area, bulleted the most essential facts, and offered high-resolution imaging to illustrate each topic. Selected references are included for further review. Full color anatomic-pathologic computer graphics model many of the actual diseases.

Each **PocketRadiologist**™ title follows an identical format. The same information is in the same place—every time—and takes you quickly from key facts to imaging findings, differential diagnosis, pathology, pathophysiology, and relevant clinical information.

PocketRadiologist™ titles are available in both print and hand-held PDA formats. Our first modules feature Brain, Head and Neck, and Orthopedic (Musculoskeletal) Imaging. Additional titles include Spine and Cord, Chest, Breast, Vascular, Cardiac, Pediatrics, Emergency, and Genital Urinary, and Gastro Intestinal. Enjoy!

Anne G Osborn MD
Editor-in-Chief, Amirsys Inc

PocketRadiologist™
Head and Neck
Top 100 Diagnoses

The diagnoses in this book are divided into 15 sections in the following order:

CPA-IAC
Skull Base
Temporal Bone
Orbit
Nose & Sinus
Pharyngeal Mucosal Space
Lymph Nodes
Larynx
Oral Cavity
Masticator Space
Parotid Space
Carotid Space
Midline Spaces
Visceral Space
Pediatric Lesions

Table of Diagnoses

Orbit

Nose & Sinus

Pharyngeal Mucosal Space

Lymph Nodes

Notice and Disclaimer

PocketRadiologist™
Head and Neck
100 Top Diagnoses

CPA - IAC

Epidermoid Cyst, CPA

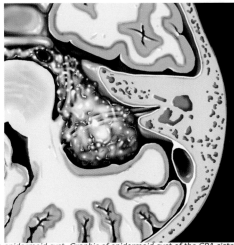

CPA cistern epidermoid cyst. Graphic of epidermoid cyst of the CPA cistern illustrates the "bed of pearls" seen by the surgeon. The tendency of this lesion to engulf the cisternal portions of cranial nerves VII and VIII is depicted.

Key Facts
- Synonyms: Epidermoid tumor; non-neoplastic inclusion cyst
- Definition: Congenital lesion that arises from inclusion of ectodermal epithelial elements at the time of neural tube closure during the 3rd to 5th week of embryonic life, resulting in migration abnormalities of epiblastic cells
- Classic imaging appearance: Signal shows an **insinuating cisternal lesion** with low T1, high T2 close to that of CSF
  - FLAIR shows incomplete or absent attenuation
  - Diffusion-weighted imaging shows epidermoid cyst (EpC) has restricted diffusion (high-signal lesion)
- Other key facts
  - 3rd most common CPA-IAC mass
  - 1% of all intracranial tumors

Imaging Findings
General Imaging Features
- Best imaging clue: Cisternal insinuation
  - Engulfs cranial nerves and vessels
- Mass **insinuates** into cisterns, engulfs cranial nerves and vessels
- Margins usually scalloped or irregular
CT Findings
- Resembles CSF on NECT scans
- Calcification in 20%
- No enhancement is rule; sometimes margin of cyst minimally enhances
- "Dense epidermoid" = rare variant
MR Findings
- Signal close to CSF on all standard MR sequences
  - T1 low, T2 high signal
  - T1 C+ images show EpC **does not enhance**
- "Dirty CSF" = MR description

1

Epidermoid Cyst, CPA

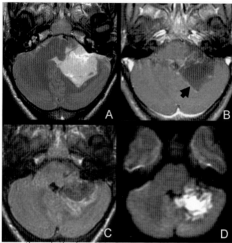

Axial MR images through the low CPA cistern. T2 (A), T1 C+ (B), FLAIR (C) and diffusion (D) sequences are shown. High T2 signal, non-attenuation on FLAIR and diffusion restriction (high lesion signal in D) is characteristic of EpC. Insinuating margins and thin rim enhancement (arrow in B) also typical.

- FLAIR/CISS and diffusion MR are diagnostic
  - Does not null on FLAIR or CISS
  - High signal on diffusion scans (restricted diffusion)
- "White EpC" (high signal on T1) rare

Imaging Recommendations
- Begin with routine enhanced MR imaging
- FLAIR and diffusion sequences added to confirm diagnosis
- Follow-up imaging looking for recurrence must include FLAIR and diffusion sequences

Differential Diagnosis: Cystic CPA Mass
Arachnoid Cyst
- Pushes broadly on adjacent structures, does not insinuate
- Attenuates on FLAIR sequence
- Shows no restriction on diffusion weighted imaging

Benign Cystic Neoplasm
- Cystic meningioma and schwannoma will show some areas of enhancement on T1 C+ MR

Malignant Cystic Neoplasm
- Ependymoma and astrocytoma pedunculate from brainstem and 4th ventricle respectively
- Will show some foci of enhancement on T1 C+ MR

Pathology
General
- Etiology-Pathogenesis
  - From inclusion of **ectodermal elements** during neural tube closure
- Epidemiology

Epidermoid Cyst, CPA

- o   Posterior fossa most common site
- o   CPA 75%, 4th ventricle 25%

Gross Pathologic, Surgical Features
- Pearly white, "the beautiful tumor"
- Lobulated, cauliflower-shaped surface features
- Insinuating growth pattern in cisterns, engulfs vessels and nerves

Microscopic Features
- Cyst wall: Simple stratified cuboidal squamous epithelium
- Cyst contents: Solid crystalline cholesterol, keratinaceous debris
    - o   Does not contain hair follicles, sebaceous glands or fat in contrast to dermoid
- Grows in successive layers by desquamation from the cyst wall

Clinical Issues

Presentation
- Principal presenting symptom: Dizziness
- Broad presentation from 20 to 70: Peak age = 40
- Other symptoms: Depend on location, growth pattern
    - o   Headache
    - o   Trigeminal neuralgia (tic douloureux)
    - o   Facial neuralgia (hemifacial spasm)
    - o   Sensorineural hearing loss

Natural History
- Grows slowly, remains clinically silent for many years

Treatment
- Complete surgical removal is goal
- If recurs, takes many years to grow

Prognosis
- Smaller cisternal lesions are readily cured with surgery
- Larger lesions where upward supratentorial herniation has occurred are more difficult to completely remove

Selected References
1. Dechambre S et al: Diffusion-weighted MRI postoperative assessment of an epidermoid tumor in the cerebellopontine angle. Neuroradiology 41:829-31, 1999
2. Ikushima I et al: MR of epidermoids with a variety of pulse sequences. AJNR 18:1359-63, 1997
3. Gao P et al: Epidermoid tumor of the cerebellopontine angle. RadioGraphics 13:863-72, 1992

Arachnoid Cyst, CPA

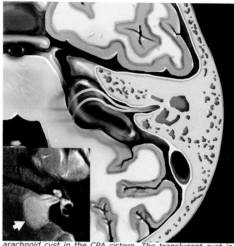

Drawing of arachnoid cyst in the CPA cistern. The translucent cyst in this case is shown displacing the 7th and 8th cranial nerves. In most cases, the AC is an incidental finding unrelated to the patient's symptoms. The insert in the left lower quadrant shows an AC (arrow) on axial T2-FSE MR image.

Key Facts

- Synonyms: Primary or congenital arachnoid cyst (AC)
- Definition: Arachnoid or collagen-lined cavities that do not communicate directly with the ventricular system or the subarachnoid space
- Classic imaging appearance: Cystic cisternal mass with almost imperceptible walls with CSF density (CT) or intensity (MR)
- Split arachnoid contains CSF
- 10% of all AC occur in posterior fossa
  - CPA = Most common infratentorial site
- Often an incidental finding on MR imaging of the brain

Imaging Findings

General Imaging Features

- Best imaging clue: **Complete fluid attenuation** (low signal) on FLAIR MR imaging with **no diffusion restriction** on diffusion sequence
- Resembles CSF in density (CT) and signal intensity (MR)
- Focal lesion that pushes cisternal structures but does not insinuate
- Sharply demarcated round or ovoid lesion

CT Findings

- Density same as CSF
- Higher density from hemorrhage or proteinaceous fluid rare
- No enhancement of cavity or wall
- Rarely causes pressure erosion of adjacent bone

MR Findings

- Signal parallels CSF on all sequences
- Suppresses completely (low signal) with FLAIR
- No restriction (low signal) on diffusion MR

Arachnoid Cyst, CPA

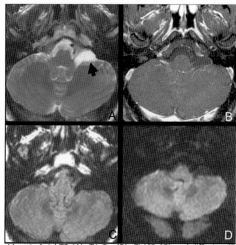

CPA arachnoid cyst. Axial T2 (A), T1 C+ (B), FLAIR (C) and diffusion (D) sequences are shown. High signal AC on T2 image (arrow in A) does not enhance (B). Low signal on FLAIR sequence (C) indicates fluid attenuation has occurred. No diffusion restriction is seen as low signal on the diffusion sequence (D).

Differential Diagnosis: Cystic CPA Mass
Epidermoid Cyst
- Shows restriction (high signal) on diffusion MR
- Insinuates adjacent CSF spaces and structures

Cystic Neoplasm
- Cystic meningioma, schwannoma, ependymoma, astrocytoma all will show some foci of enhancement on T1 C+ MR

Neurenteric Cyst
- Very rare lesion
- Often contains proteinaceous fluid (high-signal on T1 MR sequences)

Pathology
General
- Etiology-Pathogenesis
  - Embryonic meninges fail to merge
  - Noncommunicating fluid compartment surrounded by arachnoid is formed that contains CSF
- Epidemiology
  - Accounts for 1% of intracranial masses

Gross Pathology, Surgical Features
- Fluid-containing cyst with translucent membrane
- May displace but does not engulf adjacent vessels or cranial nerves

Microscopic Features
- Thin wall of flattened but normal arachnoid cells
- No inflammation or neoplastic change

Arachnoid Cyst, CPA

Clinical Issues

Presentation
- Principal presenting symptom: None, incidental finding on MR
- May be first seen at any age
  - 75% of AC occur in children
- Other symptoms: Defined by location
  - Headache
  - Dizziness, SNHL
  - Hemifacial spasm or trigeminal neuralgia

Natural History
- Usually do not enlarge over time

Treatment
- Most cases require no treatment
- Surgical removal is highly selective process
  - Reserved for cases where clear symptoms can be directly linked to AC anatomic location

Prognosis
- If surgery limited to AC where symptoms are clearly related, prognosis is excellent

Selected References
1. Choi JU et al: Pathogenesis of arachnoid cyst: congenital or traumatic? Pediatr Neurosurg 29:260-6, 1998
2. Flodmark O: Neuroradiology of selected disorders of the meninges, calvarium and venous sinuses. AJNR 13:483-91, 1992
3. Weiner SN et al: MR imaging of intracranial arachnoid cysts. JCAT 11:236-41, 1987

Aneurysm, CPA

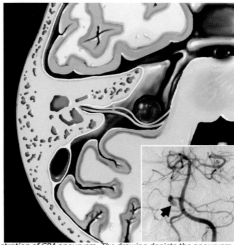

Graphic illustration of CPA aneurysm. The drawing depicts the aneurysm compressing the 7th and 8th cranial nerves in the CPA cistern. Because the 8th nerve is more sensitive to compression, aneurysms will be found when searching for a cause of SNHL. Insert shows PICA-AICA aneurysm (arrow) at angiography.

Key Facts
- Definition: CPA aneurysm is a focal ballooning of the wall of the posterior inferior cerebellar artery (PICA), vertebral artery (VA) or anterior inferior cerebellar artery (AICA)
- Classic imaging appearance: Ovoid mass with a calcified rim (CT) and complex layered signal (MR) in CPA cistern that does not enter IAC
- 10% of intracranial aneurysms are in vertebrobasilar circulation
- Aneurysms in CPA account for approximately 1% of CPA masses
- CPA aneurysms arise from **PICA > VA > AICA**

Imaging Findings
Imaging Features
- Best imaging clue: Calcified rim (CT) or layered complex signal (MR)
- Ovoid CPA mass that is in immediate proximity to an area artery

CT Findings
- Patent aneurysm
  - Well-delineated iso- to hyperdense extra-axial mass with strong, uniform enhancement
- Partially thrombosed aneurysm
  - Complex mass with central or eccentric enhancing lumen, nonenhancing mural thrombus
  - Often has **calcified rim**
- Completely thrombosed aneurysm
  - As above without enhancing lumen

MR Findings
- Signal varies from **hypointense "flow void" to complex mixed signal** appearance depending on flow rate, presence and age of luminal thrombus
- Subacute luminal clot is **high signal** on T1 MR images secondary to methemoglobin T1 shortening

Aneurysm, CPA

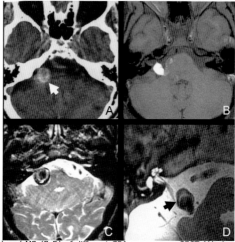

Axial CT (A) and MR (B-D) of different CPA aneurysms. CECT (A) shows an ovoid, high-density mass (arrow) in the right CPA cistern. T1 axial MR (B) reveals a fusiform high-signal mass (methemoglobin) while T2 (C) shows layered clot. T2-FSE (D) shows aneurysm bowing the 8th cranial nerve (arrow).

- **Phase artifact** across image from patent aneurysm common
- Aneurysm lumen may enhance if slow flow is present
- **MRA** delineates relationship of lesion to parent vessel

Angiographic Findings
- Visible lumen may be smaller than overall aneurysm if clot is present
  - Angiogram may underestimate aneurysm size
- Delineates precise vascular relationships

Imaging Recommendations
- Once a mass of the CPA is found on CT or MR suspected of being an aneurysm, confirmation with MRA or angiography is needed
- Most surgeons still want angiography prior to clipping an aneurysm
- A growing group of surgeons are operating on MRA alone

Differential Diagnosis: Vascular CPA Masses
Vertebrobasilar Dolichoectasia
- Imaging: MRA reprojections or source images show no aneurysm
- Clinical: Seen in elderly vasculopaths

Venous Varix
- Imaging: Dural AVF seen on angiography
  - Ovoid mass fully enhancing on T1 C+ MR
  - MR venography may help delineate
- Clinical: Objective pulsatile tinnitus

Pathology
General
- Genetics
  - Aneurysm propensity has hereditary driver

- Etiology-Pathogenesis
  - o Inherited factors + hemodynamic-induced degenerative changes in vessel wall often combine to form aneurysm
- Epidemiology
  - o Rare CPA mass; rare cause of SNHL
  - o 10% of intracranial aneurysms are in vertebrobasilar circulation
  - o Aneurysms in CPA cistern account for approximately 1% CPA masses

Gross Pathologic, Surgical Features
- Saccular: Rounded, berry-like outpouching of artery wall
- Fusiform: Enlarged, ectatic vessel with gross changes of atherosclerosis

Microscopic Features
- Lacks internal elastic lamina, smooth muscle layers
- Degenerative changes in parent vessel common
- Thrombus, atherosclerosis are common

Clinical Issues
Presentation
- Principal presenting symptom: SNHL (70%)
- Other symptoms: Facial nerve palsy (60%), subarachnoid hemorrhage (50%) and hemifacial spasm
- Peak presentation = 40-60 years

Natural History
- < 1 cm rupture less frequently than large lesions
- Partial or complete thrombosis
  - o Results in posterior fossa stroke or cranial nerve palsy

Treatment
- Surgical clipping of aneurysm base still gold standard of care
- Endovascular coiling growing as acceptable treatment

Prognosis
- Left unclipped, aneurysm rupture remains a growing possibility

Selected References
1. Bonneville F et al: Unusual lesions of the cerebellopontine angle: a segmental approach. RadioGraphics 21:419-38, 2001
2. Hancock JH et al: Spontaneous dissection of the anterior inferior cerebellar artery. Neuroradiology 42:535-8, 2000
3. Morris DP et al: Thrombosed PICA aneurysm: a rare cerebellopontine angle tumor. J Laryngol Otol 109:429-30, 1995

Acoustic Schwannoma

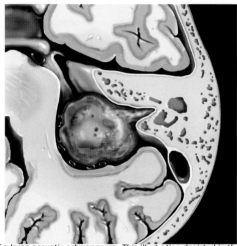

Drawing of a large acoustic schwannoma. This illustration depicted in the axial plane shows the AS filling the CPA as it flares the internal auditory canal. The lesion resembles a small ice cream cone (IAC component) with a big scoop of ice cream (CPA component) compressing the brachium pontis.

Key Facts
- Synonyms: Acoustic neuroma, vestibular schwannoma
- Definition: Benign tumor arising from the Schwann cells that wrap the vestibulocochlear nerve in the CPA-IAC
- Classic imaging appearance
  - T1 C+ MR: Focal, enhancing mass of CPA-IAC cistern
  - FSE-T2 MR: "Filling defect" in high-signal CSF of CPA-IAC cistern
- Most common CPA-IAC mass (85% of all lesions found there)
- Second most common extra-axial neoplasm in adults
- Presents in adults with unilateral sensorineural hearing loss (SNHL)

Imaging Findings
General Imaging Features
- Best imaging clue: Well-circumscribed, ovoid mass in CPA-IAC cistern
- When small and intracanalicular, looks like ovoid to tubular mass
- Larger lesions look like "ice cream (CPA) on cone (IAC)"
CT Findings
- Well-delineated, enhancing mass of CPA-IAC cistern
- Calcification not present (cf. meningioma)
- May flare IAC when larger
MR Findings
- T1 C+ MR
  - 100% enhance strongly
  - 15% with **intramural cysts** (low signal foci)
- FSE-T2 MR
  - Small lesion: Ovoid filling defect in high signal CSF of IAC
  - Large lesion: "Ice cream in cone" shaped filling defect in CPA-IAC
    - Often have mixed intensity signal as FSE more sensitive to variations in concentration of Antoni A and B cells
- Other MR findings

Acoustic Schwannoma

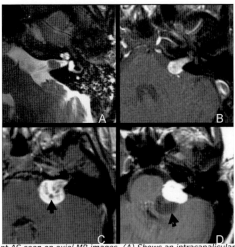

Four different AS seen on axial MR images. (A) Shows an intracanalicular AS on FSE-T2 MR as a filling defect in the high-signal CSF. (B) Axial T1 C+ MR reveals an enhancing AS in the IAC-CPA. (C) An intramural cyst is displayed (arrow) while image (D) reveals an associated arachnoid cyst (arrow).

- o 0.5% associated arachnoid cyst
- o 0.5% hemorrhagic foci; high signal on T1 unenhanced MR
- o Dural tails are rarely present (cf. meningioma)

Imaging Recommendations
- Full brain MR with T1 C+ MR imaging of CPA-IAC is gold standard
- High-resolution FSE-T2 MR imaging of CPA-IAC only can be used as screening exam for acoustic schwannoma (AS)

Differential Diagnosis: CPA-IAC Mass
Epidermoid Cyst
- May mimic the rare cystic acoustic schwannoma
- Insinuating morphology
- Does not attenuate on FLAIR; diffusion restriction on diffusion sequence

Arachnoid Cyst
- Follows CSF signal on all MR sequences; T1 C+ shows no enhancement
- Pushing lesion that does not enter IAC

Neurosarcoidosis
- Multiple meningeal enhancing nodules

Meningioma
- Calcified dural-based mass eccentric to porus acusticus
- Intracanalicular meningioma may mimic AS (rare)

Facial Nerve Schwannoma
- When confined to CPA-IAC, may exactly mimic AS
- Look for labyrinthine segment involvement (tail) to differentiate

Metastasis & Lymphoma
- May be bilateral; multifocal meningeal involvement

Pathology
General
- Genetics

- o Inactivating mutations of NF-2 tumor suppressor gene in 60% of sporadic schwannomas
- o Loss of chromosome 22q also seen
- o Multiple schwannomas = NF-2
- Etiology-Pathogenesis
  - o Slowly-growing, benign tumor arising from vestibular portion of VIII at oligodendrocyte-Schwann cell junction
- Epidemiology
  - o Most common lesion in patients with unilateral SNHL (>90%)
  - o Most common lesion of CPA-IAC (85%)

Gross Pathologic, Surgical Features
- Tan, round-ovoid, encapsulated mass
- Arises eccentrically from nerve

Microscopic Features
- Differentiated neoplastic Schwann cells
- Areas of compact, elongated cells = **Antoni A**
- Other areas less densely cellular with tumor loosely arranged, +/- clusters of lipid-laden cells = **Antoni B**
- Strong, diffuse expression of S-100 protein
- No necrosis but may have intramural cysts, rarely hemorrhage

Grading
- WHO grade I lesion

Clinical Issues

Presentation
- Principal presenting symptom: Unilateral SNHL
- Other symptoms:
  - o Small AS: Tinnitus (ringing in ear)
  - o Large AS: Trigeminal and/or facial neuropathy
- Adults (rare in children unless NF-2)
- Peak age = 40-60 years

Natural History
- 75% of AS grow at a gradual pace if left untreated
- 10% of AS grow rapidly
- 15% of AS grow very slowly and can be left alone in older patients

Treatment
- Translabyrinthine resection if no hearing preservation possible
- Middle cranial fossa approach for intracanalicular AS
- Retrosigmoid approach when CPA component present

Prognosis
- If hearing is absent or very poor, successful surgical removal of AS will not restore any hearing already lost
- Hearing preservation best when tumor < 2 cm and does not involve IAC fundus or cochlear aperture

Selected References
1. Somers T et al: Prognostic value of magnetic resonance imaging findings in hearing preservation surgery for vestibular schwannoma. Otol Neurotol 22:87-94, 2001
2. Dubrulle F et al: Cochlear fossa enhancement at MR evaluation of vestibular schwannoma: correlation with success at hearing-preservation surgery. Radiology 215:458-62, 2000
3. Allen RW et al: Low-cost high-resolution fast spin-echo MR of acoustic schwannoma: an alternative to enhanced conventional spin-echo MR? AJNR 17:1205-10, 1996

Meningioma, CPA

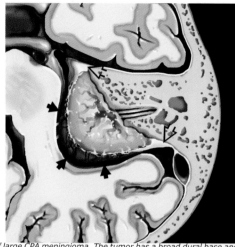

Drawing of large CPA meningioma. The tumor has a broad dural base and is eccentric to the porus acusticus of the IAC. Notice the CSF cleft (arrows) separating the tumor from the adjacent brain. Dural thickening = tails (open arrows) are found along the margins of the tumor.

Key Facts
- Definition: Benign, unencapsulated neoplasm arising from arachnoid cells associated with the dura of the CPA-IAC cistern
- Classic imaging appearance
    - T1 C+ MR shows an enhancing dural-based mass with dural tails centered along the posterior wall of the temporal bone
    - CT shows tumor calcifications
- Other key facts
    - 2nd most common CPA-IAC mass
    - 2nd most common primary intracranial tumor
    - Meningioma + schwannoma = NF-2
    - Multiple meningiomas occur in 10% of sporadic cases

Imaging Findings
General Imaging Features
- Best imaging clue: Dural-based mass
- Extra-axial mass **asymmetric to IAC** porus acusticus
- "Mushroom cap" with broad base towards temporal bone
- **CSF-vascular "cleft"** between mass and brain
CT Findings
- 75% hyperdense on NECT
- 25% calcified (sand-like or dense chunks)
- 90% strong, uniform enhancement; 10% inhomogeneous
- IAC usually not enlarged
- Hyperostotic or permeative bone changes possible
MR Findings
- 75% isointense with gray matter on all sequences
- 25% atypical appearance (necrosis, cysts, hemorrhage)
- T1 C+ MR: 95% enhance strongly; heterogeneous enhancement common especially in larger lesions

Meningioma, CPA

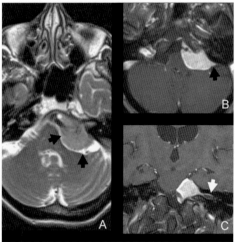

CPA meningioma with IAC penetration. (A) Axial T2 image reveals the CSF cleft as a high-signal crescent (open arrows). (B) Axial T1 C+ image shows broad dural base with a lateral "tail" (arrow). (C) Coronal T1 C+ image reveals extension into the IAC (arrow).

- o **Dural thickening ("tail")** in 60%
- T2 MR: CSF-vascular cleft
  - o Peritumoral brain edema correlates with pial blood supply
  - o Its presence signals problems with safe removal and with early recurrence
- MR and tumor grade
  - o Anaplastic meningiomas "mushroom," invade brain
  - o MR spectroscopy useful (Cho/Cr, lipid)

Angiographic Findings
- Dural vessels supply center, pial vessels supply the rim
- "Sunburst" pattern of enlarged dural feeders common
- Prolonged vascular "stain" into venous phase
- Arteriovenous shunting may occur

Differential Diagnosis: Solid CPA-IAC Area Mass

Sarcoidosis
- Often multifocal, dural-based foci
- Look for infundibular stalk involvement

Acoustic Schwannoma
- Intracanalicular 1st, then CPA extension
- Intracanalicular meningioma may mimic AS (rare)

Metastasis & Lymphoma
- May be bilateral; multifocal meningeal involvement

Idiopathic Hypertrophic Pachymeningitis (rare)
- Diffuse meningeal thickening and enhancement

Pathology

General
- Genetics
  - o Long-arm deletions of chromosome 22 common

- o NF-2 gene inactivated in 60% of sporadic cases
- o Angiogenic factors (FGF-2, VEGF, integrins) expressed
- o May have progesterone, prolactin receptors
- o May express growth hormone
- Etiology-Pathogenesis
  - o Arises from arachnoid "cap" cells, not dura
- Epidemiology
  - o Account for 15%-25% of primary intracranial tumors
  - o 1%-1.5% prevalence at autopsy or imaging
  - o 10% occur in posterior fossa
  - o 10% multiple (NF-2; multiple meningiomatosis)

Gross Surgical-Pathologic Features
- **"Mushroom cap"** or **"en plaque"** in CPA common
- Sharply circumscribed, unencapsulated
- Distinct CSF-vascular "cleft" between mass and adjacent brain
- Adjacent dural thickening (collar or "tail") is usually reactive, not neoplastic

Microscopic Pathologic Features
- WHO Grading Classification
  - o Meningioma (classic, benign) = 90%
  - o Atypical meningioma = 9%
  - o Anaplastic (malignant) meningioma = 1%
- Subtypes (wide range of histology with little bearing on outcome!)
  - o Meningothelial (lobules of meningothelial cells)
  - o Fibrous (parallel, interlacing fascicles of spindle-shaped cells)
  - o Transitional (mixed form; "onion-bulb" whorls and lobules)
  - o Psammomatous (numerous small calcifications)
  - o Angiomatous (abundant vascular channels)- Not equated with obsolete term "angioblastic meningioma"
  - o Miscellaneous forms (microcystic, chordoid, clear cell, secretory, lymphoplasmacyte-rich, etc.)

Clinical Issues
Presentation
- Principal presenting symptom: Most common to find incidentally
- Female: male = 3:1
- Middle-aged, elderly patients; peak age = 60; in children, think NF-2
Treatment
- Surgical removal if medically safe
Prognosis
- Amount of peritumoral edema, hyperintensity on T2, cortical penetration, pial vascular supply predict decreased "cleavability"

Selected References
1. Ildan F et al: Correlation of relationships of brain-tumor interfaces, magnetic resonance imaging, and angiographic findings to predict cleavage of meningiomas. J Neurosurg 91:384-90, 1999
2. Buetow M et al: Typical, atypical and misleading features in meningioma. RadioGraphics 11: 1087-1106, 1991
3. Goldsher D et al: Dural "tail" associated with meningiomas on Gd-DTPA-enhanced MR images: characteristics, differential diagnostic value and possible implications for treatment. Radiology 176:447-50, 1990

PocketRadiologist™
Head and Neck
100 Top Diagnoses

SKULL BASE

Anterior Neuropore Anomalies

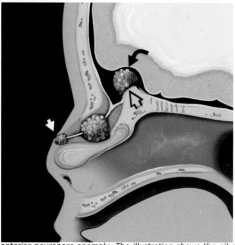

Drawing of anterior neuropore anomaly. The illustration shows the pit at tip of the nose with associated subcutaneous dermoid (arrow). The dural sinus tract has associated dermoid as it passes through an enlarged foramen cecum. Bifid crista galli (open arrow). Intracranial dermoid (curved arrow).

Key Facts
- Definition: Defective embryogenesis of the anterior neuropore resulting in any mixture of **dermoid**, **epidermoid** and/or **dural sinus tract** in the frontonasal region
- Classic imaging appearance: Focal mixed density/intensity masses (dermoid or epidermoid) seen from tip of nose to foramen cecum
  - Associated with bifid crista galli and a large foramen cecum
- A midline pit on bridge of nose sends the clinician in search of these associated anomalies
- Imaging recommendation: Thin section CT and MR imaging focused to the frontonasal area best delineates underlying pathology

Imaging Findings
General Features
- Best imaging clue: **Bifid crista galli + large foramen cecum**
- Focal mass (dermoid or epidermoid) within or deep to the nasal bridge; additional masses may be seen along the dermal sinus tract
  - Epidermoid or dermoid may be found anywhere along the course of the dural sinus tract from the tip of the nose to the intracranial side of the foramen cecum
- **Dermal sinus tract** extends from nasal bridge cephalad through enlarged foramen cecum
- If dermal sinus tract is present and reaches dura of anterior cranial fossa, crista galli is bifid and foramen cecum is large
  - Beware! Foramen cecum closes postnatally in 1st 5 years of life
  - Do not overcall a "large foramen cecum" or unnecessary craniotomy may result
  - If crista galli is not bifid and tract is not seen, foramen cecum is probably just not yet closed

Anterior Neuropore Anomalies

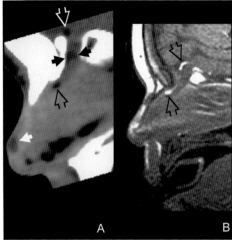

Sagittal CT (A) and MR (B) of anterior neuropore anomaly. (A) Sagittal CT reformation shows the subcutaneous dermoid on the tip of the nose (white arrow). Open arrows mark multiple sinus tract dermoids. Large foramen cecum: black arrows. (B) Sagittal T1 MR shows multiple tract dermoids (open arrows).

CT Findings
- Expansile, scalloping mass along line from tip of the nose, midline nasal bone projected to the foramen cecum just anterior to the crista galli
- Fluid density mass = **epidermoid**; fat density mass = **dermoid**
- If dural sinus tract present, enlarged foramen cecum and bifid crista galli may be seen

MR Findings
- Fluid intensity mass = **epidermoid**; fat intensity mass = **dermoid**
- If dural sinus tract associated, the tract may be seen passing from tip of nose through an enlarged foramen cecum on sagittal MR images
- Rarely an additional mass is seen on the cranial margin of foramen cecum or at the point of attachment of the falx to the crista galli

Imaging Recommendations
- Imaging "sweet spot" is small and anterior
  - Focus imaging from tip of nose to back of foramen cecum
  - Inferior end of axial imaging is hard palate
- Thin section (1-2 mm) bone-only axial and coronal CT
- If CT suggests possibility of sinus tract &/or intracranial dermoid, use thin-section (2-3 mm) MR in the axial, coronal & **sagittal** planes

Differential Diagnosis: Cranio-Nasal Masses

Nasal Cephalocele
- Bone dehiscence is larger, involving a broader area of the midline cribriform plate or frontal bone
- Direct extension of meninges, subarachnoid space and/or brain can be seen projecting into cephalocele on sagittal MR images

Nasal Glioma
- Solid mass of glial tissue separated from the brain by subarachnoid space and meninges

- Most commonly found projecting extranasally into the paramedian bridge of the nose; less commonly in anterior nasal septum

Pathology
General
- Embryology-Anatomy
  - Normal development of the **anterior neuropore** involves a dural stalk passing from the area of the future foramen cecum to the tip of the nose, then regressing completely
- Etiology-Pathogenesis
  - Failure of involution of the neuropore in the 4th gestational week may leave neuroectoderm along tract of the dural stalk
  - Dermal sinus, dermoid or epidermoid alone or in concert results
- Epidemiology
  - 60% of children with a cutaneous pit, lesion is confined to the skin
  - The dermal sinus tract reaches intracranially in a minority of cases; still fewer have intracranial epidermoid or dermoid associated

Microscopic Features
- Nasal dermal sinus is a midline epithelial-lined tract
- Epidermoid cyst contain desquamated epithelium
- Dermoid cyst contains skin adnexa

Clinical Issues
Presentation
- Principal presenting symptom: **Pit** on skin of nasal bridge
- Classic clinical presentation: Child (average age = 3) with a midline pit over the dorsum of nose occasionally containing wiry hairs
- Distal opening of the dermal sinus may be found anywhere from the anterior nasal septum to the glabella including the tip of the nose
- Intermittent sebaceous material discharge from pit
- < 50% a mass is associated with increasing size with broadening the nasal root and bridge
- If intracranial connection via dural sinus tract, recurrent meningitis or anterior cranial fossa abscess may occur (rare)

Treatment
- When multiple dermoids or epidermoids are associated with a dural sinus, combined head and neck-intracranial surgery is required
- Most cases just require facial-plastics procedure to remove pit and associated dermoid or epidermoid from the nasal bridge

Prognosis
- One time problem when surgical correction is successful

Selected References
1. Denoyelle F et al: Nasal dermoid sinus cysts in children. Laryngoscope 107:795-800, 1997
2. Castillo M: Congenital abnormalities of the nose: CT and MR findings. AJR 162:1211-17, 1994
3. Barkovich AJ et al: Congenital nasal masses: CT and MR imaging features in 16 cases. AJNR 12:105-16, 1991

Clival Chordoma

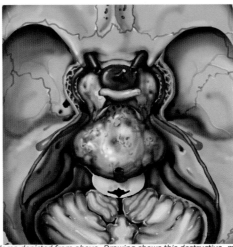

Clival chordoma depicted from above. Drawing shows this destructive, midline tumor invading the basi-sphenoid and the basi-occiput. Bone fragments characteristically float in the substance of the tumor.

Key Facts
- Synonym: Basicranial chordoma
- Definition: Rare malignant tumor of clivus that arises from remnants of the cranial end of the primitive notochord
- Classic imaging findings: Midline destructive lesion in the clivus with CT showing destroyed bone within its matrix; MR reveals mixed T1 signal and high T2 signal
- Other key facts
  - Locally invasive tumor found in **midline** from the sella to coccyx
  - 35% arise in skull base around the spheno-occipital synchondrosis
  - Presents in middle age as visual disturbance and ophthalmoplegia
  - Histologic identification of **physaliphorous cell** confirms diagnosis

Imaging Findings
General Features
- Best imaging clue: Destructive midline mass centered in clivus
  - Most commonly centered at the spheno-occipital synchondrosis within the upper clivus
- Expanding tumor invades:
  - Nasopharynx inferiorly
  - Cavernous sinus and sella superiorly
  - Jugular foramen and petrous apex laterally
  - Basilar artery and brainstem posteriorly
  - Basisphenoid, sphenoid and ethmoid sinuses anteriorly
CT Findings
- Clival mass with associated bone destruction (95%) and high attenuation foci within tumor matrix (50%)
  - High-density foci represents ossific fragments of destroyed clival bone floating in the chordoma matrix
- CECT shows mass as mixed density with areas of cystic necrosis mixed with enhancing soft tissue

Clival Chordoma

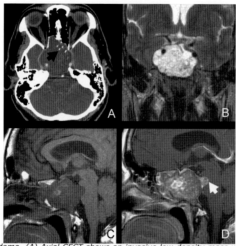

Clival chordoma. (A) Axial CECT shows an invasive low-density mass with multiple bone fragments (arrow). (B) Coronal T2 MR reveals the mass as high-signal. (C) T1 C- sagittal MR shows low-signal mass in central skull base. (D) T1 C+ reveals inhomogeneous enhancement with tumor "thumb" (arrow) indenting pons.

MR Findings
- T1 signal variable with focal areas of high T1 signal sometimes seen within the tumor secondary to focal hemorrhage or mucoid material
- **T2** signal characteristically **hyperintense**
- Sagittal images show tumor **"thumb"** indenting the anterior pons

Angiographic Findings
- Avascular mass with internal carotid artery displacement and encasement

Imaging Recommendations
- Axial & coronal bone only unenhanced CT of skull base
- Focused enhanced MR of skull base including MRA & MRV
- Angiography with test occlusion

Differential Diagnosis: Clivus-Petro-occipital Fissure Mass

Giant Pituitary Macroadenoma
- Emanation of the pituitary macroadenoma from the sella above differentiates this lesion from chordoma

Chondrosarcoma
- Centered along the lateral margin of clivus in petro-occipital fissure
- Displays chondroid calcifications (> 50%)

Plasmacytoma
- Can also be midline destructive mass of clivus
- T2 signal usually intermediate to low (cf. chordoma high T2 signal)

Pathology

General
- General Comments
  - Lateral chondroid chordoma reported in the literature is probably best dealt with as a low-grade chondrosarcoma of the petro-occipital fissure

Clival Chordoma

- Etiology-Pathogenesis
  - Rare malignant tumor of bone that arises from remnants of the cranial end of the **primitive notochord**
- Epidemiology
  - 35% of all chordoma in skull base
  - Of the rest, 50% are sacrococcygeal while 15% arise from a vertebral body

Gross Pathologic, Surgical Features
- Gross appearance is translucent, gray mass (myxoid matrix)

Microscopic Features
- The physaliphorous cell reveals large, intracellular vacuoles +/- both mucin and glycogen

Clinical Issues

Presentation
- Principal presenting symptom: Ophthalmoplegia
- Other symptoms: Orbitofrontal headache and visual complaints
- Classic patient profile: 30-50 year old with gradual onset of ophthalmoplegia and visual complaints
  - Ophthalmoplegia results from tumor proximity to cranial nerves
    - Cranial nerve VI in Dorello's canal
    - Cranial nerves III, IV and VI in the cavernous sinus
  - Visual disturbance signals optic nerve injury
- Large chordoma may reach the jugular foramen inferolaterally affecting cranial nerves 9-12
- Lateral growth can injure cranial nerves 7 or 8 in the CPA-IAC

Treatment
- Combined complete surgical resection and proton beam irradiation is currently considered the treatment of choice

Prognosis
- Once relapse occurs, 5-year survival rates are as low as 5%

Selected References
1. Meyers SP et al: Chordomas of the skull base: MR features. AJNR 13:1617-36, 1992
2. Sze G et al: Chordomas: MR imaging. Radiology 166:187-91, 1988
3. Oot RF et al: The role of MR and CT in evaluating clival chordomas and chondrosarcomas. AJNR 9:715-23, 1988

Chondrosarcoma, Skull Base

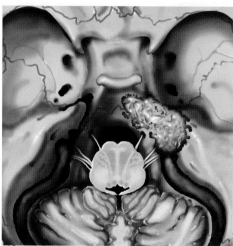

Petro-occipital fissure chondrosarcoma. Drawing shows chondrosarcoma as an invasive mass centered on the petro-occipital fissure. Typical chondroid matrix is shown as whorls of bone within the tumor parenchyma.

Key Facts
- Definition: Chondroid malignancy of the skull base
- Classic imaging appearance: T1 C+ MR shows a heterogeneously-enhancing tumor located at the petro-occipital fissure with high-signal intensity on T2 MR
  - CT often shows **chondroid mineralization**
  - Invasive bone changes in petro-occipital fissure strongly favors the diagnosis of Chondrosarcoma (CSa)
- Uncommon skull-base tumor that must be distinguished from chordoma
- Combined radical resection and proton beam irradiation has resulted in 10 year survival rate of 99%

Imaging Findings
General Features
- Best imaging clue: If present, **chondroid matrix**
- Tumor centered on **petro-occipital fissure** of posterior skull base
CT Findings
- **Unenhanced CT** shows characteristic chondroid calcification matrix (>50%) with associated bone destruction
- When no tumor matrix found, cannot tell chondrosarcoma from chordoma, plasmacytoma, non-Hodgkin lymphoma or focal metastasis
MR Findings
- MR shows low T1 and high T2 signal
- Low signal foci within the tumor may suggest the underlying coarse matrix mineralization or fibrocartilaginous elements within the tumor
- C+ T1 MR images show a heterogeneously-enhancing mass, often with whorls of enhancing lines within the tumor matrix
Angiographic Findings
- Shows avascular mass with internal carotid artery displacement and encasement

Chondrosarcoma, Skull Base

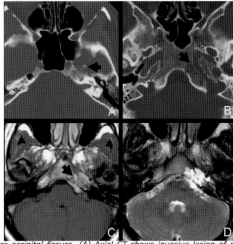

CSa of petro-occipital fissure. (A) Axial CT shows invasive lesion of petrous apex with chondroid calcifications (arrow). (B) Permeative bone changes on either side of petro-occipital fissure (arrow) mark the location of the CSa. (C) T1 C+ MR shows tumor enhancement (arrow) while T2 MR (D) shows it as high-signal lesion.

Imaging Recommendations
- Axial & coronal bone only unenhanced CT of skull base
- Focused enhanced MR of skull base including MRA & MRV
- Pre-operative angiography with test occlusion

Differential Diagnosis: Destructive Mass of POF-Clivus
Chordoma
- Midline; lacks coarse chondroid calcifications
- Key tumor to differentiate from CSa
Plasmacytoma
- Usually more midline within clivus
- T2 signal is low to intermediate
- Over 50% have concurrent multiple myeloma
Metastatic Tumor
- Destructive mass that can be anywhere in skull base
- Often multiple with known primary tumor

Pathology
General
- Etiology-Pathogenesis
  - Arises from cartilage, endochondral bone or from primitive mesenchymal cells in the meninges
- Epidemiology
  - 6% of all skull base tumors
  - Locations: Found in the more anterior basi-sphenoid (1/3) and the petro-occipital fissure (2/3)
Gross Pathologic, Surgical Features
- Smooth, lobulated mass welling up from the petro-occipital fissure
- Cut surface shows a gray-white, glistening tumor parenchyma

Chondrosarcoma, Skull Base

Microscopic Features
- Hypercellular tumor composed of **chondrocytes** with hyperchromatic, pleomorphic nuclei and prominent nucleoli
- Binucleate or multinucleate cells are the rule

Grading
- Grading is from low-grade to high-grade based on the degree of cellularity, pleomorphism, mitoses and multinucleated cells

Clinical Issues

Presentation
- Principal presenting symptom: Abducens palsy
- Age range: 10-79 years with a mean age of 39 years
- Other symptoms: Insidious onset trigeminal neuropathy

Natural History
- Slow-growing, malignant, cartilaginous tumor

Treatment
- Combined radical resection and post-operative, high-dose, fractionated precision conformal radiation therapy
- Basal subfrontal approach used for tumor that invades the clivus and extends anteriorly into the sphenoid and ethmoid sinuses
- Subtemporal and preauricular infratemporal approach used when CSa extends laterally beyond the petrous internal carotid artery

Prognosis
- Depends on tumor extent at time of diagnosis, histologic grade and the completeness of the initial resection
  - High-grade CSa metastasize to bones and lung more frequently
- Disease-specific 10-year survival rates of 99% recently reported

Selected References
1. Rosenberg AE et al: Chondrosarcoma of the base of the skull: a clinicopathologic study of 200 cases with emphasis on its distinction from chordoma. Am J Surg Pathol 23:1370-8, 1999
2. Hug EB et al: Proton radiation therapy for chordomas and chondrosarcomas of the skull base. J Neurosurg 91:432-9, 1999
3. Meyers SP et al: Chondrosarcomas of the skull base: MR imaging features. Radiology 184:103-8, 1992

Paraganglioma, Jugular Foramen

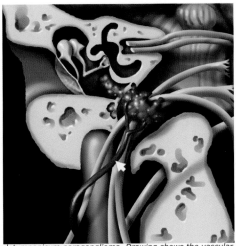

Glomus jugulotympanicum paraganglioma. Drawing shows the vascular mass of the superolateral jugular foramen invading into the middle ear cavity through the floor. The main arterial feeder is the ascending pharyngeal artery (arrow). The clinician sees only the tip of the iceberg behind the tympanic membrane.

Key Facts
- Synonym: Glomus jugulare and glomus jugulotympanicum
- Definitions: **Glomus jugulare paraganglioma** refers to paraganglioma confined to the jugular foramen (JF) area only; **glomus jugulotympanicum paraganglioma** describes paraganglioma involving both the jugular foramen and the middle ear cavity
- Classic imaging appearance
  - **Permeative bone margins** on CT
  - **High-velocity flow voids** on T1 MR
  - Rapid tumor blush and early venous egress on angiography
- Most common tumor found in the jugular foramen

Imaging Findings
General Features
- Best imaging clue: Permeative walls of JF on CT
- **Glomus jugulare paraganglioma**
  - JF mass without extension into the middle ear cavity that is "peppered" with high-velocity flow voids on T1 MR
  - CT reveals permeative bone changes along the margins of the jugular foramen with jugular spine amputation
- **Glomus jugulotympanicum paraganglioma**
  - JF mass extends superolaterally into floor of middle ear cavity
  - Vector of tumor spread in a superolateral direction into middle ear
CT Findings
- Bone-only CT provides the surgeon information about bony destruction, dehiscence, and landmarks not available from MR alone
- Shows **permeative, erosive margins** of the JF associated with jugular spine erosion
MR Findings
- **T1 MR** sequence show **"salt-and-pepper"** appearance

Paraganglioma, Jugular Foramen

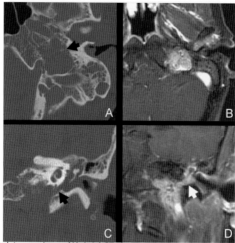

Glomus jugulotympanicum. (A) Axial CT shows permeative bony margins to JF and jugular spine (arrow). (B) T1 C+ MR reveals the avidly-enhancing tumor filling the JF. (C) Coronal CT shows the tumor has eroded the middle ear floor (arrow). (D) T1 C+ MR shows enhancing tumor entering the middle ear (arrow).

- "Salt" or high-signal areas within the tumor parenchyma rarely seen; secondary to subacute hemorrhage
- "Pepper" = low-signal foci from high-velocity flow voids
- Coronal T1 C+ MR images show tongue of tumor curving up from jugular foramen, through the floor of the middle ear cavity, terminating in a wedge of tumor between the cochlear promontory and the tympanic membrane = glomus jugulotympanicum

Angiographic Findings
- Enlarged feeding vessels with prolonged, intense, vascular blush with early draining veins seen secondary to arteriovenous shunting
- Ascending pharyngeal artery = major feeding vessel

Imaging Recommendations
- CT, MR and angiography all done before surgery
- CT shows critical bony landmarks
- MR reveals exact soft tissue extent of tumor
- Angiography provides a vascular road map for the surgeon; evaluates the collateral arterial and venous circulation of the brain; searches for multicentric tumors; embolization used for preoperative hemostasis

Differential Diagnosis: Jugular Foramen Mass

High-riding Jugular Bulb
- Jugular foramen bony margins intact
- Increased signal does not persist in all MR sequences

Dehiscent Jugular Bulb
- Sigmoid plate is focally dehiscent
- Polypoid extension into middle ear is contiguous with jugular bulb

Meningioma of JF
- Imaging findings include permeative and/or hyperostotic bony changes on CT and dural tails on MR

26

- Centrifugal spread along dural surfaces that rarely reaches middle ear
- Prolonged but mild tumor blush during angiography

Schwannoma of JF
- Imaging shows smooth enlargement of the jugular foramen (CT) with fusiform enhancing mass (T1 enhanced MR)
- Dumbbell-shaped spread along the course of the 9-11 cranial nerves
- Absence of tumor blush or enlarged feeding arteries on angiography

Pathology
General
- Etiology-Pathogenesis
  o Arise from **glomus** (L. "a ball") **bodies = paraganglia**
  o Glomus bodies composed of chemoreceptor cells derived from primitive neural crest
- Epidemiology
  o Multicentric 5% of time
  o When familial, multicentricity reaches 25%

Gross Pathologic, Surgical Features
- Lobulated, solid mass with a fibrous pseudocapsule
- External surface is reddish-purple
- Cut surface shows multiple enlarged feeding arteries

Microscopic Features
- Biphasic cell pattern composed of **chief cells** and **sustentacular cells** surrounded by fibromuscular stroma
  o Chief cells arranged in characteristic compact cell nests or balls of cells (zellballen)
- Immunohistochemistry: Chief cells show diffuse reaction to chromogranin
- Electronmicroscopy: Shows neurosecretory granules

Clinical Issues
Presentation
- Principal presenting symptom: Objective pulsatile tinnitus
- Other symptoms: 9-11 ± 12 cranial neuropathy; 7 or 8 cranial neuropathy less often
- Age: 40-60 years
- Gender: Male:Female ratio = 3:1
- Glomus jugulare: Normal tympanic membrane exam
- Glomus jugulotympanicum: Vascular retrotympanic mass

Treatment
- Surgery when smaller
- Larger lesions may require surgery and radiation therapy
- Radiation therapy alone is palliative for older patients

Prognosis
- 60% of patients have postoperative cranial neuropathy

Selected References
1. Rao AB et al: Paragangliomas of the head and neck: Radiologic-pathologic correlation. RadioGraphics 19:1605-32, 1999
2. Vogl TJ et al: Glomus tumors of the skull base: combined use of MR angiography and spin-echo imaging. Radiology 192:103-10, 1994
3. Olsen WL et al: MR imaging of paragangliomas. AJR 148:201-4, 1987

Schwannoma, Jugular Foramen

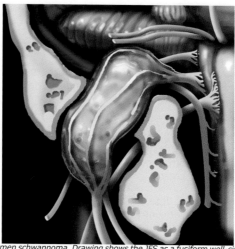

Jugular foramen schwannoma. Drawing shows the JFS as a fusiform well-circumscribed tumor within the jugular foramen. The bony margins of the jugular foramen are sharply marginated and enlarged. The vector of tumor growth is from jugular foramen to lateral medulla along the line of 9-11 cranial nerves.

Key Facts
- Synonyms: Neurilemmoma; neuroma
- Definition: Benign tumor of differentiated Schwann cells wrapping cranial nerves 9, 10 or 11
- Classic imaging appearance: Large, sharply demarcated, fusiform, enhancing mass centered in JF
- Second most common jugular foramen (JF) tumor
- Presents with sensorineural hearing loss (>90%)

Imaging Findings
General Features
- Best imaging clue: Sharply marginated, enlarged JF on CT
- **Fusiform** or dumbbell mass of JF
- Intraosseous extension may be marked
- Growth path: Along line of retro-olivary sulcus of medulla to jugular foramen inferiorly to nasopharyngeal carotid space

CT Findings
- Smooth enlargement of jugular foramen margins
  - JF with thin, sclerotic rim
- Coronal plane: Amputation of lateral jugular tubercle ("bird's beak")

MR Findings
- T1 C+ MR: Tubular or dumbbell mass with uniform enhancement ± intramural cystic components in larger tumors
- T2 signal high; compare lower T2 signal with meningioma

Angiographic Findings
- Tumor is moderately vascular
- Feeding vessels are tortuous but not enlarged
- Scattered contrast "puddles" are characteristic
  - Arteriovenous shunting or vascular encasement not present

Schwannoma, Jugular Foramen

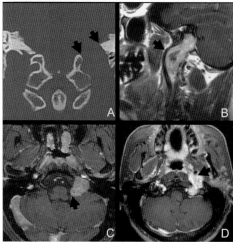

JFS. (A) Coronal CT reveals enlarged, sharply marginated left JF (arrows). (B) Sagittal T1 C+ MR shows enhancing fusiform JFS with ICA pushed anteriorly (arrow). (C) Axial SPGR C+ shows medial tumor margin pointing at lateral medulla. (D) Axial T1 C+ reveals inferior JFS in carotid space (arrow).

- Internal carotid artery is characteristically displaced over lower anteromedial margin of schwannoma, jugular foramen (JFS) in the nasopharyngeal CS

Differential Diagnosis: Jugular Foramen Mass

JF Paraganglioma
- CT: Permeative bone margins of JF
- T1 MR: High-velocity flow voids are characteristic
- Angiography: Rapidly fills and blushes
- Growth vector: Grows up and out from JF into middle ear

JF Meningioma
- CT: Permeative hyperostotic bony changes
- T1 C+ MR: Dural-based mass with dural tails
- Angiography: Prolonged blush into capillary phase
- Growth vector: Centrifugally along dural surfaces

Acoustic Schwannoma
- CT: Bone changes confined to IAC flaring
- T1 C+ MR: IAC-CPA enhancing mass
- Centered above JF
- Growth vector: Projects toward brainstem from IAC

Metastatic Tumor or NHL
- CT: Bony margins of JF are destructive
- T1 C+ MR: Mixed, enhancing, invasive mass
- Growth vector: Centrifugal away from JF

Pathology

General
- Etiology-Pathogenesis
  - Arises from Schwann cells wrapping CN 9, 10 or 11
- Epidemiology

29

Schwannoma, Jugular Foramen

- o   Glossopharyngeal nerve most common nerve of origin
- o   Multiple schwannomas = NF-2

Gross Pathologic, Surgical Features
- Smooth, lobulated mass arising from the nerve sheath
- Tan, round/ovoid, encapsulated mass
- Arises eccentrically from nerve

Microscopic Features
- Differentiated neoplastic Schwann cells
- Spindle cells with elongated nuclei
  - o   Areas of compact, elongated cells = Antoni A
  - o   Areas of less cellular loosely arranged tumor, ± clusters of lipid-laden cells = Antoni B
- Immunochemistry: Strong, diffuse immuno-staining for S-100 protein = neural crest marker antigen present in supporting cells of nervous system
- No necrosis but may have intratumoral cysts and/or hemorrhage

Clinical Issues

Presentation
- Principal presenting symptom: SNHL
  - o   > 90% have hearing loss at presentation
  - o   Clinically mixed into the "rule out acoustic schwannoma" group
- Symptoms from 9-11 cranial neuropathy occur late

Natural History
- Slowly-growing, benign tumor

Treatment
- Total surgical removal of tumor in a single operation is goal

Prognosis
- Treatment may still result in 7-12 cranial nerve injury
- CSF leak is a less common complication

Selected References
1.   Eldevik OP et al: Imaging findings in schwannomas of the jugular foramen. AJNR 21:1139-44, 2000
2.   Caldemeyer KS et al: The jugular foramen: a review of anatomy, masses, and imaging characteristics. RadioGraphics 17:1123-39, 1997
3.   Kaye AH et al: Jugular foramen schwannomas. J Neurosurg 60:1045-53, 1984

Meningioma, Jugular Foramen

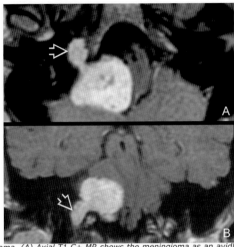

JF Meningioma. (A) Axial T1 C+ MR shows the meningioma as an avidly enhancing bilobed mass with its smaller component in the JF (open arrow). The basal cistern piece compresses the medulla. (B) Coronal T1 C+ MR reveals the jugular foramen component (open arrow) to better advantage.

Key Facts
- Definition: Meningioma arising from **arachnoid cap cells** sprinkled along the cranial nerves within the jugular foramen
- Classic imaging appearance
  - CT shows bony margins of jugular foramen (JF) are **permeative-sclerotic** while tumor may show matrix calcifications
  - T1 C+ MR shows an enhancing, **dural-based mass** with **dural tails** welling up from jugular foramen
- Meningioma is most common intracranial extra-axial neoplasm
- Meningioma, jugular foramen (MJF), clinically and radiologically mimics paraganglioma
  - Especially true when it enters the middle ear cavity and presents as vascular retrotympanic mass
- Meningioma arises from arachnoidal cells of the meninges
  - 1/3 of arachnoid cells are in the meninges of skull base
  - Arachnoidal cells can follow cranial nerves, permitting meningioma to follow the 9-11 cranial nerves into the JF and beyond into the nasopharyngeal carotid space

Imaging Findings
General Imaging Features
- Best imaging clue: Dural-based mass with dural tails
- MJF mimics glomus jugulare and jugulotympanicum paraganglioma
CT Findings
- Hyperdense, calcified, dural-based mass
- Uniform, strong enhancement
- **Permeative and/or sclerotic** bone changes at margins of MJF
MR Findings
- **Absence of high-velocity flow voids** on T1 unenhanced MR images or any other MR sequence

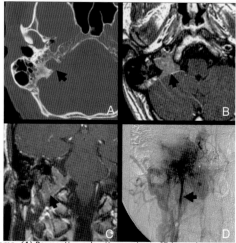

JF meningioma. (A) Permeative-sclerotic margins to JF (arrow) seen on axial CT. (B) Uniform MJF enhancement (arrow) fills the JF on T1 C+ MR. (C) Coronal T1 C+ MR shows the extent of MJF (arrow) to best advantage. (D) Angio shows ECA feeder = ascending pharyngeal artery (arrow) and prolonged tumor stain.

- Dural-based mass along with **"dural tails"** along margin of JF

<u>Angiographic Findings</u>
- External carotid artery dural branches supplying the center of tumor
- Internal carotid artery pial branches supply periphery of the MJF
- **Prolonged tumor stain** well into the venous phase of angiogram

<u>Imaging Recommendations</u>
- CT, MR and angiography all done before surgery
- CT shows critical bony landmarks
- MR reveals exact soft tissue extent of tumor
- Angiography provides a vascular road map for the surgeon
  - Evaluates the collateral arterial and venous circulation of the brain
  - Embolization used for preoperative hemostasis

Differential Diagnosis: Jugular Foramen Mass

<u>High-riding Jugular Bulb</u>
- Jugular foramen bony margins intact
- Increased signal does not persist in all MR sequences

<u>Dehiscent Jugular Bulb</u>
- Sigmoid plate is focally dehiscent
- Polypoid extension into middle ear is contiguous with jugular bulb

<u>Glomus Jugulare Paraganglioma</u>
- Mass with permeative bony margins on CT
- High-velocity flow voids on T1 MR
- Short but pronounced tumor blush on angiography

<u>9-11 Schwannoma</u>
- Mass with well-circumscribed, bony margins without hyperostotic or permeative changes on CT
- T1 C+ MR reveals an enhancing, tubular mass along the course of cranial nerves 9-11; intramural cysts may be seen
- No tumor blush or large, feeding arteries on angiography

Meningioma, Jugular Foramen

Pathology
General
- Genetics
  - Genetic drivers associated with chromosome 22
- Etiology-Pathogenesis
  - Benign, unencapsulated neoplasm arising from arachnoid cap cells sprinkled along cranial nerves 9-11 in JF
- Epidemiology
  - Paraganglioma > schwannoma > meningioma of JF

Gross Pathologic, Surgical Features
- Gray-colored mass supplied by enlarged, dural blood vessels
- **Lobulated** and **en plaque** morphotypes
- En plaque MJF more likely to infiltrate underlying dura and invade subjacent bone

Microscopic Features
- Heterogeneous, benign appearance
- Both **psammomatous calcifications** and **meningothelial cells** that cluster into whorls and lobules seen

Staging Criteria
- World Health Organization's classification
  - Typical meningioma (90%)
  - Atypical meningioma (8%)
  - Anaplastic or malignant meningioma (2%)

Clinical Issues
Presentation
- Principal presenting symptom: 9-11 cranial neuropathy
- Other symptoms
  - Pulsatile tinnitus ± vascular, retrotympanic mass
  - Cranial neuropathy may involve any of cranial nerves 7-12
- MJF when extensively invading the temporal bone may be clinically indistinguishable from glomus jugulotympanicum paraganglioma
- Occurs in 40-60 year old patients; female to male ratio of 2:1
- Risk factors: Prior radiation, NF-2 and female sex hormones

Treatment
- Surgical removal
- Preoperative embolization used for hemostasis
- Radiotherapy when too old or sick to have surgery

Prognosis
- Surgical cure results in multiple lower cranial neuropathies

Selected References
1. Harnsberger HR et al: The posterior skull base, with emphasis on the clivus, petro-occipital fissure and jugular foramen. Syllabus, RSNA Categorical Course in Diagnostic Radiology: Neuroradiology 2000: 153-66, 2000
2. Tekkok IH et al: Jugular foramen meningioma: Report of a case and review of the literature. J Neurosurg Sci 41:283-92, 1997
3. Molony TB et al: Meningiomas of the jugular foramen. Otolaryngol Head Neck Surg 106:128-36, 1992

Fibrous Dysplasia, Skull Base

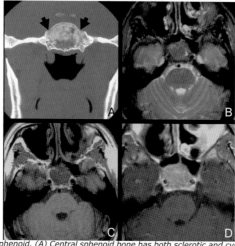

FD of basisphenoid. (A) Central sphenoid bone has both sclerotic and cystic changes on CT (arrows). (B) Axial T2 MR shows the FD as intermediate and low signal. (C) T1 C- image shows FD as low signal. (D) T1 C+ axial MR images reveals FD to uniformly enhance.

Key Facts

- Definition: Bone disorder characterized by progressive replacement of normal bone marrow by a mixture of fibrous tissue and woven bone
- Classic imaging appearance: CT shows 3 major appearances, pagetoid (ground glass), sclerotic and cystic bone changes
- Affects any bone in the body with the skull, skull base and facial bones involved 25% of time with monostotic fibrous dysplasia (FD) and 50% of polyostotic FD

Imaging Findings

General Imaging Features

- Best imaging clue: CT shows ground-glass matrix in a bone lesion
- Findings relate to relative content of fibrous versus osseous tissue
- Appearances: Ground-glass pagetoid (56%), sclerotic (23%) & cystic (21%)

CT Findings

- Expansile mass in bone with a surrounding sclerotic bone called a rind
  - **Pagetoid FD** has "ground-glass" appearance
  - **Sclerotic FD** density approaches cortical bone
  - **Cystic FD** is hypodense except along its edges
- Disease activity may relate to CT appearance
  - Cystic, pagetoid and sclerotic FD proposed to represent in order the most active to least active

MR Findings

- Expansile mass with **low signal** on both T1 and T2 images
- Heterogeneous signal pattern, especially on T2 images where patchy high signal within the lesion secondary to areas of diminished bone trabeculae can also be seen

Bone Scan Findings

- Increased radionuclide accumulation, perfusion and delayed bone phase

Fibrous Dysplasia, Skull Base

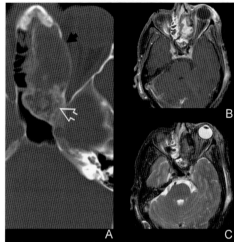

FD of ethmoid bone. (A) Axial CT shows the FD to have both a cystic-active area (solid arrow) and more bony-inactive area (open arrow). (B) Axial T1 C+ MR reveals enhancement of both areas. (C) Axial T2 MR shows most of the FD lesion to be low signal.

- Nonspecific; sensitive to extent of skeletal lesions in polyostotic FD

Differential Diagnosis: Bony Lesions of Skull Base
Paget's Disease
- Pagetoid ground-glass FD mimics Paget's disease
- Involves temporal bone and calvarium, not the craniofacial area
- "Cotton wool" CT appearance is useful clue to Paget's diagnosis
Osteomyelitis of the Skull Base
- Cystic FD may mimic
- Clinical setting of skull base infection very different from FD
Ossifying Fibroma
- Cystic form of FD mimics ossifying fibroma
- Has a typical thick, bony rim and lower density center
Intraosseous Meningioma
- Sclerotic FD mimics intraosseous meningioma or giant cell tumor
- En plaque soft tissue mass present; not so for FD
Giant Cell Tumor
- Sclerotic FD may mimic
- Giant cell tumor may be indistinguishable from monostotic FD
Histiocytosis X
- Cystic FD may mimic; usually more destructive

Pathology
General
- Genetics
  - Sporadic gene mutation
- Etiology-Pathogenesis
  - All cells descended from this mutated cell can manifest features of monostotic or polyostotic FD
- Epidemiology

- o   Monostotic FD is 6 times more common than polyostotic FD
- o   Monostotic form (75%): Found in skull and face 25% of time
- o   Polyostotic form (25%): Found in skull and face 50% of time

Gross Pathologic, Surgical Features
- •   Tan-yellow to white lesion that may have variable consistency from soft/ rubbery to gritty/firm depending on fibrous versus osseous make-up

Microscopic Features
- •   FD lesion contains fibrous tissue with intramural bone trabeculae
- •   Fibrous stroma is myxofibrous tissue of mixed vascularity
- •   Osseous metaplasia creates bone trabeculae made up of immature, **woven** bone seen as peculiar shapes floating in the fibrous stroma

Clinical Issues

Presentation
- •   Principal presenting symptom: Facial deformity
- •   Young affected (< 30 years old)
- •   Other symptoms: Incidental asymptomatic imaging observation; hemifacial deformity; visual problems and cranial neuropathy
- •   3 presentations: Monostotic, polyostotic and McCune-Albright syndrome
- •   **Monostotic FD**
  - o   70% of all FD cases; single osseous site is affected
  - o   Older children and young adults (75% present before the age 30)
  - o   Skull and face involved in 25%; maxilla (especially the zygomatic process) and mandible (molar area) >> frontal bone > ethmoid and sphenoid bones > temporal bone
  - o   May be asymptomatic, incidental imaging findings
  - o   Other symptoms nonspecific: Pain, focal swelling and tenderness
- •   **Polyostotic FD**
  - o   25% of all FD cases; involves ≥ 2 separate osseous sites
  - o   Skull and face involved in 50%
  - o   Younger patient group, mean age at diagnosis of 8 years
  - o   2/3 have symptoms by age 10 including craniofacial asymmetry
- •   **McCune-Albright syndrome**
  - o   Subtype of polyostotic FD defined by the clinical triad of polyostotic FD (usually unilateral), endocrine dysfunction and cutaneous hyperpigmentation (café-au-lait spots)
  - o   5% of all FD cases
  - o   Appears earlier and affects more bones more severely

Treatment
- •   Aggressive surgical management not recommended in most cases
- •   Non-disabling surgical intervention is utilized when safe
- •   No radiation therapy! May cause malignant transformation

Prognosis
- •   Monostotic craniofacial FD has an excellent prognosis
- •   Most spontaneously "burn out" or cease to grow in their teens and 20s
- •   Polyostotic FD rarely life threatening but poorer prognosis is present

Selected References
1.   Jee WH et al: Fibrous dysplasia: MR imaging characteristics with radiopathologic correlation. AJR 167:1523-27, 1996
2.   Casselman JW et al: MRI in craniofacial fibrous dysplasia. Neuroradiology 35:234-7, 1993
3.   Kransdorf MJ et al: Fibrous dysplasia. RadioGraphics 10:519-37, 1990

PocketRadiologist™
Head and Neck
100 Top Diagnoses

TEMPORAL BONE

EAC Atresia

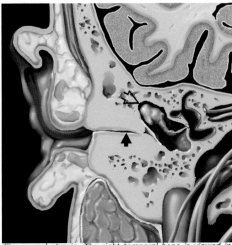

External auditory canal atresia. The right temporal bone is viewed in the coronal plane in this drawing depicting EAC atresia. The deformed auricle and lateral EAC stenosis alerts the clinician to the underlying anomaly. Bony atresia leaves behind only a seam (arrow). Ossicular fusion and rotation is present (open arrow).

Key Facts
- Synonyms: Congenital aural dysplasia; microtia
- Definition: Stenosis or atresia of the of external auditory canal (EAC) with associated auricle deformity
- May be isolated malformation, or part of a cranial-facial syndrome, such as Crouzon's, Goldenhar's or Pierre Robin
- Classic imaging appearance (CT)
  - Bony or membranous stenosis or atresia of the EAC
  - Associated with underdeveloped mastoid air cells and small middle ear cavity
  - Malformations of the malleus and incus are common

Imaging Findings
General Features
- Best imaging clue: Absent EAC (bony or membranous atresia)
- Dysplastic auricle
- Non-syndromal EAC atresia usually unilateral
- Bilateral EAC atresia seen when EAC malformation is syndromal
- **Inner ear** and IAC usually **normal**
- EAC atresia = clinical diagnosis; CT provides pre-operative roadmap

CT Findings
- Bony, membranous or mixed atresia plate
- Middle ear findings variable but include
  - **Small middle ear cavity** with fusion of the malleus and incus to the lateral middle ear cavity wall
  - Fusion of the malleolar-incudal articulation
  - **Aberrant** anterior course of mastoid segment of **facial nerve**
  - Oval window atresia may be associated
- Normal morphology and location of the stapes important for surgical reconstruction of ossicular function

EAC Atresia

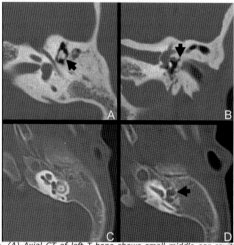

EAC atresia. (A) Axial CT of left T-bone shows small middle ear cavity and fused ossicles (arrow). (B) Coronal CT reveals a thin bony atresia plate (arrow) with stenotic EAC. (C-D) Axial CT images on another case with severe atresia show very small opacified middle ear (arrow), no ossicles and thick bony atresia plate.

- **Congenital cholesteatoma** may form behind the atresia plate or in the middle ear; check for soft tissue mass here

MR Findings
- MR may be used to confirm normal membranous labyrinth and internal auditory canal
- Usually unnecessary

Imaging Recommendations
- High resolution axial and coronal plane CT is best imaging approach

Differential Diagnosis: Narrowed External Auditory Canal

Acquired EAC Stenosis
- Usually presents later in life, with history of cold water swimming, or other local EAC trauma
- Auricle is normal

Pathology

General
- General Path Comments
  - Atresia is membranous, bony or a mix of the two
  - There is either stenosis or complete EAC atresia
- Genetics
  - 14% have positive prior family history
  - May be associated with inherited syndromes
    - Crouzon's, Goldenhar's or Pierre Robin syndromes
- Embryology-Anatomy
  - 1st and 2nd branchial arches and 1st pharyngeal pouch develop at same time
    - Associated middle ear and mastoid anomalies are commonly seen with auricular dysplasia and EAC atresia

- o Meckel's cartilage/first branchial arch forms malleus head and body, incus short process, tensor tympani muscle and tendon
- o Reichert's cartilage/second branchial arch forms manubrium of malleus, body and long process of incus, stapes (except footplate) and stapedial muscle and tendon
- o Inner ear forms earlier during gestation, so anomalies of labyrinth and IAC are rarely associated with EAC atresia
- Etiology-Pathogenesis
  - o Etiology of malformation is presumed to be an in utero insult
  - o Epithelial cells of first branchial groove fail to split and canalize, resulting in atresia
- Epidemiology
  - o 1 in 10,000 births

Clinical Issues

Natural History
- Status at birth remains unchanged through life
- Association with cholesteatoma makes temporal bone CT later in life a good idea for those with unilateral unoperated EAC atresia
- Principal clinical symptom: Conductive hearing loss

Treatment
- Unilateral atresia not treated if the other ear is normal
- Cosmetic reconstruction of auricle dysplasia usually occurs in adolescence
- Bilateral atresia is treated at 5-6 years of age, when the head has reached 90% of adult size
  - o Reconstruction of the auricle precedes surgical treatment of the middle ear and ossicular deformities
  - o Surgical reconstruction on side with mildest EAC atresia
  - o Both auricles are repaired for cosmetic reasons
- Principal clinical sign: Auricle dysplasia with EAC stenosis or atresia

Prognosis
- In unilateral atresia, the other ear has normal hearing
- Bilateral atresia may present as bilateral conductive hearing loss
  - o After surgery, hearing is adequate but generally not normal
- Auricle reconstruction may require 4-5 staged surgeries
- Auricle dysplasia; severity of auricular dysplasia parallels involvement of middle ear and ossicles
  - o Milder auricle dysplasia found with milder middle ear anomalies
  - o Severe auricle dysplasia found with severe middle ear anomalies

Selected References
1. Benton C et al: Imaging of congenital anomalies of the temporal bone. Neuroimaging Clin N Am 10:35-53, 2000
2. Mehra YN et al: Correlation between high-resolution CT and surgical findings in congenital aural atresia. Arch Otolaryngol Head Neck Surg 114:137-41, 1988
3. Swartz JD et al: Congenital malformations of the external and middle ear: high-resolution CT findings of surgical import. Am J Roentgenol 144:501-6, 1985

Cholesteatoma, Congenital

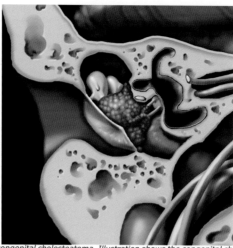

Middle ear congenital cholesteatoma. Illustration shows the congenital cholesteatoma within the middle ear cavity. Much of the cholesteatoma is medial to the ossicles compared with the typical acquired middle ear cholesteatoma. Ossicle erosion is minor given the size of the cholesteatomatous mass.

Key Facts
- Definition: Middle ear aberrant epithelial rest of exfoliated keratin within stratified squamous epithelium
- Classic imaging appearance: Focal soft-tissue mass with mild ossicular erosions behind an **intact tympanic membrane**
- Account for only 5% of all temporal bone cholesteatomas
- Occur in petrous apex, mastoid, middle ear, middle ear and mastoid, and external auditory canal
- Patients with EAC atresia may develop congenital cholesteatoma (CCh) behind the obstruction

Imaging Findings
General Features
- Best imaging clue: Sharply-marginated mass in middle ear with wall erosion or ossicular dehiscence when large
- Well-circumscribed middle ear or mastoid mass
  - Middle ear location is most common site of occurrence
- Well-pneumatized mastoids without chronic inflammatory changes
CT Findings
- Common locations of CCh
  - Anterosuperior middle ear, adjacent to eustachian tube and anterior tympanic ring, medial to the ossicles
    - Inferior but adjacent to tensor tympani muscle
  - Near the stapes
  - Posterior tympanum
- Bone erosion less common than in acquired cholesteatoma
  - Occurs late in disease
- Ossicular erosion unusual with anterior mesotympanum involvement
- Long process of incus and stapes superstructure most commonly dehisced ossicles

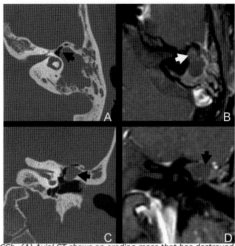

Middle ear CCh. (A) Axial CT shows an eroding mass that has destroyed all but head of malleus (arrow). (B) Axial T1 C+ MR image reveals the CCh as a non-enhancing plug of tissue (arrow). (C) Epitympanic tissue eroding (arrow) ossicles (coronal CT). (D) CCh (arrow) does not enhance on coronal T1 C+ MR.

- Labyrinthine extension may occur but only late in disease process

MR Findings
- T1 C+ MR shows rim-enhancing middle ear mass
- T2 signal is intermediate compared to inflammatory tissues

Imaging Recommendations
- Bone-only temporal bone CT is examination of choice
- T1 C+ MR is adjunctive test used when glomus tympanicum or facial nerve schwannoma are considerations

Differential Diagnosis: Middle Ear Mass

Middle Ear Effusion
- Complete middle ear mastoid opacification without ossicle erosion
- If middle ear completely opacified, may not be able to tell from CCh from effusion if no ossicle erosion present
- Clinical: Fluid behind tympanic membrane (TM)

Cholesterol Granuloma of Middle Ear
- Imaging: Middle ear mass with ossicular erosion common
  - T1 high signal on MR
- Clinical: Blue TM

Glomus Tympanicum Paraganglioma
- Imaging: Stuck on cochlear promontory
  - No bony erosions on CT; focal enhancing mass on T1 C+ MR
- Clinical: Vascular mass (red) behind TM ± pulsatile tinnitus

Facial Nerve Schwannoma
- Imaging: Tubular mass emanating from tympanic facial nerve canal
  - Enlarged facial nerve canal on CT; enhancing mass on T1 C+ MR
- Clinical: Also white mass behind intact TM

Cholesteatoma, Congenital

Pathology

General
- Embryology-Anatomy
  - Congenital ectodermal rest is left behind in middle ear cavity
- Etiology-Pathogenesis
  - This aberrant congenital epithelial rest occurs when there is abnormal migration of external canal ectoderm beyond the tympanic ring
  - Becomes a mass-like middle ear accumulation of stratified epithelial squamous cells = congenital cholesteatoma
    - The epidermoid formation, the point of transformation between the tympanic cavity and eustachian tube, is a rest of stratified squamous epidermal cells where many CCh arise
    - The posterior epitympanum, at the tympanic isthmi, an area contiguous between the middle ear cavity and the attic, is another common location where CCh arise

Gross Pathologic, Surgical Features
- Circumscribed, **pearly-white mass** with capsular sheen

Microscopic Features
- Identical to epidermoid inclusion cyst
- Stratified squamous epithelium, with progressive exfoliation of keratinous material
- Contents rich in cholesterol crystals

Clinical Issues

Presentation
- Principal presenting symptom: **White mass behind an intact TM**
- Other symptoms: Unilateral conductive hearing loss
- No preceding history of recurrent, chronic, middle ear infections
- Facial nerve canal invasion is a rare manifestation
- More common in boys
- Average age of presentation
  - Anterior or anterosuperior: 4 years
  - Posterosuperior and mesotympanum: 12 years
  - Attic and antral involvement: 20 years

Treatment
- Complete surgical extirpation is treatment of choice
- Ossicle chain reconstruction may be necessary

Prognosis
- Large lesions or posterior epitympanic CCh have high recurrence rate

Selected References
1. Yeo SW et al: The clinical evaluations of pathophysiology for congenital middle ear cholesteatoma. Am J Otolaryngol 22:184-9, 2001
2. Zappia JJ et al: Congenital cholesteatoma. Arch Otolaryngol Head Neck Surg 121:11-22, 1995
3. Friedberg J: Congenital cholesteatoma. Laryngoscope 104:1-24, 1994

Cholesteatoma, Acquired

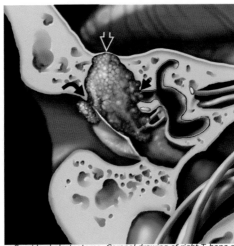

Acquired pars flaccida cholesteatoma. Coronal drawing of right T-bone shows a large cholesteatoma welling up from a pars flaccida perforation, amputating the scutum (curved arrow), dehiscing the tegmen tympani (open arrow) and eroding through the cortex of the lateral semicircular canal (arrow).

Key Facts

- Definition: Attempted "healing" of a perforated tympanic membrane (TM) leads to exfoliated keratin within stratified squamous epithelium = ball of **"skin in the wrong place"**
  - "Wrong place" = middle ear-mastoid
- Classic imaging appearance: Non-dependent mass centered in lateral epitympanic recess associated with **scutum and ossicular erosion**
- History of recurrent or chronic middle ear infections common
- TM perforation or retraction (retraction pocket) precede development of acquired cholesteatoma

Imaging Findings

General Features

- Best imaging clue: CT evidence of scutum, ossicular or middle ear wall **erosion** in association with a non-dependent middle ear mass
  - Alternatively, if referring clinician can see a cholesteatoma in or through a perforated TM, then your job is made easier as you only need to define the associated findings, not make the diagnosis

CT Findings

- CT diagnosis established when middle ear mass is associated with ossicular erosion and/or bony scalloping (scutum or bony walls)
- Radiologist must evaluate images to detect the following
  - Relationship of cholesteatoma to ossicles
  - Integrity of ossicles
  - Erosion of the scutum
  - Tegmen tympani dehiscence
  - Dehiscence of any part of facial nerve canal
  - **Dehiscence of lateral semicircular canal** or other point on lateral wall of otic capsule
  - Extension of cholesteatoma into the mastoid antrum

Cholesteatoma, Acquired

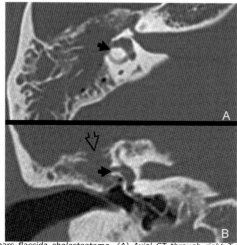

Acquired pars flaccida cholesteatoma. (A) Axial CT through right T-bone shows opacification of middle ear and mastoid with associated lateral semicircular canal dehiscence (arrow). (B) Coronal CT reveals both lateral semicircular canal (arrow) and tegmen tympani (open arrow) dehiscence.

- Mastoid air cells may be small and underpneumatized from chronic infections in child

MR Findings
- T1 C+ MR: Rim-enhancing **low-signal** mass in middle ear
- Bony dehiscence poorly seen on MR

Imaging Recommendations
- Bone-only T-bone **CT** is best 1st radiologic examination
- CT is imaging modality of choice to identify ossicular destruction & bony scalloping that make this imaging diagnosis
  - Pars flaccida cholesteatoma best evaluated on coronal CT
  - Pars tensa cholesteatoma best evaluated on axial CT
- Enhanced MR is adjunctive test used when cephalocele, middle cranial fossa infection or cholesteatoma extratemporal extent is at issue

Differential Diagnosis: Middle Ear Mass

Congenital Cholesteatoma
- Ossicles and other bony erosions may occur
- Clinical: Focal mass behind intact TM

Chronic Inflammatory Disease with Post-inflammatory Ossicular Erosion
- May be indistinguishable from acquired cholesteatoma by CT
- Clinical: Must rely on clinical exam and history

Cholesterol Granuloma of Middle Ear
- May have ossicular, scutal and other bony erosions like cholesteatoma
- Clinical: Clinical presentation different with no TM perforation & blue hue to intact TM

Glomus Tympanicum Paraganglioma
- Focal mass on cochlear promontory without significant erosions
- Clinical: Intact TM with pulsatile vascular retrotympanic mass

Cholesteatoma, Acquired

Pathology
General
- General Comments
  - **Pars flaccida cholesteatoma** occur in Prussak's space, lateral to the malleus head and above the lateral mallear ligament
    - Mass can fill the antrum and mastoid air cells
    - Scutum erosion is characteristic
    - Erosion of lateral aspect of malleus head and incus body
  - **Pars tensa cholesteatoma** results from posterosuperior TM retractions or perforation
    - Sinus tympani and facial recess may be involved
    - Extension into attic may push ossicles laterally
- Etiology-Pathophysiology
  - TM perforation or retraction results in middle ear accumulation of stratified epithelial squamous cells
  - Mass-like collection continually enlarges, eroding adjacent bones
- Epidemiology
  - Most common lesion imaged in the middle ear-mastoid

Gross Pathologic, Surgical Features
- Circumscribed, capsular sheen (the "pearly tumor")
- Filled with soft, waxy, white material

Microscopic Features
- Identical to epidermoid cyst
- Stratified squamous epithelium, with progressive exfoliation of keratinous material
- Contents rich in cholesterol crystals

Clinical Issues
Presentation
- Principal presenting symptom: Conductive hearing loss
- Other symptoms: Painless otorrhea; larger lesions that dehisce lateral semicircular canal have vertigo
- Typical patient profile: Adult with long history of chronic ear problems; children with history of recurrent or chronic middle ear infections

Treatment
- Mastoidectomy with cholesteatoma removal and ossicular reconstruction
- Radical mastoidectomy when cholesteatoma goes down eustachian tube, invades deeply into inner ear or petrous apex

Prognosis
- Smaller cholesteatoma: Excellent after full removal
- Larger cholesteatoma: Residual conductive or sensorineural hearing loss and peripheral facial nerve paralysis possible

Selected References
1. Watts S et al: A systematic approach to interpretation of computed tomography scans prior to middle ear cholesteatoma. J Laryngol Otol 114:248-53, 2000
2. Mafee MF et al: Epidermoid cyst (cholesteatoma) and cholesterol granuloma of the temporal bone and epidermoid cysts affecting the brain. Neuroimaging Clin N Am 4:561-78, 1994
3. Swartz JD: Cholesteatomas of the middle ear: Diagnosis, etiology and complications. Radiol Clin North Am 22:15-35, 1984

Aberrant Internal Carotid Art.

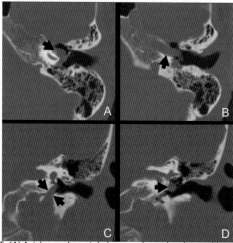

AbICA on CT. (A) Axial scan shows tubular mass (arrow) on low cochlear promontory. (B) Just below (A) the AbICA is seen re-entering posterior margin of horizontal petrous ICA (arrow). (C) Coronal CT, large inferior tympanic canaliculus (arrows). (D) En face view of AbICA crossing cochlear promontory (arrow).

Key Facts
- Definition: Aberrant Internal Carotid Artery (AbICA) = congenital vascular anomaly resulting from **regression of the cervical ICA** during embryogenesis
- Classic imaging appearance: AbICA enters posterior middle ear cavity from below, hugs the cochlear promontory as it crosses the middle ear, then joins the posterior lateral margin of the horizontal petrous ICA
- Otoscopic appearance of this vascular-appearing retrotympanic lesion mimics glomus tympanicum and jugulotympanicum paraganglioma
- Radiologist must hold onto correct imaging diagnosis against clinical impression of paraganglioma
- Disaster lurks if misdiagnosis results in biopsy!

Imaging Findings
General Features
- Best imaging clue: **Tubular** nature of AbICA
- Tubular lesion crossing middle ear cavity from posterior to anterior
- Absent normal vertical segment of the petrous ICA
CT Findings
- **CT** appearance of AbICA is **diagnostic**
- AbICA enters posterior middle ear through an **enlarged inferior tympanic canaliculus**
- Courses anteriorly across the cochlear promontory to join the horizontal carotid canal through a dehiscence in the carotid plate
- Stenosis at the point where it rejoins the horizontal carotid canal sometimes occurs and can lead to pulsatile tinnitus
- **Aberrant stapedial artery** is often associated with AbICA
- Coronal CT shows a round soft-tissue density on cochlear promontory
  - On a single slice looks disturbingly like paraganglioma
  - Viewing multiple slices reveals tubular nature

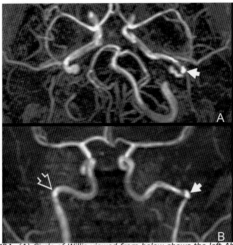

AbICA on MRA. (A) Circle of Willis viewed from below shows the left AbICA is more posterior and lateral than the opposite right ICA. Irregular lumen can be seen (arrow). (B) Anterior view of AbICA reveals a more angular and irregular vessel (arrow) than smoother curve on normal right side (open arrow).

MRA & Angiography Findings
- Conventional MR does not reliably identify aberrant ICA
- Lack of MR signal contrast between the low signal of mobile proton poor bone and the low signal from AbICA blood flow precludes MR diagnosis
- MRA source and reprojected images show aberrant arterial nature of this lesion
  - Side-to-side comparison shows the AbICA enters the skull base posterolateral to the opposite normal side
  - On a frontal reprojection, the AbICA looks like a 7 or a reverse 7 depending on the side of involvement
- Angiography no longer necessary to confirm this imaging diagnosis

Imaging Recommendations
- Bone-only temporal bone CT makes this diagnosis
- If MR done, MRA source and reprojection images are diagnostic

Differential Diagnosis: Vascular Retrotympanic Mass

Dehiscent Jugular Bulb
- Focal absence of sigmoid plate
- Bud from superolateral jugular bulb enters middle ear mass

Cholesterol granuloma, middle ear
- CT appearance often identical to acquired cholesteatoma
- T1 MR non-contrasted high signal is highly suggestive

Paraganglioma
- Glomus tympanicum
  - Focal mass on cochlear promontory
  - No tubular shape
- Glomus jugulotympanicum
  - Mass enters middle ear through medial floor
  - CT shows permeative bone changes between jugular foramen and middle ear mass

Aneurysm, Petrous Internal Carotid Artery
- Bone-only CT shows focal smooth expansion of petrous ICA canal
- MRA is diagnostic of aneurysm

Pathology

General
- Embryology-Anatomy
  - Regression of cervical ICA during embryogenesis triggers a secondary anastomosis to occur between the **inferior tympanic artery** and the **caroticotympanic artery**
  - No normal vertical segment of petrous ICA is present
  - The **inferior tympanic canaliculus** enlarges to accommodate the enlarged inferior tympanic artery
  - Bony margin of posterolateral horizontal petrous IAC canal is dehiscent to allow the AbICA to rejoin the ICA at this point
- Etiology-Pathogenesis
  - Occurs when **enlarged inferior tympanic artery** anastomoses with enlarged **caroticotympanic artery** resulting from regression of cervical ICA during embryogenesis
- Epidemiology
  - Very rare vascular anomaly
  - 30% have aberrant stapedial artery associated

Clinical Issues

Presentation
- Principal presenting symptom: Vascular retrotympanic mass
- Other symptoms
  - Objective or subjective pulsatile tinnitus (PT)
    - Objective PT when stenosis is present at junction of AbICA and normal horizontal petrous ICA
  - Conductive hearing loss
- Otoscopic exam: **Vascular retrotympanic mass** behind inferior TM
- Important clinical observation: Vascular-appearing retrotympanic mass may exactly mimic paraganglioma

Treatment
- Most patients have minor symptoms that do not require treatment
- A clinical-radiologic mistake in diagnosis with resultant surgical intervention can be disastrous and must be avoided at all cost!

Prognosis
- No long term sequelae reported with AbICA
- Poor prognosis results only if misdiagnosis leads to biopsy
- If PT is loud, can be debilitating

Selected References
1. Botma M et al: Aberrant internal carotid artery in the middle-ear space. J Laryngol Otol 114:784-7, 2000
2. Davis WL et al: MR angiography of an aberrant internal carotid artery. AJNR 12:1225, 1991
3. Lo WW et al: Aberrant carotid artery: Radiologic diagnosis with emphasis in high-resolution computed tomography. RadioGraphics 5:985-993, 1985

Glomus Tympanicum

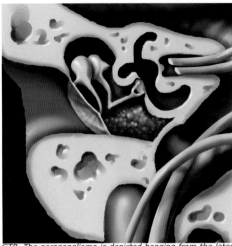

Drawing of GTP. The paraganglioma is depicted hanging from the lateral margin of the cochlear promontory. Its lateral margin abuts the tympanic membrane. No ossicle erosion is present. The floor of the middle ear cavity is intact.

Key Facts
- Synonym: Glomus tympanicum paraganglioma (GTP)
- Definition: Benign tumor that arises in glomus bodies situated on the cochlear promontory of the medial wall of the middle ear cavity
- Classic imaging appearance: Round mass with base on cochlear promontory; CT shows no bone erosion and T1 C+ MR shows intense enhancement
- GTP may be clinically indistinguishable from glomus jugulotympanicum paraganglioma or AbICA; imaging must differentiate these diagnoses
- Most common tumor of the middle ear

Imaging Findings
General Imaging Features
- Best imaging clue: MR shows enhancing mass on cochlear promontory
- Floor of middle ear cavity is intact (if eroded, jugulotympanicum)
CT Findings
- Focal mass on cochlear promontory is characteristic
- Small lesions: Fills lower middle ear, just reaches medial border of TM
- Large lesions: Fills middle ear cavity, creating attic block resulting in fluid collection in mastoid; margins of tumor not visible on CT
- Bone erosion **not** usually present with GTP, even with larger lesions
- Rare involvement of air cells along the inferior cochlear promontory may be mistaken for invasion
MR Findings
- T1 C+ MR shows focal enhancing mass on cochlear promontory
- Small GTP will be missed if slice thickness exceeds 3 mm
Angiographic Findings
- Unnecessary if GTP diagnosis clearly established by CT
- GTP supplied by enlarged ascending pharyngeal artery and its inferior tympanic branch, via the inferior tympanic canaliculus

Glomus Tympanicum

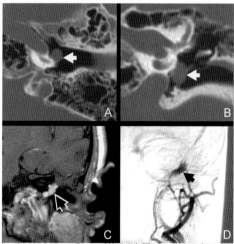

Glomus tympanicum paraganglioma. (A) Axial CT shows round mass with base on cochlear promontory (arrow). (B) Coronal CT reveals the GTP abuts the TM (arrow). (C) A slightly larger GTP fills the middle ear cavity (open arrow) and obstructs the attic. (D) Angio shows GTP in (C) vascular blush (arrow).

Imaging Recommendations
- Bone-only CT without contrast best if GTP suspected clinically
- MR and angiography only used if glomus jugulotympanicum found by CT

Differential Diagnosis: Middle Ear Mass
Aberrant Internal Carotid Artery
- Imaging: Tubular mass crosses middle ear cavity to rejoin horizontal petrous ICA; large inferior tympanic canaliculus
- Clinical: Vascular mass behind TM ± pulsatile tinnitus
Dehiscent Jugular Bulb
- Imaging: CT shows sigmoid plate is dehiscent; venous protrusion into middle ear cavity from superolateral jugular bulb
- Clinical: Asymptomatic incidental otoscopic observation
Congenital Cholesteatoma of Middle Ear
- Imaging: C+ T1 MR shows no enhancement
- Clinical: "White" mass behind intact TM
Glomus Jugulotympanicum Paraganglioma
- Imaging: CT shows permeative change in bony floor of middle ear
- Clinical: Identical to GTP

Pathology
General
- Etiology-Pathogenesis
  - Arise from glomus (L. "a ball") bodies (paraganglia) found along inferior tympanic nerve (Jacobson's nerve) on cochlear promontory
    - Chemoreceptor cells derived from primitive neural crest
  - Nonchromaffin (nonsecretory) in this location
- Epidemiology
  - GTP = most common tumor of middle ear
  - GTP not associated with multicentric paragangliomas

Glomus Tympanicum

Gross Pathologic, Surgical Features
- Glistening, red polypoid mass with base on cochlear promontory
- Fibrous pseudocapsule

Microscopic Features
- Biphasic cell pattern composed of chief cells and sustentacular cells surrounded by fibromuscular stroma
- Chief cells arranged in characteristic compact cell nests or balls of cells (zellballen)
- Immunohistochemistry: Chief cells show a diffuse reaction to chromogranin
- Electronmicroscopy: Shows neurosecretory granules

Glasscock-Jackson Classification of GTP
- Type I: Small mass limited to cochlear promontory
- Type II: Tumor completely filling middle ear space
- Type III: Tumor filling middle ear and extending into mastoid air cells
- Type IV: Tumor filling middle ear, extending into the mastoid or through tympanic membrane to fill the external auditory canal; may extend anterior to carotid artery

Clinical Issues

Presentation
- Principal presenting symptom: Vascular retrotympanic mass
- Other symptoms: Pulsatile tinnitus (90%), conductive hearing loss (50%), facial nerve paralysis (5%) and asymptomatic (5%)
- 3 times more common in women than in men
- 66% are between 40-60 years of age at diagnosis
- Vascular (red) retrotympanic mass
  - Posteroinferior quadrant of tympanic membrane

Natural History
- Slow-growing, non-invasive tumor
- Average time from onset of symptoms to surgical treatment is 3 years

Treatment
- Tympanotomy for smaller lesions; mastoidectomy for larger lesions
- Incomplete surgery of glomus jugulotympanicum paraganglioma or biopsy of an AbICA may result in serious patient complications
- The radiologist must correctly interpret the pretreatment images!

Prognosis
- Complete resection yields a permanent surgical cure

Selected References
1. Mafee MF et al: Glomus faciale, glomus jugulare, glomus tympanicum, glomus vagale, carotid body tumors, and simulating lesions: Role of MRI. Radiol Clin North Am 38:1059-76, 2000
2. Larson TC et al: Glomus tympanicum chemodectomas: Radiographic and clinical characteristics. Radiology 163:801-6, 1987
3. Lo WW et al: High-resolution CT in the evaluation of glomus tumors of the temporal bone. Radiology 150:737-42, 1984

Cochlear Dysplasia

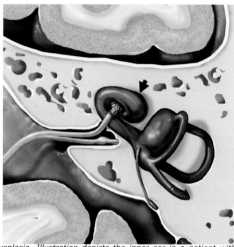

Cochlear dysplasia. Illustration depicts the inner ear in a patient with ChD. With incomplete partition form of ChD, the modiolus is deficient and only the basal turn of the cochlea is normally formed. The second and apical turns of the cochlea are dysmorphic and bulbous (arrow).

Key Facts
- Synonym: Mondini malformation
- Definition: Arrested development of the cochlea short of the expected 2½ turns of the normal cochlea
- Classic imaging appearance of cochlear dysplasia (ChD): CT or FSE-T2 MR show a cystic cochlea (severe ChD), incomplete partition (moderate ChD) or apical turn dysmorphism (mild ChD)
  - Imaging appearance depends on the time when cochlear development is arrested
  - Usually associated with large endolymphatic sac anomaly
- Second most common imaging diagnosis in congenital SNHL

Imaging Findings
General Imaging Features
- Best diagnostic clue: Cochlea lacks normal 2½ turns
- Imaging appearance depends on how early in inner ear development cochlear arrest occurs
- **Severe dysplasia** = Cystic cochlea ~ 6 week gestational arrest
  - No internal architecture to cochlea
  - Modiolus absent and cochlear nerve is hypoplastic
- **Moderate dysplasia** = Incomplete partition (aka, Mondini malformation) ~ 7 week gestational arrest
  - Incomplete development of the middle + apical turns of cochlea
  - Modiolar deficiency with scalar chamber asymmetry
- **Mild dysplasia** = Incomplete development of the apical turn of the cochlea ~ 8 week gestational arrest
  - Modiolar deficiency
  - Scalar chamber asymmetry
    - Scala vestibuli larger than scala tympani
    - ChD often associated with large, endolymphatic sac anomaly

Cochlear Dysplasia

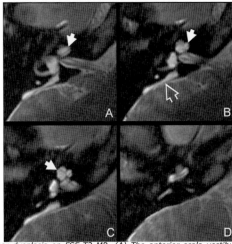

Mild cochlear dysplasia on FSE-T2 MR. (A) The anterior scala vestibuli (arrow) is asymmetrically enlarged compared to the more posterior scala tympani. (B) Large scala vestibuli (arrow); large endolymphatic sac (open arrow). (C) Bulbous apical turn (arrow). (D). Normal basal turn of cochlea.

CT Findings
- Severe dysplasia = Cystic cochlea: No turns seen in cochlea; cochlear aperture large; often associated with cystic vestibule
- Moderate dysplasia = Incomplete partition: Basal turn well delineated; middle and apical turns poorly defined
- Mild dysplasia = Apical turn bulbous; may be difficult to diagnosis on CT

MR Findings
- Severe dysplasia = Cystic cochlea: No turns seen in cochlea; cochlear aperture large with no modiolus visible; cochlear nerve may be hypoplastic
- Moderate dysplasia = Incomplete partition: Basal turn well delineated; middle and apical turns poorly defined; modiolus deficient; scalar chambers asymmetric with the anterior scala vestibuli larger than the posterior scala tympani
- Mild dysplasia = Apical turn bulbous; modiolar deficiency and asymmetric scalar chambers more subtle or absent

Imaging Recommendations
- Can be readily diagnosed with 1 mm temporal bone CT or focused high-resolution FSE-T2 MR
- If available, high-resolution MR defines modiolar anomalies, scalar chamber asymmetry and cochlear nerve hypoplasia not visible on CT

Differential Diagnosis: Cochlear Abnormality
Cochlear Aplasia (Michel's Aplasia)
- Imaging: No cochlea or vestibule present
  - Thought to be secondary to inner ear development arrest in the 4th gestational week
- Clinical: Dead ear from birth
Cystic Vestibule
- Imaging: Vestibule itself is large with lateral semicircular canal evident

Cochlear Dysplasia

- o Semicircular canals may be hypoplastic
- • Clinical: If isolated vestibule anomaly, may have normal hearing

Vestibule and Lateral Semicircular Canal Common Chamber
- • Imaging: Shape looks like "master lock" on its side on axial view
- • Clinical: May not have any hearing loss associated

Pathology
General
- • Embryology-Anatomy
  - o Embryogenesis of the inner ear begins with otic placode becoming the otic pit, then migrating deep to the middle and external ear to become the **otic vesicle**
  - o Medial elongation of the otic vesicle occurs with protrusions for the endolymphatic sac and semicircular canals
  - o Anterior protrusion becomes the **cochlear duct** which by the 9th gestational week spirals fully to form the normal **"nautilus" configuration** of the cochlea
- • Etiology-Pathogenesis
  - o Arrest of cochlear spiral development creates an anomalous cochlea with less than the normal 2½ turns
  - o Cystic cochlea: Arrested development at 6 weeks gestation
  - o Incomplete partition: Arrested development at 7 weeks gestation
  - o Mild cochlear dysplasia: Arrested development at 8 weeks gestation

Microscopic Features
- • Modiolar aplasia or hypoplasia accompanied by absence or pronounced reduction of the spiral ganglion cells respectively

Clinical Issues
Presentation
- • Principal presenting symptom: SNHL
  - o Often bilateral

Treatment
- • Cochlear implantation used when bilateral profound sensorineural deafness occurs

Prognosis
- • An increased risk of perilymph or CSF fistulae have been reported

Selected References
1. Graham JM et al: Congenital malformations of the ear and cochlear implantation in children; review and temporal bone common cavity. J Laryngol Otol Suppl 25:1-14, 2000
2. Phelps PD et al: Cochlear dysplasia and meningitis. Am J Otol 15:551-7, 1994
3. Urman SM et al: Otic capsule dysplasia: clinical and CT findings. RadioGraphics 10:823-38, 1990

Labyrinthine Ossificans

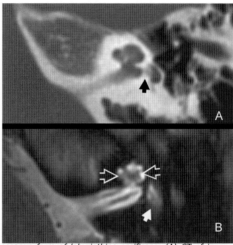

Early fibro-osseous form of labyrinthine ossificans. (A) CT of inner ear shows a normal cochlea and an ossific plaque in the vestibule (arrow). (B) FSE-T2 MR at same level as (A) shows cochlear fibro-osseous LO as an enlarged modiolus (open arrows) and low signal in the vestibule (arrow).

Key Facts
- Synonym: Labyrinthine ossification
- Definition: Membranous labyrinth ossification as a healing response to infectious, inflammatory or surgical insult to inner ear
- Classic imaging appearance
  - CT: High density bone deposition within membranous labyrinth
  - MR: Low intensity foci within high signal fluid of inner ear
- Post-meningitis labyrinthine ossificans (LO) = primary cause of acquired childhood deafness
- Bilateral cochlear LO can be a serious detriment to cochlear implantation, requiring a rethink of treatment options

Imaging Findings
General Features
- Best imaging clue: Bony encroachment on membranous labyrinth
- Radiologist should describe LO as "cochlear" or "non-cochlear"
  - Just describing LO of inner ear does not help the cochlear implant surgeon decide what can be done
    - Cochlear LO makes implant problematic
  - Next be specific about what non-cochlear portions of the membranous labyrinth are involved

CT Findings
- Mild LO: Fibro-osseous changes seen as a hazy increase in density within fluid spaces of membranous labyrinth and a prominent modiolus
- Moderate LO: Focal areas of bony encroachment on fluid spaces of membranous labyrinth; may be cochlear or non-cochlear
- Severe LO: Membranous labyrinth is completely obliterated by bone replacement of its fluid spaces

Labyrinthine Ossificans

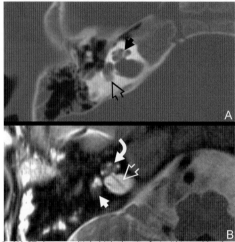

Moderate LO. (A) CT shows multiple high-density foci within cochlea (arrow) and one large bony LO foci in posterior vestibule (open arrow). (B) FSE-T2 MR reveals mixed osseous and fibro-osseous LO foci in cochlea (curved arrow), bony LO foci in posterior vestibule (arrow) and small cochlear nerve (open arrow).

MR Findings
- Mild LO: Intermediate and low signal fibro-osseous plugging of the high signal fluid spaces of membranous labyrinth with enlargement of modiolus
- Moderate LO: Focal areas of low signal bone encroaching on high signal fluid spaces of membranous labyrinth; may be cochlear or non-cochlear
- Severe LO: High signal membranous labyrinth is absent as it is completely replaced by low signal bone

Imaging Recommendations
- High resolution FSE-T2 MR imaging best tool
- If unavailable, 1 mm temporal bone CT is exam of choice for LO
- FSE-T2 MR imaging can demonstrate fibrous obliteration of the membranous labyrinth whereas CT cannot

Differential Diagnosis: Bony Obliteration of Membranous Labyrinth

Cochlear Hypoplasia or Aplasia
- Cochlear edifice is small or absent (< 2½ turns seen)
- SNHL present from birth

Cochlear Otosclerosis
- Involves the bony labyrinth
- Does not encroach on membranous labyrinth even in healing phase
- Adult disease

Pathology

General
- Etiology-Pathogenesis
  - Suppurative membranous labyrinthitis sets up a cascading inflammatory response in membranous labyrinth
  - Begins with fibrosis, progresses to ossification
  - LO arises from suppurative labyrinthitis from multiple sources

Labyrinthine Ossificans

- Meningitis => **Meningogenic LO**, bilateral
- Middle ear => **Tympanogenic LO**, unilateral
- Blood born => **Hematogenic LO** (Measles, mumps), bilateral
  - LO may also arise after severe trauma or temporal bone surgery
- Epidemiology
  - Meningogenic labyrinthitis is the most common cause of acquired childhood deafness

Gross Pathologic, Surgical Features
- At surgery for cochlear implantation, bony obstruction to implant entry into the round window niche is observed

Microscopic Features
- Fibrous stage shows fibroblast proliferation
- Ossific stage seen as osteoblasts forming abnormal bony trabeculae with the membranous labyrinthine spaces

Clinical Issues
Presentation
- Principal presenting symptoms: Bilateral SNHL
- History of meningitis is usually present
  - Profound bilateral SNHL developing 6-18 months after the acute infectious episode
- Severe vertigo is infrequent but devastating symptom

Treatment
- Labyrinthectomy used in cases of intractable vertigo
- Cochlear implantation used for SNHL correction
  - Bilateral severe cochlear LO is a contraindication to cochlear implantation

Prognosis
- Prognosis for SNHL is completely defined by possibility of and response to cochlear implantation

Selected References
1. Johnson MH et al: CT of postmeningitic deafness: observations and predictive value for cochlear implants in children. AJNR 16:103-9, 1995
2. Harnsberger HR et al: Cochlear implant candidates: assessment with CT and MR imaging. Radiology 164:53-7, 1987
3. Swartz JD et al: Labyrinthine ossification: etiologies and CT findings. Radiology 157:395-9, 1985

Inner Ear Schwannoma

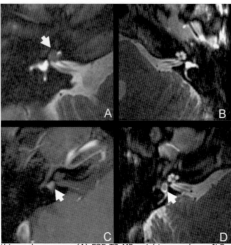

Intralabyrinthine schwannoma.(A) FSE-T2 MR axial image shows ILS as soft-tissue intensity mass in cochlear membranous labyrinth (arrow). (B) Normal comparison opposite ear. (C) T1 C+ MR image reveals another ILS as focal enhancement of vestibule (arrow). (D) T2-FSE shows ILS as focal mass in vestibule (arrow).

Key Facts
- Definition: Benign tumor arising from Schwann cells within the structures of the membranous labyrinth
- Classic imaging appearance: Focal mass within the membranous labyrinth of the inner ear on MR images
  - T1 C+ MR: Focal enhancing mass in membranous labyrinth
  - FSE-T2 MR: "Filling defect" within high-signal perilymph
- Intralabyrinthine schwannoma (ILS) is a missed diagnosis by excellent radiologists because they are not aware of its existence
- If serviceable hearing remains in the setting of ILS, conservative management of the lesion is prudent

Imaging Findings
General Features
- Best imaging clue: Focal mass within membranous labyrinth
- Focal intralabyrinthine mass named by location
  - Intravestibular = **Intravestibular schwannoma**
  - Intracochlear = **Cochlear schwannoma**
  - Vestibulocochlear in location = **Vestibulocochlear schwannoma**
  - Middle ear, inner ear, IAC = **Translabyrinthine schwannoma**
- ILS may project multiple directions from inner ear
  - Through round window into middle ear
  - Along vestibular nerve branches into fundus of IAC
  - Through the modiolus and cochlear aperture into IAC
CT Findings
- Normal CT is rule unless mass projects into middle ear through round window niche
- CT usually not helpful in making this diagnosis
MR Findings
- T1 C+ MR shows focal enhancement of ILS

Inner Ear Schwannoma

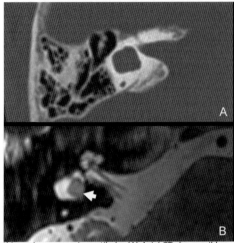

Intralabyrinthine schwannoma in vestibule. (A) Axial CT shows mild congenital inner ear anomaly where lateral semicircular canal and vestibule are combined. (B) Axial FSE-T2 MR shows an intravestibular schwannoma (arrow) within the anomalous vestibule-lateral semicircular canal.

- FSE-T2 MR shows focal low-signal mass within the high-signal fluids of the membranous labyrinth

Imaging Recommendations
- Use focused T1 C+ or FSE-T2 imaging of the CPA-IAC-Inner ear to make the diagnosis of ILS
- Careful examination of all "rule out acoustic" MR scans for the presence of intralabyrinthine mass is critical
- Observe precise location of tumor
  - Does it involve the vestibule, cochlea or both?
  - Does it project into middle ear ± IAC fundus?
- All patients undergoing surgery for Meniere's disease should undergo preoperative focused MR imaging to exclude ILS

Differential Diagnosis: Intralabyrinthine Lesion
Labyrinthitis
- Enhancement of most or all of membranous labyrinth
- FSE-T2 MR images shows fluid, not a low-signal mass
Labyrinthine Ossificans
- Encroachment on fluid of membranous labyrinth by bone
- Directly visible on both CT and MR
Acoustic Schwannoma of IAC Invading Membranous Labyrinth
- IAC fundal mass is the dominant observation
- Extension into inner ear is seen but is subtle compared to IAC mass
Facial Schwannoma with Secondary Erosion Into Inner Ear
- Tubular mass enlarges intratemporal facial nerve canal
- Involvement of inner ear is secondary

Inner Ear Schwannoma

Pathology

General
- Etiology-Pathogenesis
  - Tumor arises from Schwann cells wrapping distal vestibular or cochlear nerve axons within the membranous labyrinth
  - Secondary endolymphatic hydrops thought to explain Meniere's disease symptoms
- Epidemiology
  - Rare lesion
  - Perhaps 1/100th as common as acoustic schwannoma of CPA-IAC

Gross Pathologic, Surgical Features
- Tan-gray, round/ovoid encapsulated mass found within labyrinth

Microscopic Features
- Differentiated neoplastic Schwann cells
- Areas of compact, elongated cells = Antoni A
- Other areas less densely cellular with tumor loosely arranged, ± clusters of lipid-laden cells = Antoni B
- Strong, diffuse expression of S-100 protein

Clinical Issues

Presentation
- Principal presenting symptom: SNHL
- Presenting symptoms different from classic acoustic schwannoma involving the CPA-IAC
- Tumor location-specific symptoms
  - Vestibule
    - Tinnitus, episodic vertigo with nausea and vomiting, mixed hearing loss (tumor impedes stapes footplate, creating an element of conductive hearing loss)
  - Cochlea
    - Slowly progressive sensorineural hearing loss

Natural History
- **Very slow-growing, benign tumor** of the membranous labyrinth
- History of progressive hearing loss may date back 20 years
- May grow to fill inner ear, then stop growing

Treatment
- When symptoms are minor (serviceable hearing maintained) and tumor is confined to inner ear, watchful waiting is prudent
- If symptoms are disabling (intractable vertigo), translabyrinthine surgery undertaken to remove tumors in the vestibule while transotic surgery completed for tumors involving the cochlea or middle ear

Prognosis
- Total deafness in ear will result eventually if left alone and certainly if tumor removed

Selected References
1. Deux JF et al: Slow-growing labyrinthine masses: contribution of MRI to diagnosis, follow-up and treatment. Neuroradiology 40:684-9, 1998
2. Green JD et al: Diagnosis and management of intralabyrinthine schwannomas. Laryngoscope 109:1626-31, 1999
3. Mafee MF et al: CT and MR imaging of intralabyrinthine schwannoma: report of two cases and review of the literature. Radiology 174:395-400, 1990

Endolymphatic Sac Tumor

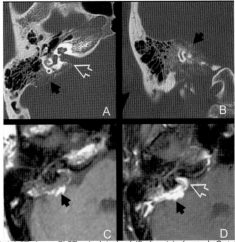

ELST. (A) Axial CT shows ELST spiculated calcified matrix (arrow). Ca++ enters IAC (open arrow). (B) Coronal CT reveals ELST surrounding posterior semicircular canal (arrow). (C) T1 C- MR depicts high signal blood in tumor (arrow). (D) ELST enhances on C+ MR (arrow); extends to IAC (open arrow).

Key Facts
- Synonym: Adenomatous tumor of the endolymphatic sac
- Definition: Papillary cystadenomatous tumor of the endolymphatic sac
- Classic imaging appearance: Distinctive retrolabyrinthine location as well as CT and MR findings
  - CT: **Intratumoral bone spicules**
  - MR C- T1: **High-signal foci** (blood); flow voids

Imaging Findings
General Imaging Features
- Best imaging clue: High-signal foci within tumor matrix on unenhanced T1 MR images
- Centered in fovea of endolymphatic sac (retrolabyrinthine) in the presigmoid, posterior surface of petrous temporal bone
- Enlarges to involve the entire posterior wall of the T-bone, CPA cistern and jugular foramen
- Large lesions (> 3 cm) involve the middle ear
  - Spread is from endolymphatic sac area through inner ear (semicircular canals and vestibule) to middle ear
CT Findings
- Aggressive, soft-tissue mass that erodes posterior wall of T-bone
- **Central spiculated calcifications** within tumor matrix (100%)
- Most have thin rim of calcification along the posterior margin of tumor
MR Findings
- Foci of **increased signal intensity** on T1 C- MR images seen along tumor margin when < 3 cm, within tumor matrix when > 3 cm
- 80% of endolymphatic sac tumors (ELST) have these foci of increased signal intensity
- Heterogeneous enhancement on T1 C+ MR images
- Flow voids (focal low-signal areas on T1 C- MR) when tumors > 2 cm

Endolymphatic Sac Tumor

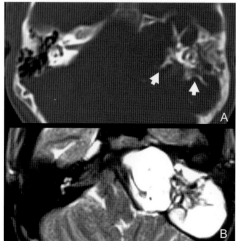

Enormous ELST. (A) Axial CT shows large ELST engulfing inner ear. Large residual bony spurs (arrows) are seen within tumor parenchyma. (B) FSE-T2 MR image reveals the bulk of the tumor is high signal. Lacy low-signal central area represents residual inner ear and tumor bony matrix.

Angiographic Findings
- Small tumors (< 3 cm) supplied by branches of external carotid artery only, larger tumors (> 3 cm) supplied by ECA branches, ± ICA, ± posterior circulation
- ECA branches serving tumor = ascending pharyngeal, stylomastoid and petrosal branch of middle meningeal arteries
- **Hypervascular tumor blush** is norm

Imaging Recommendations
- Both CT & T1 C+ MR are necessary to fully work up this lesion, especially when large
- MRA & MRV help in defining vascular relationships
- Larger lesions will benefit from pre-operative embolization

Differential Diagnosis: Deep T-Bone Lesions

Cholesterol Granuloma of Petrous Apex
- Centered in petrous apex
- High-signal on T1 C- MR involves entire lesion

Glomus Jugulare and Jugulotympanicum Paraganglioma
- Involve jugular foramen, then middle ear, not retrolabyrinthine temporal bone
- High signal foci on T1 C- MR rare

Schwannoma of Jugular Foramen
- Centered in jugular foramen
- Does not involve retrolabyrinthine temporal bone

Metastasis, Renal Cell or Papillary Thyroid Carcinoma
- More destructive appearing
- No posterior rim calcification
- Lack internal high-signal foci on T1 C- MR

Endolymphatic Sac Tumor

Pathology

General

- Genetics
  - Most ELST are sporadic
  - Mutations and allelic deletions of the von Hippel-Lindau tumor suppressor gene play a role in generating these sporadic tumors
  - 7% of von Hippel-Lindau patients will develop ELST
  - If ELST is bilateral, von Hippel-Lindau disease is present
- Etiology-Pathogenesis
  - Slow-growing tumor arising from cells lining the endolymphatic sac

Gross Pathologic, Surgical Features

- Heaped up tumor on posterior wall of temporal bone with foci of old hemorrhage within the substance of the tumor

Microscopic Features

- Histopathologic variability is common, causing ELST to be referred to as adenoma, adenocarcinoma, and adenomatous or carcinoid tumors
- Complex, interdigitating papillary processes that infiltrate the surrounding connective tissue and bone
  - Papillary processes embedded in sheets of dense fibrous tissue with evidence of recent and previous hemorrhage
  - Papillary processes lined with a single layer of cuboidal epithelial cells that resembles cells that line endolymphatic sac
    - These lining cells are low columnar to cuboidal with deeply eosinophilic homogeneous cytoplasm and small, centrally placed ovoid nuclei

Clinical Issues

Presentation

- Principal presenting symptom: SNHL (100%)
- Other symptoms: Facial nerve palsy (60%), pulsatile tinnitus (50%) or vertigo (20%)

Treatment

- Complete surgical resection with wide margins
- Patients with sporadic ELST should be systematically investigated for clinical and molecular evidence of **von Hippel-Lindau disease**

Prognosis

- Prognosis is excellent if complete surgical resection achieved
- Late recurrence is possible given slow growth rate of tumor

Selected References
1. Richard S et al: Central nervous system hemangioblastomas, endolymphatic sac tumors and von Hippel-Lindau disease. Neurosur Rev 23:1-22, 2000
2. Mukherji SK et al: Papillary endolymphatic sac tumors: CT, MR imaging, and angiographic findings in 20 patients. Radiology 202:801-8, 1997
3. Lo WW et al: Endolymphatic sac tumors: radiologic appearance. Radiology 189:199-204, 1993

Fenestral Otosclerosis

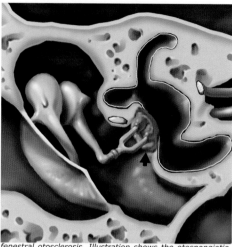

Drawing of fenestral otosclerosis. Illustration shows the otospongiotic process has surrounded the oval window margins (arrow), fixing the stapes footplate. It comes as no surprise that such a patient would present with conductive hearing loss.

Key Facts
- Synonym: **Otospongiosis**
- Definition: Pathologic condition of the bony labyrinth of unknown cause where focal areas of spongy bone are formed on the margins oval and round windows
- Classic imaging appearance: Imaging shows **otospongiotic plaques** along the oval and round window margins
- **Otospongiosis** is a better term than otosclerosis as it describes the active disease process
- Presents with tinnitus and bilateral progressive conductive hearing loss

Imaging Findings
General Imaging Features
- Best imaging clue: Lytic foci on anterior margin of oval window
- Earliest finding is a focus of otospongiotic bony growth along anterior margin of oval window = **fissula ante fenestrum**
- Disease spreads from fissula posteriorly along the oval window margins to the round window
- If the disease spreads to include the otic capsule, both FOt and cochlear otosclerosis (COt) are diagnosed
CT Findings
- Early: Radiolucent focus heaping up at anterior margin of oval window
- Spreads to involve the margins of the oval and round window
- Healing phase new bone in these areas indicated fenestral otosclerosis (Fot) is chronic; oval and/or round window may become occluded by healed plaque
MR Findings
- T1 C+ MR shows enhancing punctate foci in medial wall of middle ear
- In more chronic, severe cases, multiple enhancing foci can be seen in the region of the oval and round window

Fenestral Otosclerosis

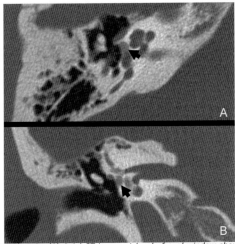

Fenestral otosclerosis. (A) Axial CT image at level of oval window shows an active otospongiotic plaque at the anterior margin of the oval window (arrow) = fissula ante fenestrum. (B) Coronal CT through anterior margin of oval window again shows this same plaque (arrow).

Imaging Recommendations
- Temporal bone CT best imaging tool for diagnosing FOt

Differential Diagnosis: Abnormal Bony labyrinth
Tympanosclerosis, Post-Inflammatory New Bone Deposition
- Imaging: Post-inflammatory new bone deposition is not limited to oval window
  - Seen in TM, middle ear, ossicles and mastoids
  - New bone deposition is irregular, not smooth in oval window area
- Clinical: Obvious inflammatory middle ear-mastoid disease
Paget's Disease
- Imaging: Diffuse skull base involvement is the rule
  - Diffuse involvement of bony labyrinth, not confined to lateral wall
  - Usually seen as a diffuse temporal bone cotton-wool appearance
- Clinical: Elderly patient
Fibrous Dysplasia
- Imaging: Involves all parts of the temporal bone
  - Relative sparing of inner ear is the rule
  - Usually sclerotic, ground glass in appearance
- Clinical: Bone disease of the young (<30 year old)
Otosyphilis
- Imaging: CT shows diffuse, permeative lucencies of otic capsule
- Clinical: Adults with systemic syphilitic infection

Pathology
General
- Genetics
  - Sporadic or autosomal dominant gene transmission
- Pathophysiology of conductive hearing loss
  - Active FOt fixes the stapes footplate in the oval window niche

Fenestral Otosclerosis

- Epidemiology
  - Occurs in 1.0% of the population
  - Most common type of otosclerosis is FOt (85%) vs. COt (15%)
  - If COt present, FOt also is present; look for it

Gross Pathologic, Surgical Features
- Otoscopic vascular hue behind tympanic membrane=**Schwartze's sign**
  - Represents the active otosclerotic areas along the margins of the oval and round windows
- **Bony ankylosis** of the stapes footplate is reflected as stapes immobilization when tension is exerted during surgery

Microscopic Features
- Spongy, vascular, decalcified, irregular bone formation in the enchondral layer of the labyrinth along the margins of the oval and round windows
- Three pathologic phases
  - Acute phase: Deposition of islets of osteoid tissue
  - Subacute phase: Spongiotic remodeling with osteoclasts causing resorption of bone and creating large cavities
  - Chronic-sclerotic phase: Osteoblasts create new bone with irregular features that resemble a mosaic

Clinical Issues

Presentation
- Principal presenting symptom: Conductive hearing loss
- Other symptoms: Tinnitus (ringing in ears)
- Appears in 2nd to 3rd decades of life
- 2:1 female to male

Treatment
- Stapedectomy followed by prosthesis insertion
- Fluoride treatment

Prognosis
- Conductive hearing loss is progressive
- Fluoride treatment early in disease may stabilize hearing loss

Selected References
1. Chole RA et al: Pathophysiology of otosclerosis. Otol Neurotol 22:249-57, 2001
2. Mafee MF et al: Use of CT in stapedial otosclerosis. Radiology 156:709-714, 1985
3. Swartz JD et al: Fenestral otosclerosis: significance of preoperative CT evaluation. Radiology 151:703-7, 1984

Cochlear Otosclerosis

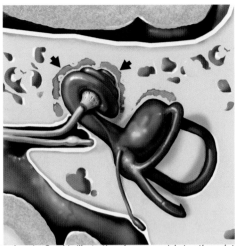

Cochlear otosclerosis. Graphic illustration shows an axial view through the inner ear with active otospongiotic plaques in the bony otic capsule (arrows) surrounding the cochlea.

Key Facts
- Synonym: Cochlear otospongiosis = retrofenestral otosclerosis = Beethoven's malady
- Definition: Primary lytic disease of the enchondral layer of the bony labyrinth of unknown cause
- **Otospongiosis** is a better term than otosclerosis, since it describes the active disease process, not the healing phase of the disease
- Presents with tinnitus and bilateral, progressive, mixed hearing loss
- CT shows **otospongiotic plaques** in a pericochlear distribution

Imaging Findings
General Features
- Best imaging clue: Focal lytic plaques in the bony labyrinth
- Bilaterally symmetric in 85% of cases
- Fenestral otosclerosis (FOt) concurrent in most cases of cochlear otosclerosis (COt)

CT Findings
- Active disease seen as low-density foci within the bony labyrinth giving a "halo" appearance to the bony pericochlear labyrinth
- Low-density foci first surround the basal turn of the cochlea but may be seen affecting the lateral walls of the IAC and the cochlear promontory
- When severe, the **"double-ring sign"** appears = low-density ring surrounding cochlea
- Lucencies around oval and round window signal concurrent FOt
  - Healing phase new bone in these areas indicated FOt is chronic

MR Findings
- T1 C+ MR shows enhancing pericochlear lines marking lesions in the enchondral layer of the bony labyrinth

Imaging Recommendations
- Temporal bone CT best imaging tool for diagnosing COt

Cochlear Otosclerosis

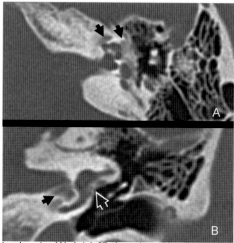

Cochlear otosclerosis. (A) Axial CT through cochlea demonstrates multiple otospongiotic plaques in the bony otic capsule ringing the cochlea (arrows). Heaped up healing bone can be seen covering the oval window. (B) Coronal CT shows otic capsule plaques (arrow) and overgrown oval window (open arrow).

Differential Diagnosis: Otic Capsule Lesion
Osteogenesis Imperfecta Tarde
- Imaging: Findings may be indistinguishable from COt
  - Looks like very severe form of COt with more generalized involvement
- Clinical: Children with brittle bones and blue sclerae

Paget's Disease
- Imaging: More diffuse involvement of the skull base than COt
  - Diffuse involvement of bony labyrinth not confined to enchondral layer
  - Usually seen as a diffuse, T-bone, cotton-wool appearance
- Clinical: Elderly patients

Fibrous Dysplasia
- Imaging: Involves all parts of the temporal bone
  - Relative sparing of the otic capsule is the rule
  - Usually sclerotic, ground glass in appearance
- Clinical: Bony disease of the young (< 30 years old)

Otosyphilis
- Imaging: Lytic lesions of otic capsule may mimic COt
- Clinical: Adults with systemic syphilitic infection

Pathology
General
- Genetics
  - Sporadic or autosomal dominant gene transmission
- Etiology-Pathogenesis
  - COt etiology unknown
  - SNHL in COt results from compromise of the spiral ligament and/or toxic proteases affecting the nerve cells of the cochlea

Cochlear Otosclerosis

- Epidemiology
  - Occurs in 1.0% of the population
  - Two types of otosclerosis, fenestral (85%) and cochlear (15%)
  - COt usually seen **with** FOt

Gross Pathologic, Surgical Features
- Otoscopic vascular hue behind tympanic membrane=**Schwartze's sign**
  - Schwartze's sign represents the active otosclerotic area just beneath the surface of the cochlear promontory

Microscopic Features
- Spongy, vascular, decalcified, irregular bone formation in the enchondral layer of the bony labyrinth
- Three pathologic phases
  - **Acute phase**: Deposition of islets of osteoid tissue
  - **Subacute phase**: Spongiotic remodeling with osteoclasts causing resorption of bone and creating large cavities
  - **Chronic-sclerotic phase**: Osteoblasts create new bone with irregular features that resemble a mosaic

Clinical Issues

Presentation
- Principal presenting symptom: Progressive mixed CHL and SNHL
- Other symptoms: Tinnitus (ringing)
- Appears in 2nd to 3rd decades of life
- 2:1 female to male
- Disease may become worse during pregnancy and lactation

Treatment
- For fenestral otosclerosis, stapedectomy followed by prosthesis insertion
- COt treated early with fluoride therapy
  - If treated early enough, can arrest progression of SNHL

Prognosis
- Gradual, progressive, mixed hearing loss leads to deafness
- Early treatment with fluoride can interrupt this decline

Selected References
1. Ziyeh S et al: MRI of active otosclerosis. Neuroradiology 39:453-7, 1997
2. Mafee MF et al: Use of CT in the evaluation of cochlear otosclerosis. Radiology 156:703-8, 1985
3. Swartz JD et al: Cochlear otosclerosis (Otospongiosis): CT analysis with audiometric correlation. Radiology 155:147-50, 1985

Large Endolymphatic Sac Anomaly

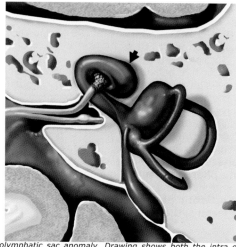

Large endolymphatic sac anomaly. Drawing shows both the intra osseous and intradural portions of the endolymphatic sac are enlarged in this congenital inner ear anomaly. Mild cochlear dysplasia is also present with modiolar deficiency and apical turn bulbous dysmorphism (arrow).

Key Facts
- Synonym: Large vestibular aqueduct syndrome
- Definition: Arrested development of inner ear leaves a large endolymphatic sac and mild cochlear dysplasia
- Classic imaging appearance: CT shows large, bony, vestibular aqueduct while FSE-T2 MR shows large endolymphatic sac
- Large Endolymphatic Sac Anomaly (LESA) is most common congenital anomaly of inner ear found by imaging
- Congenital anomaly with acquired sensorineural hearing loss
  - ○ Child hears at birth but hearing deteriorates over early years of life

Imaging Findings
General Imaging Findings
- Best imaging clue: Large endolymphatic sac
- Bilateral anomaly (90%)
- Associated cochlear dysplasia (>75%)
- Associated vestibular &/or semicircular canal anomaly (50%)
CT Findings
- Bone-only temporal bone CT
  - ○ Enlargement of the bony vestibular aqueduct
    - >1.5 mm, mid-aqueduct
    - Alternatively, vestibular aqueduct diameter exceeding that of posterior semicircular canal diameter
- CT less sensitive associated anomalies
MR Findings
- FSE-T2 high-resolution MR of inner ear
  - ○ Shows an enlarged endolymphatic sac
  - ○ Associated cochlear dysplasia
    - Subtle (modiolar deficiency, scalar chamber asymmetry, apical turn dysmorphism)

Large Endolymphatic Sac Anomaly

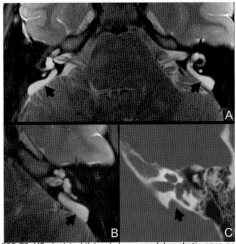

LESA. (A) FSE-T2 MR depicts bilateral, large, endolymphatic sacs as high-signal bags of fluid along posterior margins of the temporal bones (arrows). (B) Different case of LESA again shows high-signal sac (arrow) and cochlear dysplasia. (C) CT of image (B) reveals large, bony, vestibular aqueduct (arrow).

- ▪ Intermediate (incomplete partition)
- ▪ Gross (cystic cochlea)

Imaging Recommendations
- Thin-section temporal bone CT (1 mm) can make diagnosis of LESA routinely as long as large, bony, vestibular aqueduct is recognized
- Thin-section FSE-T2 MR (0.8-1 mm) can easily identify the enlarged endolymphatic sac

Differential Diagnosis
- LESA imaging appearance is diagnostic
- No differential diagnosis for CT or MR appearance of this lesion exists

Pathology
General
- Embryology-Anatomy
  - ○ Congenital anomaly resulting from arrest of normal inner ear development
  - ○ Arrested inner ear development seen as large endolymphatic sac and cochlear dysplasia
  - ○ Arrest occurs at ~ 8-9th week of fetal development
- Genetics
  - ○ Familial lesion with autosomal recessive inheritance
- Etiology-Pathogenesis
  - ○ SNHL develops as a post-natal event (often following head trauma)
  - ○ Best hypotheses for SNHL in this anomaly:
    - ▪ The cochlea is "fragile" and susceptible to injury from mild trauma as a result of microscopic infrastructural deficiencies

Gross-Surgical Pathologic Features
- Enlarged endolymphatic sac is found in the dural sleeve in the fovea in the posterior wall of the temporal bone

Large Endolymphatic Sac Anomaly

Clinical Issues

Presentation
- Principal presenting symptom: Bilateral SNHL in child
- Infant or child usually hears in the first few years of life
- Progressive SNHL may be accelerated by minor head trauma
- **Bilateral SNHL** in most cases (90%)

Natural History
- Progressive, bilateral SNHL loss that cascades after minor head trauma
- Inevitably leads to profound SNHL in affected ear(s)
- SNHL develops with variable speed; in some, hearing loss may not be present until early adult life

Treatment
- Avoidance of contact sports or other activities that may lead to head trauma is essential
- Cochlear implantation now used when bilateral profound sensorineural deafness occurs
- An increased risk of perilymph gusher during cochlear implantation has been reported

Prognosis
- Prognosis is best in those where hearing loss is either unilateral or delayed into early adult life

Selected References
1. Naganawa S et al: MR imaging of the enlarged endolymphatic duct and sac syndrome by use of a 3D fast asymmetric spin-echo sequence: volume and signal-intensity measurement of the endolymphatic duct and sac and area measurement of the cochlear modiolus. AJNR 21:1664-9, 2000
2. Davidson HC et al: MR evaluation of Vestibulocochlear anomalies associated with large endolymphatic duct and sac. AJNR 20:1435-41, 1999
3. Dahlen RT et al: Overlapping thin-section fast spin-echo MR of large vestibular aqueduct syndrome. AJNR 18:67-75, 1997

Apical Petrositis

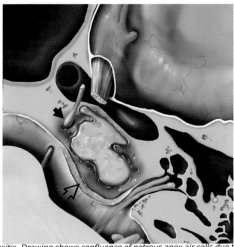

Apical petrositis. Drawing shows confluence of petrous apex air cells due to trabecular osteomyelitis. An abscess has formed in this location, affecting the surrounding bone and secondarily the 6th cranial nerve (arrow). Thick adjacent dura (open arrow) indicates one of the body's attempts to wall off this infection.

Key Facts
- Synonyms
  - Confluent apical petrositis (AP)
  - Apical petrositis associated with the clinical triad, otomastoiditis, 6th nerve palsy and deep facial pain (5th nerve palsy) is known as **Gradenigo's syndrome**
- Definition: Infectious nidus in petrous apex air cells with trabecular disintegration and meningeal involvement
- Classic imaging appearance
  - CT shows "confluent apical petrositis"
  - T1 C+ MR reveals meningeal, Meckel's cave and cavernous sinus thickening and enhancement with rim-enhancing confluent low signal in the petrous apex (PA)
- AP is rare in the post-antibiotic era
- Although aggressive antibiotic treatment has cured patients with AP, surgical intervention is generally warranted

Imaging Findings
General Features
- Best imaging clue: **Trabecular breakdown** in PA air cells
- Pneumatized petrous apex is necessary for AP to occur
- Phlegmon or abscess can be present in confluent apical air cells
CT Findings
- Destructive expansion of a PA air cells
- PA trabeculae break-down = **confluent apical petrositis**
- Cortical margins become permeative with advanced disease
- Middle ear and mastoid are also usually opacified (infected)
MR Findings
- T1 C+ MR shows rim-enhancing fluid in confluent apical air cells
- Adjacent meninges are thickened and enhance avidly

Apical Petrositis

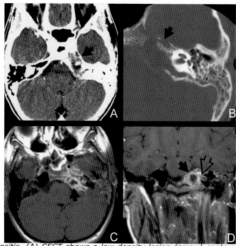

Apical petrositis. (A) CECT shows a low-density lesion (arrow) centered in PA. (B) Magnified bone CT reveals dissolution of bony PA (arrow). (C) T1 C+ MR axial shows the pocket of pus (arrow) in the confluent PA air cells. (D) Coronal T1 C+ depicts the PA pus (arrow) and meningeal thickening in IAC (open arrow).

- Ipsilateral Meckel's cave and cavernous sinus are usually more prominent and enhance asymmetrically

Imaging Recommendations
- Initial diagnosis best made with thin section temporal bone CT
- T1 C+ MR important in evaluating intracranial complications of AP

Differential Diagnosis: Petrous Apex Lesions

Congenital Cholesteatoma in PA
- CT shows smooth, expansile PA mass
- T1 MR signal is low and no meningeal enhancement is present

Trapped Fluid in PA
- PA air cell trabeculae maintained; no cortical expansion
- Bland fluid trapped in PA air cells

Cholesterol Granuloma in PA
- CT shows trabecular breakdown ad cortical expansion in PA
- T1 MR signal is high as is T2 signal

Primary Malignancy of PA Area (Chondrosarcoma, Chordoma)
- CT shows destructive mass of clivus, petro-occipital fissure or PA
- Clinical setting lacks acute infectious symptoms

Metastatic Disease of PA Area (Metastasis, NHL)
- CT shows permeative-destructive mass of PA
- Often with systemic tumor history or other lesions associated
- Clinical setting lacks acute infectious symptoms

Pathology

General
- Embryology-Anatomy
  - Pneumatized petrous apex present about 35% of time
  - PA pneumatization required for AP to occur

Apical Petrositis

- Etiology-Pathogenesis
  - o Acute or chronic suppurative otomastoiditis spreads via air cells or venous channels to the PA
  - o Infection of PA air cells causes coalescence with breakdown of trabeculae = **"coalescent apical petrositis"**
  - o Thrombophlebitis or direct infection extension involves adjacent structures including meninges, Meckel's cave, and cavernous sinus causing 5th and/or 6th nerve palsies
- Epidemiology
  - o Rare in post-antibiotic era

Gross Pathologic, Surgical Features
- Soft osteomyelitic bone with pus filling confluent air cells of PA
- Phlegmon thickens and inflames adjacent meninges

Microscopic Features
- Offending organism often not cultured as patients are already being treated with multiple antibiotics

Clinical Issues

Presentation
- Principal clinical symptom: Ear and retro-orbital pain
- Classic clinical presentation: Child or adolescent with acute otomastoiditis, develops acute 6th cranial nerve palsy and/or deep facial (retro-orbital) or ear pain
- Complete clinical syndrome = Gradenigo's syndrome
  - o Acute otomastoiditis
  - o **6th nerve palsy**: Injury in medial PA (Dorello's canal)
  - o Deep facial (retro-orbital) or ear pain = Trigeminal nerve distribution pain

Natural History
- Rapid onset of deep facial (retro-orbital) pain, 6th and/or 5th cranial nerve palsy that progresses to obtundation and death if untreated

Treatment
- Aggressive surgical intervention with mastoidectomy accompanied by PA drainage is the treatment of choice
- Cases of intravenous antibiotics precluding surgical intervention have been reported

Prognosis
- Excellent given adequate surgical drainage and aggressive antibiotics

Selected References
1. Gadre AK et al: Venous channels of the petrous apex: their presence and clinical importance. Otolaryngol Head Neck Surg 116:168-74, 1997
2. Murakami T et al: Gradenigo's syndrome: CT and MRI findings. Pediatr Radiol 26:684-5, 1996
3. Allam AF et al: Pathology of petrositis. Laryngoscope 78:1813-32, 1968

Trapped Fluid, Petrous Apex

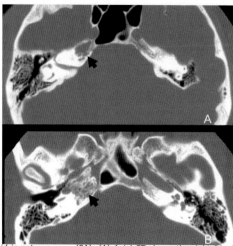

Trapped fluid in petrous apex (PA). (A) Axial CT shows the right PA air cells to be opacified (arrow). Trabeculae are present and no expansion of the area has occurred. (B) Axial CT inferior to (A) reveals continued opacification of PA air cells. Maintenance of trabeculae more obvious at this level.

Key Facts
- Synonyms: Petrous apex effusion; "leave-me-alone lesion of the PA"
- Definition: Sterile residual fluid collection in PA air cells left behind from remote otomastoiditis
- Classic imaging appearance
  - CT shows non-expansile, non-destructive opacified PA air cells
  - MR reveals PA air cell fluid (low T1, high T2) in most cases
- Included in 100 Top ENT Diagnoses because is a very common incidental finding on brain MR that can be misdiagnosed as cholesterol granuloma or apical petrositis
  - Misguided aggressive medical or surgical therapy may result
- No therapy or follow-up is warranted for classic trapped fluid in the petrous apex (TF-PA)

Imaging Findings
General Features
- Best imaging clue: Opacified PA air cells without trabecular loss
- TF-PA does not occur unless the PA is pneumatized (33%)
- No destructive or expansile bony changes
CT Findings
- Unilateral opacification of PA air cells usually in absence of middle ear or mastoid inflammatory changes
- Air cell margins may be sclerotic from previous inflammation but there is no evidence for expansion or destruction of trabeculae or cortical margins
MR Findings
- Most common appearance: Non-enhancing low T1, high T2 fluid in otherwise normal appearing PA air cells

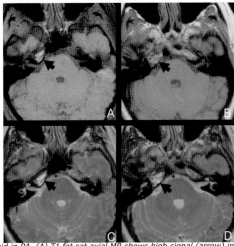

Trapped fluid in PA. (A) T1 fat sat axial MR shows high signal (arrow) in PA air cells. (B) T1 below (A) shows high signal (arrow) and maintained trabeculae. (C-D) Two axial T2 MR images to match A. and b. reveals high signal within these PA air cells only.

- Less common appearance: Non-enhancing intermediate or high T1 and high T2 signal fluid in otherwise normal PA air cells
  - When the T1 signal is intermediate to high in TF-PA, high protein content is the cause

Imaging Recommendations
- As TF-PA is most commonly an incidental finding on brain MR, temporal bone CT is recommended to assess the importance of the MR finding
- Bone-only CT through the T-bone is used to sort out the rare surgical lesions of the PA from the far more common but incidental TF-PA
- Remote (3 year) follow-up CT is recommended for the TF-PA lesion with normal air cells but high T1 signal on MR to exclude the remote possibility of transformation into cholesterol granuloma

Differential Diagnosis: Petrous Apex Lesion
Congenital Cholesteatoma, PA
- Smooth, expansile lesion of PA on CT
- T1 C+ MR signal is low with rim enhancement present
- No meningeal enhancement present
Mucocele, PA
- Rare expansile lesion of PA with low T1 MR signal
- Rim enhancement on T1 C+ MR
Cholesterol Granuloma, PA
- Expansile lesion of PA on CT
- High T1 and high T2 MR signal

Pathology
General
- Embryology-Anatomy
  - 33% of people have pneumatized petrous apices

- o   5% of these are asymmetrically pneumatized
- o   Amount of PA pneumatization correlates exactly with the degree of mastoid pneumatization
- Etiology-Pathogenesis
  - o   TF-PA is a sterile residual fluid collection in PA air cells left behind from remote otomastoiditis
- Epidemiology
  - o   Residual fluid in PA air cells is present in ~1% of all head MR
  - o   TF-PA is the most common lesion found in the PA
  - o   TF-PA: Cholesterol granuloma of PA ratio is approximately 500:1

Gross Pathologic, Surgical Features
- Clear to xanthochromic fluid discovered in bland PA air cells
- Adjacent cortical bone is not soft and meninges are not thickened

Microscopic Features
- Sterile fluid
- No micro-organisms or tumor cells present

Clinical Issues
Presentation
- Principal presenting symptom: None!
- Patient is undergoing brain MR for unrelated symptoms
- Incidental MR finding of a PA lesion described as "suspicious for cholesterol granuloma or apical petrositis" in the radiology report
- Patient is referred for surgical assessment
- Temporal bone CT reveals normal but opacified PA air cells

Natural History
- True TF-PA remain unchanged throughout the patient's life
- A theoretical possibility that one of the rare intermediate or high T1 signal lesions will transform into a cholesterol granuloma exists
- No case report or series has been published as yet showing this transformation can occur

Treatment
- Classic TF-PA requires no treatment or follow-up

Prognosis
- Great if it is just left alone!

Selected References
1.   Moore KR et al: "Leave me alone" lesions of the petrous apex. AJNR 19:733-8, 1998
2.   Virapongse C et al: Computed tomography of temporal bone pneumatization, 1: normal pattern and morphology. AJR 145:473-81, 1985
3.   Flood LM et al: The investigation and management of petrous apex erosion. J Laryngol Otol 99:439-50, 1985

Cholesterol Granuloma, ME

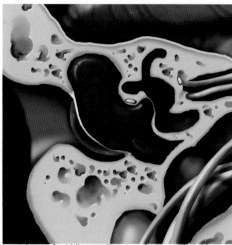

Cholesterol granuloma of middle ear. Drawing depicts a dark blue mass filling the middle ear cavity with loss of ossicles. The lesion fills the middle ear without eroding the lateral semicircular canal or tegmen tympani.

Key Facts
- Synonyms: Cholesterol cyst, "chocolate ear"
- Definition: Specialized granulation tissue forms from recurrent hemorrhage in middle ear cavity
- Classic imaging appearance
  - CT: Smoothly expansile mass of the middle ear and/or mastoid
  - MR shows **high T1 and T2** signal
- Cholesterol granuloma (CG) of the middle ear mastoid is much more common than the rarer CG of the petrous apex
- Clinical setting: "Blue eardrum" with conductive hearing loss

Imaging Findings
General Features
- Best imaging clue: **High T1 signal** on MR imaging
- Early, smaller CG: Lesion within middle ear and/or mastoid cavity without bone remodeling or ossicular loss
- Late, larger CG: Expansile lesion scallops surrounding bone; ossicular loss present
CT Findings
- Opacified middle ear and mastoid with expansile bony changes and ossicular erosions
MR Findings
- High T1 and T2 signal is characteristic
- High T1 signal secondary to paramagnetic effect of hemoglobin breakdown products derived from micro-hemorrhages around cholesterol crystals
- Very low signal may be present along the margins or within the lumen of the mass = areas of hemosiderin deposition

Cholesterol Granuloma, ME

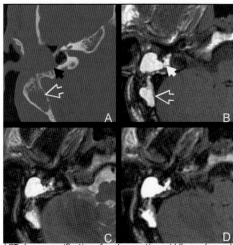

CG. (A) Axial CT shows opacification of post-operative middle ear (arrow) and mastoid (open arrow). (B) T1 C- MR shows true nature of lesion by defining high T1 signal in middle ear (arrow) and mastoid (open arrow). (C) T2 and (D) FLAIR sequences both show these areas as high signal.

Differential Diagnosis: Vascular-Appearing Middle Ear Mass

Dehiscent Jugular Bulb
- Mass contiguous with superolateral jugular bulb

Aberrant Internal Carotid Artery
- Tubular "mass" enters middle ear through enlarged inferior tympanic canaliculus
- Passes across cochlear promontory and reconnects to horizontal petrous ICA anteromedially

Chronic Otitis Media with Hemorrhage
- Inflammatory tissue and blood fill middle ear and mastoid without expansile bony changes

Post-traumatic Hemotympanum
- History compelling; associated fractures

Post-traumatic or Surgical Encephalocele
- Can mimic CG strongly at surgery
- Imaging shows dehiscent tegmen with brain herniation into middle ear or mastoid cavity

Paraganglioma
- Glomus tympanicum paraganglioma: Confined to cochlear promontory
- Jugulotympanicum paraganglioma: Permeative bone changes from jugular foramen below through floor of middle ear cavity

Pathology

General
- Etiology-Pathogenesis (Current hypothesis)
  - Chronic otitis media, cholesteatoma or previous surgery obstructs the air cells of the middle ear and/or mastoid air cells with negative pressure developing in these cells

- o Decrease in atmospheric pressure induces mucosal engorgement, leading to rupture of blood vessels and resultant hemorrhage
- o Red blood cell degradation to cholesterol crystals incites a multinucleated foreign giant cell response to this irritant with subsequent inflammation and initial small vessel proliferation followed by vessel rupture
- o Granulation tissue forms secondary to repeated hemorrhage leading to an expansile lesion of the middle ear or mastoid
- • Epidemiology
  - o CG is far more common than CG of the petrous apex

Gross Pathologic, Surgical Features
- • Cystic mass with fibrous capsule filled with brownish liquid containing old blood and cholesterol crystals
- • Fluid has been described as "crankcase oil"

Microscopic Features
- • Red blood cells
- • Multinucleated giant cells surrounding cholesterol crystals embedded in fibrous connective tissue along with hemosiderin-laden macrophages, chronic inflammatory cells and blood vessels

Clinical Issues

Presentation
- • Principal clinical symptom: Slowly progressive conductive hearing loss
- • Other symptoms: Pulsatile tinnitus, pressure
- • Otoscopy: Non-pulsating bluish discoloration of the retracted tympanic membrane = **"blue eardrum"**

Natural History
- • Great variability in the rate of growth of CG exists, depending on the frequency and severity of the micro-hemorrhages within the lesion
- • Most take decades to grow with symptoms showing up years after the initial episodes of chronic otitis media

Treatment
- • Surgical resection of the wall and contents is treatment of choice

Prognosis
- • Because of the accessibility of CG, recurrence rates are much lower than with cholesterol granuloma of petrous apex air cells

Selected References
1. Campos A et al: Cholesterol granuloma of the middle ear: report of 5 cases. Acta Otorhinolaryngol Belg 50:125-9, 1996
2. Martin N et al: Cholesterol granuloma of the middle ear cavities: MR imaging. Radiology 172:521-5, 1989
3. Palva T et al: Large cholesterol granuloma cysts in the mastoid. Arch Otolaryngol 111:786-91, 1985

Cholesterol Granuloma, PA

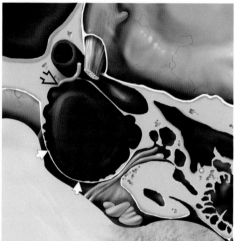

Cholesterol granuloma of the petrous apex. Drawing depicts a "chocolate cyst" enlarging the air cells of the petrous apex. The medial expansile margin of the lesion is "egg-shell" thin (arrows). Old blood is found in the cystic mass. The 6th cranial nerve is involved (open arrow).

Key Facts
- Synonyms: Cholesterol cyst, "chocolate" cyst
- Definition: Expansile mass of the PA resulting from air cell isolation from the middle ear with edema leading to recurrent hemorrhage
- Classic imaging appearance
  - CT shows a **smoothly expansile mass** with trabecular breakdown and cortical thinning and dehiscence
  - MR shows **high T1** and high **T2** signal
- PA Cholesterol Granuloma (PACG) is the most common lesion found in the petrous apex (PA)

Imaging Findings
General Features
- Best imaging clue: High T1 and T2 signal in expansile mass of PA
- Smooth, sharply marginated expansile lesion centered in PA
- When large, extends into surrounding area
  - Medially into clivus
  - Posteriorly to involve meninges and prepontine-CPA cisterns
  - Laterally into inner and middle ear
CT Findings
- Smoothly expanding petrous apex cortical margins
- Trabecular breakdown within PA expected
- When large, focal smooth erosion into clivus and inner ear present
MR Findings
- High T1 and T2 signal
  - Secondary to presence of hemorrhage, blood break-down products and cholesterol crystals
- When small, petrous apex smooth expansion
- When large, appear multilobular

Cholesterol Granuloma, PA

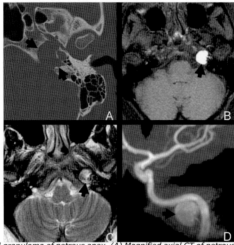

Cholesterol granuloma of petrous apex. (A) Magnified axial CT of petrous apex shows a sharply marginated expansile lesion (arrows). (B) T1 fat sat MR reveals the lesion contents to be high signal (arrow). (C) T2 signal is mixed to high (arrow). (D) MRA falsely depicts the lesion as possible aneurysm (arrow).

Imaging Recommendations
- Bone only CT of T-bone usually is first exam that identifies PACG
- MR then reveals the correct diagnosis in the characteristic high T1 and T2 signal (contrast is not helpful)

Differential Diagnosis: Petrous Apex Lesion
Congenital Cholesteatoma
- CT: Smooth, expansile margins
- T1 MR: Low to intermediate signal; T2 MR: Intermediate to high
- T1 C+ MR: Rim enhancement
- Gross path: White tissue
- Micro path: Squamous epithelium with desquamated keratin
Apical Petrositis
- CT: Permeative, destructive changes of cortex and trabeculae
- T1 MR: Low signal: T2 MR: High signal
- T1 C+ MR: Thick, enhancing rim; meninges thick and enhancing
- Gross path: Yellow-green pus
- Micro path: WBCs, bacteria if not on antibiotics
Trapped Fluid, Petrous Apex (Effusion)
- CT: Opacified air cells; nonexpansile; cortex and trabeculae intact
- T1 MR: Low to intermediate signal (rarely high signal); T2 MR: High
- T1 C+ MR: No contrast enhancement of lesion or meninges
- Gross path: Sterile, xanthochromic (yellow-colored) fluid
- Micro path: A few chronic inflammatory cells; no bacteria

Pathology
General
- Embryology
  - PA pneumatization occurs normally in 30% of people
- Etiology-Pathogenesis (Current hypothesis)

Cholesterol Granuloma, PA

- o Chronic otitis media, cholesteatoma or previous surgery obstructs the PA air cells with negative pressure developing
- o Decrease in luminal pressure induces mucosal engorgement, leading to rupture of blood vessels and hemorrhage
- o RBC degradation to cholesterol crystals incites a multinucleated foreign giant cell response to this irritant with inflammation and initial small vessel proliferation followed by vessel rupture
- o Granulation tissue forms secondary to repeated hemorrhage leading to an expansile lesion of the PA
- Epidemiology
  - o 60% of all lesions of the PA are PACG
  - o CG of middle ear-mastoid more common than PACG

Gross Pathologic, Surgical Features
- Cystic mass with fibrous capsule filled with brownish liquid containing old blood and cholesterol crystals
- Fluid has been described as "crankcase oil"

Microscopic Features
- RBCs in various stages of degradation
- Multinucleated giant cells surrounding cholesterol crystals embedded in fibrous connective tissue along with hemosiderin-laden macrophages, chronic inflammatory cells and blood vessels

Clinical Issues
Presentation
- Principal presenting symptom: SNHL
- Other presenting symptoms: Tinnitus, hemifacial spasm, facial numbness, trigeminal neuralgia
- Age of onset: Young to middle age adults

Natural History
- Great variability in the rate of growth of PACG exists
- Depends on the frequency and severity of the micro-hemorrhages
- Most take decades to grow with symptoms showing up years after the initial episodes of chronic otitis media

Treatment
- Traditional treatment: Drainage and stent placement via a transtemporal approach; associated high recurrence rate
- Extended middle cranial fossa approach with extradural removal of PACG and obliteration of its cavity decreases recurrence rates

Prognosis
- If adequately drained, excellent

Selected References
1. Chaljub G et al: Magnetic resonance imaging of petrous tip lesions. Am J Otolaryngol 20:304-13, 1999
2. Greenberg JJ et al: Cholesterol granuloma of the petrous apex: MR and CT evaluation. AJNR 9:1205-14, 1988
3. Lo WW et al: Cholesterol granuloma of the petrous apex: CT diagnosis. Radiology 153:705-11, 1984

Hemangioma, Facial Nerve

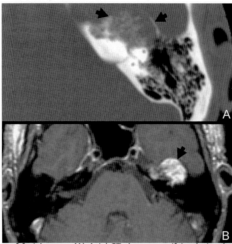

Hemangioma of facial nerve. (A) Axial CT shows a ossifying lesion (arrows) in the enlarged geniculate fossa. (B) Axial T1 C+ MR at the same level as (A) reveals an avidly enhancing mass (arrow) in the geniculate fossa.

Key Facts
- Synonyms: Intratemporal benign vascular tumor; **ossifying hemangioma**; vascular malformation
- Definition: Benign vascular tumor growing in the capillary bed of the facial nerve; capillary, cavernous or ossifying types defined
- Classic imaging appearance: **"Honeycomb" matrix** on CT highly characteristic when present (100% of large lesions)
- Facial nerve hemangioma (FNH) produces facial nerve paralysis early in its natural history
- Early detection while still extraneural may save VII at surgery

Imaging Findings
General Features
- Best imaging clue: **Ossific honeycomb tumor matrix**
- Site of occurrence
  - Geniculate fossa >> IAC fundus > posterior genu of facial nerve
- Small at presentation, often < 1 cm
- Irregular, invasive-appearing margins

CT Findings
- Amorphous "honeycomb" bone changes are distinctive
- Seen in 100% of larger lesions

MR Findings
- T1 C+ MR shows avid contrast enhancement
- Perineural spread along proximal facial nerve may be present
- If in fundus of IAC, may exactly mimic acoustic schwannoma
  - Ovoid, well-demarcated, enhancing mass on T1 C+ MR

Imaging Recommendations
- Thin section T1 C+ MR imaging focused to CPA-IAC-temporal bone-parotid best for patients with peripheral facial nerve paralysis
  - Axial and coronal planes recommended

Hemangioma, Facial Nerve

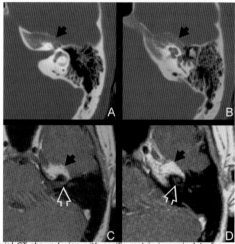

FNH. (A) Axial CT shows lesion with ossific matrix in geniculate fossa (arrow). (B) Slightly lower CT shows same lesion surrounding anterior cochlea (arrow). (C) T1 C+ MR reveals enhancing lesion (arrow) with IAC extension (open arrow). (D) Enhancing FNH (arrow); cochlea (open arrow).

- Bone-only 1 mm thickness temporal bone CT should be used to further evaluate any small areas of enhancement along facial nerve found by T1 C+ MR imaging

Differential Diagnosis: Intratemporal Facial Nerve Lesion
Congenital Cholesteatoma
- T1 C+ MR shows a non-enhancing middle ear mass tracking along the facial nerve canal
- Rare appearance of this lesion

Bell's Palsy (Herpetic Facial Paralysis)
- T1 C+ MR shows prominent enhancement of the entire intratemporal facial nerve
- No focal mass; CT normal

Facial Nerve Schwannoma
- T1 C+ MR reveals a tubular mass smoothly enlarging the VII canal
- Most commonly centered on the geniculate ganglion

Perineural Parotid Malignancy
- Invasive parotid mass is present
- Stylomastoid foramen is tissue filled
- VII enlarged from distal to proximal + mastoid air cell invasion

Pathology
General
- Etiology-Pathogenesis
  - Benign tumor arising out of sites of anastomoses between feeding arteries in the temporal bone
- Epidemiology
  - Rare (about as common as facial nerve schwannoma)

Gross Pathologic, Surgical Features
- Richly vascular mass without large feeding vessels

Hemangioma, Facial Nerve

Microscopic Features
- Nonencapsulated benign tumor composed of vascular channels-vessel walls of varying size
- Capillary type: Small vascular channels
- Cavernous type: Large vascular channels
- Ossifying type: Tumor produces spicules of lamellar bone
  - When seen called **ossifying hemangioma**
- All three histologic types can be seen in same tumor

Clinical Issues
Presentation
- Principal presenting symptom: **Peripheral facial nerve paralysis**
  - Occurs early because of intimate relationship between facial nerve and FNH
  - Can be acute, slowly progressive or intermittent
- Hemifacial spasm may progress to facial nerve paralysis
- When in fundus of IAC, may present with SNHL

Natural History
- FNH is a slowly-growing, benign tumor that presents when small as a result of location adjacent to facial nerve

Treatment
- Small FNH are extraneural
  - May be resected with preservation of facial nerve function
- Larger FNH invade the facial nerve
  - Segmental facial nerve resection with primary or cable repair yields poorer outcome

Prognosis
- Full facial nerve function is generally not regained

Selected References
1. Gavilan J et al: Ossifying hemangioma of the temporal bone. Arch Otolaryngol Head Neck Surg 116:965-7, 1990
2. Curtin HD et al: "Ossifying" hemangiomas of the temporal bone: evaluation with CT. Radiology 164:831-5, 1987
3. Lo WW et al: Intratemporal vascular tumors: evaluation with CT. Radiology 159:181-5, 1986

Bell's Palsy

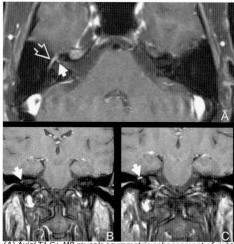

Bell's palsy. (A) Axial T1 C+ MR reveals asymmetric enhancement of right labyrinthine (arrow) and tympanic (open arrow) segments of VII. (B) Coronal T1 C+ MR shows enhancement of right tympanic VII (arrow). (C) Coronal T1 C+ MR anterior to (B) shows geniculate ganglion enhancing on right (arrow).

Key Facts
- Synonym: Herpetic facial paralysis
- Definitions
  - Term Bell's palsy (BsP) was originally used to describe idiopathic acute onset lower motor neuron facial paralysis
  - Now commonly called herpetic facial paralysis because of evidence linking **herpes simplex virus** and Bell's palsy
- Classic imaging appearance: T1 C+ MR shows intense, asymmetric, linear enhancement of holotemporal VII
- MR imaging reserved for "atypical" presentations only

Imaging Findings
General Features
- Best imaging clue: Fundal and labyrinthine segment VII enhancement
- 7th cranial nerve normally enhances at its anterior and posterior genus
- Circumneural arteriovenous plexus is most robust in these two locations
CT Findings
- CT normal in BsP
MR Findings
- T1 C+ MR shows uniform, contiguous enhancement of the facial nerve
  - VII is either normal in size or mildly enlarged
  - Enhancement pattern is linear, not nodular
- Enhancement is usually present from the distal internal auditory canal through labyrinthine segment, geniculate ganglion and anterior tympanic segment
  - A **tuft** of enhancement in the fundus of the IAC (premeatal segment) along with enhancement of the labyrinthine segment of the facial nerve are distinctive MR findings in BsP
  - The distal intratemporal facial nerve (distal tympanic, mastoid segments) enhances less frequently

Bell's Palsy

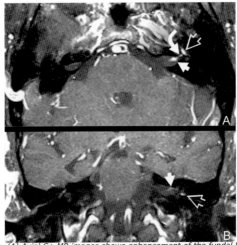

Bell's palsy. (A) Axial C+ MR images shows enhancement of the fundal VII = fundal tuft (arrow), labyrinthine segment (curved arrow) and geniculate ganglion (open arrow). (B) Coronal T1 C+ MR reveals linear enhancement in anterior superior IAC (arrow) and mid-tympanic VII (open arrow).

- Abnormal facial nerve enhancement may persist well beyond clinical improvement or full recovery
- Not all intratemporal facial nerves enhance in BsP

Imaging Recommendations
- Classic rapid onset BsP requires **no imaging** in the initial stages
  - 90% recover facial nerve function spontaneously < 2 months
  - If decompressive surgery is anticipated, MR imaging is warranted to ensure that no other lesion is causing the facial nerve paralysis
- **Atypical Bell's palsy** requires a search for an underlying lesion
  - Defined as slowly progressive palsy, facial hyperfunction (spasm) preceding the palsy, recurrent palsies, unusual degrees of pain, multiple cranial neuropathies, or peripheral facial nerve paralysis persisting or deepening beyond two months
- Thin section (3 mm) enhanced T1 MR images through the IAC and temporal bone is the examination of choice
- Temporal bone CT has a role in further defining lesions found on enhanced MR imaging and searching for the subtle intratemporal hemangioma of the facial nerve

Differential Diagnosis: Intratemporal Facial Nerve Lesion
Normal Enhancement of the Intratemporal Facial Nerve
- Mild, linear, discontinuous enhancement of the anterior and posterior genus of intratemporal VII
- Premeatal and labyrinthine segments of VII uninvolved

Facial Nerve Schwannoma
- Well-circumscribed tubular, enhancing mass within VII canal most commonly centered on the geniculate ganglion

Hemangioma of the Facial Nerve
- Poorly-circumscribed, enhancing mass on T1 C+ MR most commonly found in the geniculate fossa; CT shows intratumoral bone spicules

Bell's Palsy

Perineural Parotid Malignancy
- Invasive parotid mass is present
- Stylomastoid foramen is tissue filled; facial nerve is enlarged from distal to proximal with mastoid air cell invasion associated

Pathology
General
- Etiology-Pathogenesis (Current Hypothesis)
  - A latent herpes simplex infection of the geniculate ganglion with reactivation and spread of the inflammatory process along the proximal and distal facial nerve fibers
  - Pathophysiology: Formation of intraneural edema in the neuronal nerve sheaths caused by breakdown of the blood-nerve barrier and by venous congestion in the epineural and perineural venous plexus
- Epidemiology
  - Herpetic facial paralysis is responsible for > 50% of all cases of peripheral facial nerve paralysis

Gross Pathologic, Surgical Features
- Facial nerve edema peaks at 3 weeks following onset of symptoms

Microscopic Features
- Herpes simplex DNA has been recovered from facial nerve specimens in patients with BsP

Clinical Issues
Presentation
- Principal clinical symptom: Acute onset peripheral facial nerve paralysis
- Frequently a **viral prodrome** is reported
- 70% have alterations in taste days before the facial paralysis
- 50% have pain in or around the ipsilateral ear
- 20% have numbness in the ipsilateral face

Treatment
- Medical: Steroids +/- acyclovir
- Surgical: Profound denervation (>95%) treated with facial nerve decompression from IAC fundus to stylomastoid foramen
  - Decompression must be performed within 2 weeks of onset of total paralysis for it to be maximally effective
- The intensity, pattern and/or location of enhancement seen on T1 C+ MR not helpful in predicting outcome for an individual patient
- The older the patient, the lower the percentage of complete recovery of their facial nerve function

Prognosis
- > 90% of patients spontaneously recover all or part of their facial nerve function without therapy in first 2 months

Selected References
1. Grogan PM et al: Practice parameter: steroids, acyclovir, and surgery for Bell's palsy (an evidence-based review): report of the Quality Standards Subcommittee of the American Academy of Neurology. Neurology 56:830-6, 2001
2. Tien R et al: Contrast-enhanced MR imaging of facial nerve in 11 patients with Bell's palsy. AJNR 11:735-41, 1990
3. Daniels DL et al: MR imaging of facial nerve enhancement in Bell palsy or after temporal bone surgery. Radiology 171:807-9, 1989

Facial Nerve Schwannoma

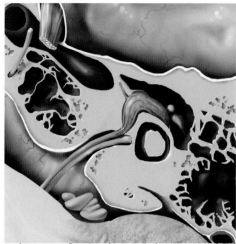

Facial nerve schwannoma. Drawing shows typical appearance of FNS as a facial nerve mass involving the geniculate ganglion and anterior tympanic segment of VII. Since the tumor bulges into the middle ear cavity, it is not surprising that this patient would present with conductive hearing loss.

Key Facts
- Synonyms: Facial neuroma; facial neurilemmoma
- Definition: Facial nerve schwannoma (FNS) is a rare benign tumor of Schwann cells that invest the peripheral facial nerve
- Classic imaging appearance: **Tubular mass** following the course of the facial nerve, enlarging the bony facial nerve canal (CT) and homogeneously enhancing (T1 C+ MR)
- Other key facts:
  - Geniculate ganglion area most frequently affected
  - Slowly-progressive facial nerve paralysis and hearing loss are the two most common presenting symptoms

Imaging Findings
General Features
- Best imaging clue: Facial nerve canal smooth enlargement
- **CPA-IAC FNS**: Exactly mimics acoustic schwannoma if no extension into labyrinthine segment occurs
  - If extension into labyrinthine segment is present, this "tail" makes imaging diagnosis
- **Intratemporal FNS**: Segmental, tubular enlargement of VII canal
  - Has distinctive imaging findings depending on the segment of the facial nerve involved (see below)

CT Findings
- CT appearance is dictated by where tumor is along VII
  - Geniculate ganglion FNS: Enlarged, remodeled geniculate fossa with thin bony walls
  - Tympanic segment FNS: Pedunculated mass emanates from tympanic segment of VII into the middle ear cavity
    - Presents as avascular retrotympanic mass

Facial Nerve Schwannoma

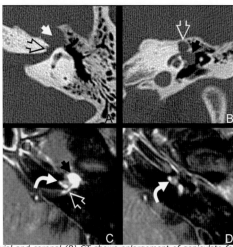

FNS. (A) Axial and coronal (B) CT shows enlargement of geniculate fossa (arrow) and labyrinthine VII canal (open arrow). (C-D) Axial T1 C+ MR reveals enhancing FNS involving geniculate ganglion (arrow) and labyrinthine VII (open arrow). Labyrinthine fistula: Cochlear (curved arrow) enhancement.

- o Mastoid segment FNS: Either tubular with sharp margin or globular with irregular margins depending on whether FNS breaks into surrounding mastoid air cells

MR Findings
- Geniculate ganglion FNS: T1 C+ MR shows an enhancing mass in the enlarged geniculate fossa
- Greater superficial petrosal nerve schwannoma: Diagnosed when an enhancing mass is seen in the location of the GSPN, just anteromedial to the geniculate fossa, projecting cephalad into middle cranial fossa
- Tympanic segment FNS: Pedunculates into the middle ear cavity
- Mastoid segment FNS: Either tubular with sharp margins or globular with irregular margins depending on whether it breaks into surrounding mastoid air cells

Differential Diagnosis: Intratemporal Facial Nerve Lesion
Congenital Cholesteatoma
- T1 C+ MR shows a non-enhancing middle ear mass tracking along the facial nerve canal; rare appearance of this lesion

Bell's Palsy (Herpetic Facial Paralysis)
- T1 C+ MR shows prominent enhancement of the entire intratemporal facial nerve; no focal mass; CT normal

Hemangioma of the Facial Nerve
- Poorly-circumscribed, enhancing mass on T1 C+ MR most commonly found in the geniculate fossa; CT shows intratumoral bone spicules

Perineural Parotid Malignancy
- Parotid mass is present; stylomastoid foramen is tissue filled; facial nerve is enlarged from distal to proximal with mastoid air cell invasion associated

Facial Nerve Schwannoma

Pathology

General
- Genetics
  - Multiple schwannomas = NF-2
- Etiology-Pathogenesis
  - Slowly-growing, benign tumor arising from Schwann cells investing the facial nerve
- Epidemiology
  - FNS is a rare tumor (< 1% of intrapetrous tumors)

Gross Pathologic, Surgical Features
- Tan, ovoid-tubular, encapsulated mass
- Arises from the outer nerve sheath layer of the facial nerve, expanding eccentrically away from the nerve

Microscopic Features
- Benign encapsulated tumor that is microscopically composed of bundles of spindle-shaped Schwann cells that usually form a whorled pattern
- Cellular architecture consists of densely cellular (Antoni A) areas and/or loose, myxomatous (Antoni B) areas

Clinical Issues

Presentation
- Principal presenting symptom: Varies with location of FNS
- Gradual onset of peripheral facial nerve paralysis occurs < 50%
- Ear and/or facial pain, hemifacial spasm, and acute onset Bell's palsy-like facial nerve paralysis = symptoms unrelated to location
- CPA-IAC FNS: SNHL, vertigo and tinnitus
- Tympanic or mastoid segment FNS
  - Conductive hearing loss
  - Retrotympanic mass behind an intact tympanic membrane

Treatment
- Surgical goal: Complete removal of the tumor with preservation of hearing and restoration of facial nerve function
- Combined with cable grafting of the facial nerve or, when tumor is small, (< 1 cm) facial nerve transposition with primary anastomosis
- If VII paralysis absent or mild at the time of diagnosis, the surgical cure can appear worse than the disease
  - Incomplete recovery of full facial nerve function despite the surgical restoration of facial nerve continuity may occur
- Location specific surgery
  - CPA-IAC FNS: Suboccipital transmeatal approach superior
    - If hearing is nonserviceable, translabyrinthine approach
  - Labyrinthine or geniculate FNS: Middle cranial fossa and transmastoid approaches combined
  - Tympanic and mastoid FNS: Transmastoid approach alone

Selected References
1. Kumon Y et al: Greater superficial petrosal nerve neurinoma: case report. J Neurosurg 91:691-6, 1999
2. Fagan PA et al: Facial neuroma of the cerebellopontine angle and the internal auditory canal. Laryngoscope 103:442-46, 1993
3. Inoue Y et al: Facial nerve neuromas: CT findings. JCAT 11:942-7, 1987

PocketRadiologist™
Head and Neck
100 Top Diagnoses

ORBIT

Orbital Dermoid

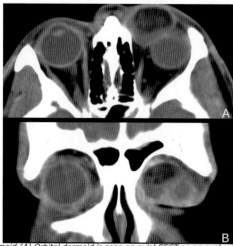

Orbital dermoid.(A) Orbital dermoid is seen on axial CECT as an oval mixed-density mass in the anteromedial orbit. The lesion is located in the pre- and post-septal extraconal space. (B) Coronal CECT shows the mixed density dermoid nestled in the superomedial orbit without underlying bone changes.

Key Facts
- Synonym: Developmental orbital cyst
- Definition: Cystic choristomatous mass lesion of the orbit resulting from congenital dermal inclusion
- Characteristic imaging appearance: Well-demarcated focal mixed density, sometimes fatty intraorbital or periorbital mass
- Spectrum of lesions including **dermoid**, **epidermoid** and **teratoma**
- Typical location at **medial canthus**

Imaging Findings
General Features
- Best imaging clue: Partially or completely fatty parenchyma
- Imaging identifies lipid components in 50% of lesions
- Well-defined mass at superior aspect of lateral orbit
  - Most common location = **frontozygomatic suture**
- Cystic and/or solid components
CT Findings
- Low density with definable wall
- Dermoid: Hypodense fat if present with density in −30 to -80 HU
  - Occasionally shows punctate calcification
- Epidermoid cyst: Uniform low density with no enhancement
- Scalloping and remodeling of the orbital wall sometimes present
MR Findings
- Dermoid
  - **Hyperintense T1** signal if **fat** present
  - Infrequently shows fluid levels
- Epidermoid cyst
  - Uniformly T1 hypointense, T2 hyperintense
- Hyperintense T2 signal for both dermoids and epidermoids

Orbital Dermoid

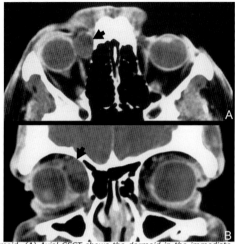

Orbital dermoid. (A) Axial CECT shows the dermoid in the immediate post- septal extraconal orbit as a mixed density mass (arrow). (B) On coronal CECT through the dermoid (arrow), no underlying bone remodeling is present.

Imaging Recommendations
- CT without contrast often adequate for diagnosis
- Pursue contrast exam and MR if imaging features not characteristic

Differential Diagnosis: Extraconal Orbital Mass
Idiopathic Orbital Pseudotumor
- Imaging: Intraconal-conal infiltrating mass
- Clinical: Painful proptosis
Lacrimal Gland Malignancy (Minor Salivary Gland Ca, NHL)
- Imaging: Invasive mass centered in superolateral quadrant of extraconal orbit
- Clinical: Painless proptosis
Non-Hodgkin Lymphoma
- Imaging: Can involve any area of orbit; a great mimic
- Clinical: Often with systemic NHL
Rhabdomyosarcoma
- Imaging: Invasive mass arising out of any rectus muscle
- Clinical: Malignancy of children and young adults

Pathology
General
- Embryology-Anatomy
  - Both dermoid and epidermoid result from inclusion of ectodermal elements during closure of the anterior neuropore of neural tube
- Etiology-Pathogenesis
  - Congenital inclusion of dermal elements at site of embryonic suture closure
- Epidemiology
  - Present from birth; spontaneous occurrence

Orbital Dermoid

Gross Pathologic, Surgical Features
- Whitish, well-delineated mass
  - ○ Connected to orbital periosteum by fibrovascular tissue
- Oily or cheesy material that is tan, yellow, or white

Microscopic Features
- **Dermoid**
  - ○ Contains dermal structures, including sebaceous glands and hair follicles, as well as blood vessels, fat and collagen within a fibrous capsule
- **Epidermoid cyst**
  - ○ Inner surface of fibrous capsule lined by keratinizing, stratified epithelium

Clinical Issues

Presentation
- Principal presenting symptom: Mass at superolateral orbital rim
  - ○ Nontender, fixed to underlying bone (cf: sebaceous cyst)
- If ruptured, inflammation similar to cellulitis will occur
- Rarely compromises globe or optic nerve unless very large
- Childhood presentation
  - ○ Most common to see dermoid present in child
  - ○ Subcutaneous nodule near orbital rim
- Adult presentation
  - ○ Lesion most commonly arises deep to orbital rim
  - ○ Often near the lacrimal gland in the extraconal orbit

Natural History
- Very slow growth, usually dormant for years
  - ○ Present during childhood but small and dormant
  - ○ Becomes symptomatic during rapid growth phase in young adult
- Sudden growth or change may occur following traumatic rupture

Treatment
- Surgical resection is curative
  - ○ Entire cyst must be removed to prevent recurrence
- Steroid therapy useful to calm inflammation in ruptured lesions

Prognosis
- Benign lesion, usually cosmetic considerations
- Large or ruptured lesions may cause significant symptoms

Selected References
1. Chawda SJ et al. Computed tomography of orbital dermoids: a 20-year review. Clin Radiol 54:821-5, 1999
2. Gunalp I et al: Cystic lesions of the orbit. Int Ophthalmol 20:273-7, 1997
3. Bartlett SP et al: The surgical management of orbitofacial dermoids in the pediatric patient. Plast Reconstr Surg 91:1208-15, 1993

Orbital Cavernous Hemangioma

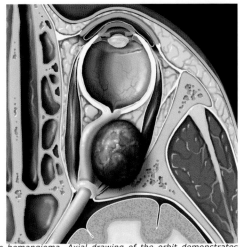

Cavernous hemangioma. Axial drawing of the orbit demonstrates cavernous hemangioma as a sharply-marginated intraconal mass that displaces the optic nerve-sheath complex.

Key Facts
- Synonym: Cavernous malformation of the orbit
- Definition: Non-neoplastic orbital tumor composed of dilated vascular channels
- Classic imaging appearance
  - CECT: Homogeneous, well-demarcated **intraconal orbital mass** with avid enhancement
  - MR with contrast: Isointense on T1, hyperintense on T2, prominent enhancement on T1 C+ MR images
- **Most common orbital tumor in adults**

Imaging Findings
<u>General Features</u>
- Best imaging clue: Focal, enhancing intraconal mass in adult
- 80% intraconal
  - Other locals include extraconal, intramuscular or intraosseous
- Sharply marginated
  - **Pseudocapsule** of compressed surrounding tissue
- Vascular lesion with intense homogeneous enhancement

<u>CT Findings</u>
- Homogeneous, slightly hyperdense
  - Hyperdensity due to **microcalcifications**
  - Coarse, punctate calcification uncommon
- Benign remodeling of bone if large

<u>MR Findings</u>
- T1 signal isointense to muscle
- T2 signal hyperintense to muscle
- Hypointense rim is pseudocapsule
- T1 C+ MR shows early, central, patchy enhancement that fills in homogeneously with time

Orbital Cavernous Hemangioma

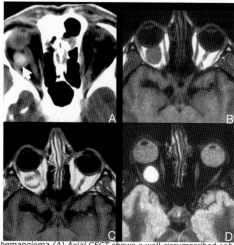

Cavernous hemangioma.(A) Axial CECT shows a well-circumscribed enhancing mass (arrow) in the intraconal space. (B) T1 MR reveals cavernous hemangioma has signal similar to muscle. (C) T1 C+ MR shows inhomogeneous enhancement. (D) STIR MR reveals the mass as homogeneous high signal.

Ultrasound Findings
- Hyperechoic, heterogeneous retrobulbar mass
- Doppler shows small areas of very slow flow and low resistance

Imaging Recommendations
- CECT is diagnostic in appropriate clinical setting
- Get coronal plane to show relationship to optic nerve and muscles
- MR useful in indeterminate lesions
  - Early patchy enhancement that fills in is a characteristic imaging feature that is similar to hemangiomas elsewhere
- **Hypointense pseudocapsule** is characteristic

Differential Diagnosis: Intraconal Mass

Lymphangioma
- Imaging: Multilocular orbital mass with fluid inside
  - Fluid-fluid levels can occur

Orbital Varix
- Imaging: Solitary intraconal ovoid or lenticular mass
  - Uniform, immediate enhancement
- Clinical: Enlarges with Valsalva maneuver

Orbital Pseudotumor
- Imaging: Infiltrating orbital mass of intraconal and conal structures
- Clinical: Painful exophthalmos

Optic Nerve Sheath Meningioma
- Imaging: Fusiform enhancing mass surrounding optic nerve
  - Tram-track calcifications are characteristic

Lymphoma & Metastasis
- Invasive mass that can involve any area of orbit

Optic Glioma
- Imaging: Sausage-shaped mass along course of optic nerve
  - Optic nerve cannot be identified in area of mass

Orbital Cavernous Hemangioma

- Clinical: NF-1 often present

Pathology
<u>General</u>
- Etiology-Pathogenesis
  - ○ Non-neoplastic dilatation of vascular spaces
- Epidemiology
  - ○ Most common isolated orbital mass in adults
<u>Gross Pathologic, Surgical Features</u>
- Discrete, well-defined, reddish vascular mass
- Lacks a prominent arterial supply
- Distinct, fibrous pseudocapsule surrounding compressed tissue
<u>Microscopic Features</u>
- Dilated vascular channels, larger than capillaries
- Thin-walled sinusoidal spaces lined with attenuated endothelial cells, filled with red blood cells
- No evidence of neoplasia

Clinical Issues
<u>Presentation</u>
- Principal presenting symptom: Painless proptosis
- Other symptoms: Diplopia, vision loss
- Increased intraocular pressure
- Retinal striae on fundoscopic exam
- Age range 10 to 60 years
<u>Natural History</u>
- Slow, progressive enlargement
  - ○ Compare capillary hemangiomas, which spontaneously regress
- Eventually compress orbital structures and remodel bone
- More rapid growth during pregnancy
<u>Treatment</u>
- Surgical resection for visual disturbance, cosmesis or other significant mass effect
  - ○ Lateral orbitotomy is conventional surgical approach
  - ○ Transorbital and maxillofacial approaches have been developed
  - ○ More extensive surgery for apex lesions
- Intralesional laser, cryosurgical and radiosurgical techniques are alternatives
- Observation only for stable lesions or poor surgical candidates
<u>Prognosis</u>
- Excellent prognosis given complete surgical removal
  - ○ Pseudocapsule promotes easy extraction
- Orbital apex lesions require more extensive surgery
  - ○ Higher complication rate
- Alternative surgical approaches and therapy considerations

Selected References
1. Thorn-Kany M et al: Cavernous hemangiomas of the orbit: MR imaging. J Neuroradiol 26:79-86, 1999
2. Koeller KK et al: Orbital masses. Semin Ultrasound CT MR 19:272-91, 1998
3. Acciarri N et al: Orbital cavernous angiomas: surgical experience on a series of cases. J Neurosurg Sci 39:203-9, 1995

Orbital Capillary Hemangioma

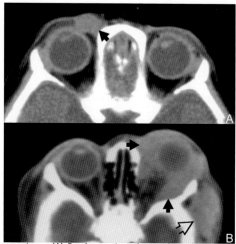

Capillary hemangioma. (A) Poorly-marginated mass (arrow) seen in anteromedial preseptal orbit with uniform enhancement on CECT is typical of capillary hemangioma. (B) A second-larger lesion is seen to involve much of the orbit (arrows) as well as the suprazygomatic masticator space (open arrow).

Key Facts
- Synonyms: Benign hemangioendothelioma; infantile periocular hemangioma; congenital or juvenile hemangiomas
- Definition: Benign endothelial cell neoplasm of the orbit
- Classic imaging appearance: Poorly-marginated, uniformly-enhancing mass involving any area of the orbit in infant
- Seen in patients under 3 years of age
  - This is a **tumor of infants**
  - Grows during first years of life
- Most lesions **spontaneously regress**
- Steroid therapy is effective

Imaging Findings
General Features
- Best imaging clue: Poorly-marginated, uniformly-enhancing mass
- Sites of orbital involvement
  - Most commonly superomedial extraconal location
  - May involve eyelid or eyebrow
  - May extend intraconal and into superior orbital fissure
- Intense contrast enhancement is the rule
CT Findings
- Intensely-enhancing, poorly-marginated mass
- May involve any area of orbit or multiple contiguous areas
MR Findings
- T1 signal is variable, may be hyperintense
- T2 signal is hyperintense
- When on the vascular end of spectrum, small flow voids visible
- MRA usually normal since vascular component is at capillary level
Ultrasound Findings
- Irregular contour

Orbital Capillary Hemangioma

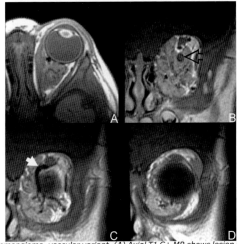

Capillary hemangioma, vascular variant. (A) Axial T1 C+ MR shows lesion in intraconal space. (B-D) Back-to-front coronal T1 C+ images reveal lesion is extraconal, conal and intraconal. Intraconal component surrounds optic nerve-sheath (open arrow, B). Ophthalmic artery is major feeding vessel (arrow).

- Mild-to-moderate internal echogenicity

Imaging Recommendations
- CT for initial evaluation of infant as no sedation required
- Larger lesions: MR with T1 C+ fat saturated images in axial and coronal planes to assess critical structure involvement

Differential Diagnosis: Pediatric Orbital Masses
Lymphangioma
- Non-enhancing, fluid density (CT)/intensity (MR) mass

Cephalocele
- Associated with skull base dehiscence
- Meninges ± brain may be seen herniating into orbit

Rhabdomyosarcoma
- Invasive orbital mass
- Bone destruction present when large

Pathology
General
- Etiology-Pathogenesis
  - Hamartomatous proliferation of vascular endothelial cells
  - Two distinct phases
    - Growth phase: First 12-24 months
    - Involutional phase: After 2 years of age
- Epidemiology
  - Most common benign orbital tumor of infancy
  - 1% of neonates
  - 50% of all capillary hemangiomas occur in head and neck

Gross Pathologic, Surgical Features
- Lobulated, blood-red tumor in the 2-8 cm size range

- If superficial, overlying skin will have bluish hue, accentuated by crying incidents
- May have external or internal carotid arterial supply
- Capable of profuse bleeding

Microscopic Features
- Unencapsulated cellular neoplasm with lobulated growth
- Proliferation of endothelial and mast cells
- Capillary-sized vascular spaces
  o Cavernous hemangioma has larger vascular spaces
- Immunohistochemical staining
  o Positive for factor VIII

Clinical Issues

Presentation
- Principal presenting symptom: Cutaneous bluish hue
  o Present in 80%; blanches with pressure
- Loss of visual acuity (noted by parents)
- Mass lesion may be found anywhere in orbit
  o Ptosis if eyelid involved
  o Proptosis if retroseptal, especially if intraconal
- Mass enlarges with crying (50%)
- Gender preference: Female > Male (3:1)

Natural History
- Manifest in only 30% of cases at birth; 100% by 6 months
  o Cf. **Cavernous malformations** and **lymphangiomas** present at birth and grow slowly with age
- Rapid growth during first 6 to 18 months of life
- 50% spontaneously involute by 5 years, 70% by 7 years

Treatment
- Observation initially, unless vision is threatened
- Corticosteroid treatment very effective
  o Topical, intralesional, or systemic administration
- Intratumoral laser therapy now being employed in larger lesions
- Interferon treatment for recalcitrant lesions
- Intravascular embolization contraindicated for intraorbital lesions
- Surgical ligation or laser ablation options, variable results

Prognosis
- Spontaneous regression in majority of patients
- Very responsive to steroid therapy
- Kasabach-Merritt syndrome
  o Rare condition in patients with extensive hemangiomas
- Hemorrhagic complications due to thrombocytopenia and coagulopathy

Selected References
1. Yap EY et al: Periocular capillary hemangioma: a review for pediatricians and family physicians. Mayo Clin Proc 73:753-9, 1998
2. Haik BG et al: Capillary hemangioma (infantile periocular hemangioma). Surg Ophthalmol 38:399-426, 1994
3. Haik BG et al: Capillary hemangioma of the lids and orbit: an analysis of the features and therapeutic results in 101 cases. Ophthalmology 86:760-92, 1979

Orbital Lymphangioma

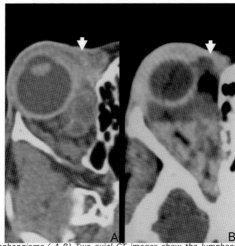

Orbital lymphangioma.(A-B) Two axial CT images show the lymphangioma filling portions of the extraconal, conal and intraconal spaces of the orbit. Preseptal involvement is also evident (arrows).

Key Facts

- Synonyms: Vascular hamartoma, venolymphatic malformation
- Definition: Congenital, benign, vascular tumor consisting of dilated vascular channels surrounded by lymphoid tissue
- Classic imaging appearance: Poorly-marginated, **multilocular,** extraconal mass, pre- or post-septal, with multiple cystic regions
  - Lesions confined to the conjunctivae are most common
- Other key facts
  - Orbital lymphangioma lesions will continue to expand in size; do **not** involute
    - Cf. capillary hemangioma which often involutes
  - Less than 5% of childhood orbital tumors
  - May be associated with lymphangiomas in other locals of H & N
  - Lymphatic tissue is not normally found in the orbit

Imaging Findings

General Imaging Features

- Best imaging clue: Fluid-fluid levels from spontaneous hemorrhage
- Poorly-marginated, enhancing, extraconal > intraconal mass

CT Findings

- Extraorbital (usually, may be conal or extraconal), multicystic, multilocular mass with irregular margins
- Crossing anatomic borders, with increased density compared with muscle tissue, somewhat heterogeneous
- Variable wall enhancement
- Edge enhancement algorithms may show slight bony remodeling
- Small calcifications or phleboliths may be seen

MR Findings

- May see **fluid-fluid levels** of hemorrhage into cystic regions
  - May be different ages of hemorrhage
- T1 signal variable from low to high signal; T2 signal high

Orbital Lymphangioma

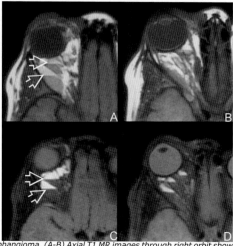

Orbital lymphangioma. (A-B) Axial T1 MR images through right orbit shows a proptotic globe caused by a transpatial mixed signal mass that is found in extraconal, conal and intraconal spaces. Fluid-fluid levels (arrows) indicate previous hemorrhage. (C-D) Axial T2 MR: Hemorrhage (arrows).

Imaging Recommendations
- Brain and orbital MR including T1 C+ fat saturated images best for surgical road mapping
  - May be associated intracranial abnormalities
- Lesions will not increase in size with Valsalva maneuver

Differential Diagnosis: Intraconal Mass
Cavernous Hemangioma
- Imaging: Ovoid, well-circumscribed, intraconal mass
- Clinical: Proptosis; most common orbit vascular tumor in adults
Capillary Hemangioma
- Imaging: Poorly-marginated, diffusely-enhancing orbital mass
- Clinical: Lesion of infancy and childhood
Idiopathic Orbital Pseudotumor
- Imaging: Intraconal-conal, poorly-marginated mass
- Clinical: Painful proptosis
Rhabdomyosarcoma
- Imaging: Invasive mass arising out of any rectus muscle
- Clinical: Malignancy of children and young adults
NHL or Metastases
- Imaging: Invasive mass; often multiple; both are mimics
- Clinical: Known primary tumor or systemic NHL involvement

Pathology
General
- General Path Comments
  - Orbital lymphangioma consists of dysplastic venous and/or lymphatic channels, smooth muscle fibers and loose connective tissue

Orbital Lymphangioma

- Embryology-Anatomy
  - Hamartomas from vascular mesenchymal anlage that develop with no direct connection to vascular or lymphatic systems
- Etiology-Pathogenesis
  - Lesions likely associated with relative hemodynamic isolation
- Epidemiology
  - Incidence 3:100,000
  - 8% of all expanding orbital tumors

Gross Pathologic, Surgical Features
- Thin-walled cystic structure with clear or chocolate-colored fluid from prior hemorrhage
- Not well encapsulated allowing invasion of surrounding tissues
- Cysts usually contain blood and serous fluid

Microscopic Features
- Unencapsulated group of multiple, irregularly-shaped lymphatic channels, lined with flattened endothelial cells
- Lesions may have collections of lymphoid cells within the walls or large follicles

Classification schemes
- Lymphangiomas can be classified by the size of the dysplastic channels:
  - Simple (capillary): Lymphatic channels of similar size
  - Cavernous: Dilated microscopic channels
  - Cystic: Macroscopic cystic regions of various size
- Lesions sometimes graded by location: Superficial, deep, combined

Clinical Issues
Presentation
- Principal presenting symptom: Intermittent proptosis
- Other symptoms include diplopia, ptosis, restricted EOM movement, compressive optic nerve findings and periorbital ecchymosis
- May be associated with lesions on face/eyelid and/or lymphangiomatous cysts in oral mucosa
- If spontaneous hemorrhage, acute onset of proptosis may be seen
- Usually presents in 1st decade

Natural History
- Lesions will increase and decrease in size, especially in conjunction with upper respiratory infection
- Lesion may rapidly increase in size with acute hemorrhage
- Generally, lesions will continue to enlarge until after puberty; however, optic nerve function is usually spared until large

Treatment
- Difficult to treat surgically
  - Complex interdigitation with normal orbital tissues
- Systemic steroids decrease proptosis

Prognosis
- Infiltrating nature results in frequent recurrences (up to 50%)
- Poor visual acuity is associated with multiple surgical resections

Selected References
1. Koeller KK et al: Orbital masses. Seminars US CT MR 19:272-91, 1998
2. Hopper KD et al: CT and MR imaging of the pediatric orbit. RadioGraphics 12:485-503, 1992
3. Graeb DA et al: Orbital lymphangiomas: Clinical, radiologic and pathologic characteristics. Radiology 175:417-21, 1990

Orbital Subperiosteal Abscess

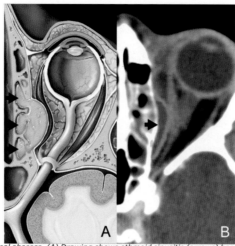

Subperiosteal abscess. (A) Drawing shows ethmoid sinusitis (arrows) has suppurated, causing an expanding subperiosteal abscess to push into orbit. (B) In this axial CECT the lenticular subperiosteal pus (arrow) can be seen pushing the medial rectus laterally.

Key Facts
- Definition: Accumulation of pus between lamina papyracea and orbital periosteum usually in medial orbital wall
- Classic imaging appearance: CECT shows hypodense lentiform fluid collection with enhancing rim along medial orbital wall
- Phases of orbital subperiosteal abscess (OSPA) from ethmoid sinusitis
  - Acute: Ethmoid sinusitis creates **periostitis** of lateral sinus wall
  - If untreated, evolves to **orbital phlegmon**
  - Next phase is **subperiosteal abscess** with purulent material
- OSPA complications
  - Optic nerve ischemia with blindness
  - Superior ophthalmic vein ± cavernous sinus thrombosis
  - Meningitis, cerebritis, subdural empyema or brain abscess
- Treatment: IV antibiotics may suffice in phlegmon phase of infection; surgical/endoscopic drainage if visual changes
- **Disease of childhood** with mean age at presentation of 9 years

Imaging Findings
General Features
- Best imaging clue: CECT shows lentiform, rim-enhancing, low-density lesion along medial orbit with adjacent ethmoid sinusitis
- Imaging may depend on stage of infection
  - Early: Solidly-enhancing phlegmon along medial orbit wall
- Late: Rim-enhancing fluid density collection ± gas
CT Findings
- Rim-enhancing fluid density lesion along orbital wall (medial >> superior wall); lateral displacement of medial rectus muscle
- Ethmoid sinusitis associated
- Cellulitic changes in orbital muscle and fat associated

Orbital Subperiosteal Abscess

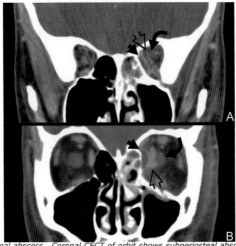

Subperiosteal abscess. Coronal CECT of orbit shows subperiosteal abscess (arrow) displacing and compressing medial rectus muscle (open arrow) and optic nerve (curved arrow) in posterior orbit (A) and in mid-orbit (B) Optic nerve compression makes this lesion a surgical emergency.

MR Findings
- T1 C+ MR shows rim-enhancing fluid collection in medial orbit
- "Blind" to air and bone changes
- T2 shows lentiform high-signal area

Imaging Recommendations
- CECT in axial and coronal planes best tool
  - Fast; better defines air and subtle bony changes
- T1 C+ MR is adjunctive; used when complications may be present
- Complications: Cavernous sinus thrombosis, cerebritis, brain abscess and subdural empyema

Differential Diagnosis: Inflammatory Orbital Diseases

Orbital Pseudotumor
- Imaging: Inflammatory mass can involve all areas of orbit
- Clinical: Painful proptosis without fever or increased WBC

Wegener's granulomatosis
- Imaging: Enhancing orbital mass; often intraconal and extraconal
  - Associated with chronic sinonasal granulomas in most cases
- Clinical: Necrotizing granulomas of upper and lower respiratory tracts, necrotizing vasculitis and glomerulonephritis

Myositis
- Imaging: Enlargement and enhancement of muscle cone

Pathology

General
- Embryology-Anatomy
  - Infection has 2 mechanisms of spread from ethmoid sinuses
    - Through valveless ophthalmic venous system
    - Directly through congenital dehiscences in lamina papyracea

Orbital Subperiosteal Abscess

- Etiology-Pathogenesis
  - ○ Acute sinusitis of ethmoid and maxillary complex is initiator
  - ○ Rarely bacterial septicemia, skin infection, penetrating injury
  - ○ Pathogenesis
    - ▪ Ethmoid sinusitis creates periostitis of lateral sinus wall
    - ▪ Evolves to **orbital phlegmon** and **orbital cellulitis**
    - ▪ Next phase is **subperiosteal abscess**
    - ▪ First extraconal, then intraconal
  - ○ Mixed infection common; Staphylococcus, Streptococcus, Haemophilus influenzae, Pneumococcus, anaerobics
- Epidemiology
  - ○ Orbital cellulitis is commonly associated with sinusitis
  - ○ OSPA is an uncommon sequela of sinusitis

Gross Pathologic, Surgical Features
- Thick, fibrous wall surrounds a pocket of yellow-green fluid

Microscopic Features
- Pus = necrotic debris with inflammatory cells (polymorphonuclear leukocytes, lymphocytes, macrophages); micro-organisms

Clinical Issues

Presentation
- Principal presenting symptom: Painful proptosis
- Other presenting symptoms
  - ○ Sinusitis, upper respiratory infection, fever
  - ○ Eye swelling with erythema and gaze restriction
- Age at presentation: Child (< 15 yrs); mean age 9 yrs

Natural History
- Visual disturbances occur from optic neuritis (extension of infection) or ischemia related to increased intraorbital pressure and retinal ischemia from central artery occlusion or thrombophlebitis
  - ○ Delay in treatment may result in blindness in up to 10%
- 15-30% of patients develop visual sequelae despite therapy

Treatment
- Controversial when to operate
  - ○ Orbital cellulitis treated with IV antibiotics
  - ○ OSPA without visual compromise also treated with IV antibiotics
  - ○ If visual changes and OSPA is medial: Endoscopic drainage
  - ○ If visual changes and OSPA is superior: External drainage
- Immediate surgical drainage recommended if: impaired vision, systemic manifestation, inability to perform reliable ophthalmologic exam, immunocompromised patient, lack of response of antibiotic therapy

Prognosis
- IV antibiotics ± drainage creates excellent prognosis in most cases
- 15-30% develop visual sequelae despite therapy

Selected References
1. Rahbar R et al: Management of orbital subperiosteal abscess in children. Arch Otolaryngol Head Neck Surg 127:281-6, 2001
2. Harris GJ: Subperiosteal abscess of the orbit: Age as a factor in the bacteriology and response to treatment. Ophthalmology 101:585-95, 1994
3. Arjmand EM et al: Pediatric sinusitis and subperiosteal orbital abscess formation: diagnosis and treatment. Otolaryngol Head Neck Surg 109:886-94, 1993

Optic Neuritis

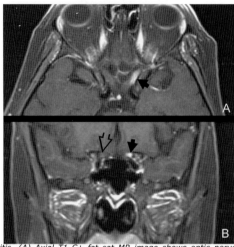

Optic neuritis. (A) Axial T1 C+ fat sat MR image shows optic nerve segmental enhancement (arrow) as it passes into the optic canal in the orbital apex. (B) Coronal T1 C+ fat sat MR image reveals the enhancing optic nerve (arrow) en face. Open arrow marks the normal opposite optic nerve.

Key Facts
- Definition: Acute inflammatory process involving the optic nerve
- Classic imaging appearance: T1 C+ MR shows enhancing, slightly enlarged optic nerve with hyperintensity on T2 or STIR
- May be first presentation of **multiple sclerosis** (MS) (25%)
- Patients with optic neuritis (ON) develop MS ~60% of time
- Clinical presentation: Acute visual loss, afferent pupillary defect & pain on globe movement

Imaging Findings
General Features
- Best imaging clue: Enhancing optic nerve on T1 C+ coronal fat sat MR
- Bilateral in up to 30%
- Associated white matter MS plaques on FLAIR (~50%)

CT Findings
- Often normal
- Rarely: Enlarged, enhancing optic nerve on coronal CECT

MR Findings
- T1 C+ fat sat: Enhancing, mildly enlarged optic nerve
  - Best seen on coronal images
  - On axial images may have "tram-track" enhancement pattern simulating optic nerve sheath meningioma
- FSE T2 with fat sat or STIR: Mildly enlarged, hyperintense optic nerve

MR Spectroscopy
- May aid in diagnosis of MS
  - Increased choline; decreased NAA

Imaging Recommendations
- **MR** is imaging **tool of choice** in suspected ON
- T1 C+ fat sat orbital images at 3mm, skip 0mm
  - Coronal and axial planes

Optic Neuritis

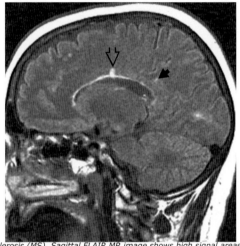

Multiple sclerosis (MS). Sagittal FLAIR MR image shows high signal areas (arrow) in the brain of the patient in the previous page image. Callosal marginal lesion (open arrow) is distinctive for diagnosis of multiple sclerosis. Patients with optic neuritis need full brain MR to evaluate for MS.

- Axial T2 with fat sat (3 mm skip 0 mm)
- Coronal STIR (3 mm skip 0 mm)
- Sagittal/Ax FLAIR images of brain to look for MS lesions

Differential Diagnosis: Optic Nerve-Sheath Lesions

Pseudotumor Affecting Optic Nerve-Sheath (Idiopathic Perineuritis)
- Imaging: Enlarged, enhancing optic nerve-sheath complex
  - May involve all orbital structures
- Clinical: Presents with orbital pain, pain with extraocular motility, decreased visual acuity, disc edema & mild proptosis

Granulomatous Optic Neuropathy (Orbital Sarcoid)
- Imaging: Indistinguishable when enhancing optic nerve only seen
  - When meningeal enhancement, involvement of lacrimal gland ± extraocular muscles present, easily differentiated from ON

Radiation Induced Optic Neuropathy
- Imaging: Bilateral optic nerve enhancement acutely
- Clinical: History of head or skull base XRT is key

Infectious Optic Neuropathy
- Imaging: May be indistinguishable from ON
- Clinical: Antecedent viral infection in children may be reported

Optic Nerve Sheath Meningioma
- Imaging: Thickened, enhancing optic nerve sheath
  - Tram-track calcifications are diagnostic

Optic Nerve Glioma
- Imaging: Tubular enlarged enhancing optic nerve
- Clinical: NF-2 often present

Pathology

General
- Genetics

Optic Neuritis

- o Human leukocyte antigen-DR2 allele is associated with ON
- o Increased odds ratio of MS development when present
- Etiology-Pathogenesis
  - o Demyelinating disease (MS >> ADEM) most common
  - o Other associated diseases
    - Ischemia, viral, syphilis, TB, toxoplasmosis, Lyme disease, sarcoid, systemic lupus erythematosis, radiation therapy
- Epidemiology
  - o ON occurs in up to 85% of patients with MS

Gross Pathologic, Surgical Features
- Chronic MS: Optic nerve atrophy

Microscopic Features
- Acute MS: Inflammatory cells, loss of myelin and axonal damage
- Chronic MS: Atrophy, gliosis, axonal/myelin loss; may cavitate

Clinical Issues

Presentation
- Principal presenting symptom: **Monocular visual loss** (visual acuity/ field defect/color) evolving over hours to days
- Other symptoms: Pain on eye movements, globe tenderness, afferent pupillary defect
- Females >>Males; mean age of onset 33 years
- Devic's disease (neuromyelitis optica): MS with ON & myelitis
- Pediatrics: Bilateral disease common (60%), often follows a viral illness; less likely to develop MS
- ON presenting symptom in 25% patients with MS
- ~60% of patients with ON develop MS

Natural History
- Vision begins to recover over 2-3 weeks
- Residual visual defects persist in 15%
- Recurrent attacks in same eye 20-30%
- If > 3 lesions on brain MR at time of ON, increased risk of MS

Treatment
- Steroid treatment (IV) accelerates short-term recovery

Prognosis
- Majority of patients (85%) have resolution of symptoms
- ~60% of patients develop MS

Selected References
1. Brusaferri F et al: Steroids for multiple sclerosis and optic neuritis: a meta-analysis of randomized controlled clinical trials. J Neurol 6:435-42, 2000
2. Hauser SL et al: Interaction between HLA-DR2 and abnormal brain MRI in optic neuritis and early MS. Optic Neuritis Study Group. Neurology 9:1859-861, 2000
3. Sorensen TL et al: Optic neuritis as onset manifestation of multiple sclerosis. Neurology 3:473-82, 1999

Idiopathic Orbital Pseudotumor

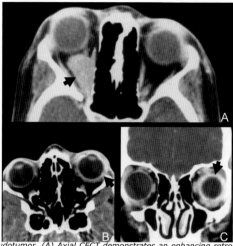

Orbital pseudotumor. (A) Axial CECT demonstrates an enhancing retroocular mass involving the intraconal, conal and extraconal spaces (arrow). Axial (B) and coronal (C) CECT in another patients shows uveal-scleral pseudotumor (arrows).

Key Facts
- Synonym: Idiopathic, nonspecific, orbital inflammatory disease
- Definition: Mixed inflammatory infiltrate in any area of the orbit
- Classic imaging appearance: Infiltrating orbital mass primarily centered in the intraconal fat but involving the conal muscles
- Other key facts
  - Most common cause of orbital mass in adults
  - Most common symptoms = painful proptosis, red eye

Imaging Findings
General Imaging Features
- Best imaging sign = Diffusely, infiltrating intraconal-conal mass
- Multiple sites can be affected; different anatomic patterns
  - "Tumefactive"
  - Myositic
  - Uveal-scleral
  - Lacrimal gland
- Invasive (rare)
CT Findings
- **"Tumefactive" pseudotumor**
  - Two-thirds of cases
  - Diffusely infiltrating >> focal
  - Often multicompartmental, crosses anatomic boundaries
    - 75% retrobulbar ± muscle cone involvement
    - Usually spares conjunctiva
    - Often extends outside orbit
- **Myositic pseudotumor**
  - 2nd most common pattern
  - Unilateral involvement
  - Single or multiple muscles
  - **Involves tendinous insertions**

Idiopathic Orbital Pseudotumor

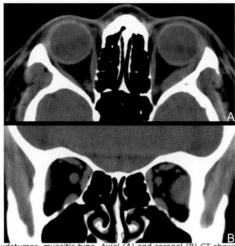

Orbital pseudotumor, myositic type. Axial (A) and coronal (B) CT shows a large left lateral rectus muscle. Concern over possible metastatic tumor infiltration resulted in biopsy revealing myositic pseudotumor.

- **Lacrimal gland pseudotumor**
  - Diffusely-enlarged lacrimal gland
  - Often occurs with myositic form
- Uncommon patterns
  - Uveal-scleral pseudotumor
    - Thickened sclera with "shaggy" enhancement
  - Optic nerve-sheath pseudotumor
  - Invasive pseudotumor
    - Invades bony orbit, erodes SOF/optic canal
    - May extend intracranially
    - Can mimic neoplasm or aggressive infection

Imaging Recommendations
- Contrast-enhanced, fat-suppressed MR is best tool
- U/S-guided fine-needle aspiration biopsy may be helpful

Differential Diagnosis
Myositis
- Usually viral etiology
- Often affects only one muscle (lateral rectus common)
Idiopathic Sclerotic Inflammation of the Orbit
- Often bilateral, may extend into adjacent sinuses (no erosion)
- Very hypointense on T1 and T2 MR
Other Benign Orbital Lymphoproliferative Disorders
- Benign (reactive) lymphoid hyperplasia
- Atypical lymphoid hyperplasia (borderline with lymphoma)
- Fibrotic inflammatory pseudotumor
Thyroid Ophthalmopathy
- Common cause of proptosis in adults
- Most patients hyperthyroid (10% euthyroid)
- 80% bilateral; 90% involve > one muscle

- Affects muscle belly, spares tendons
- Inferior > medial > lateral > superior rectus

Non-Hodgkin Lymphoma
- The "great pretender" (can mimic many orbit diseases)
- Accounts for >50% of malignant orbital tumors in adults
- May be bilateral, ± bone erosion
- Often diffuse, affecting anterior superior orbit (conjunctiva, superior rectus/levator muscles)
- May require biopsy for differentiation

Pathology
General
- General Path Comments
  - Can involve any/all parts of orbit
- Epidemiology
  - Third most common ophthalmic disorder (after Grave's, lymphoproliferative disorders)
  - 5%-8% of all orbital masses

Gross Pathologic, Surgical Features
- Common = soft, compressible mass
- Occasionally hard, fibrotic

Microscopic Features
- **Not** a true lymphoid tumor
- Histologic hallmarks
  - Mixed inflammatory infiltrate
  - Varying degrees of fibrosis

Clinical Issues
Presentation
- Principal presenting symptom: **Painful proptosis**
- Other symptoms: Visual loss; red eye
- Can occur at any age (mean age = 45 years)

Natural History
- 5%-10% resolve spontaneously

Treatment
- High-dose steroids are mainstay
- Resistant cases may require radiotherapy, chemotherapy ± decompressive orbitotomy

Prognosis
- Most respond to steroid therapy

Selected References
1. Valvassori GE et al: Imaging of orbital lymphoproliferative disorders. Radiol Clin North Am 37:135-50, 1999
2. Dehner LP et al: Idiopathic fibrosclerotic disorders and other inflammatory pseudotumors. Semin Diagn Pathol 15:161-73, 1998
3. Asao C et al: Orbital lymphoproliferative diseases: MRI and pathologic findings. IJNR 4:439-44, 1998

Thyroid Ophthalmopathy

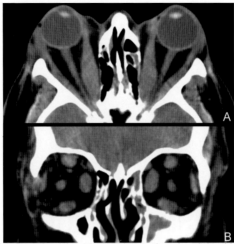

Thyroid ophthalmopathy. (A) Axial CECT shows enlarged medial and lateral rectus muscles bilaterally. As expected, coronal images show lateral rectus and oblique muscles are least involved. (B) Coronal CT reveals all rectus muscles are enlarged.

Key Facts
- Synonyms: Graves' ophthalmopathy, thyroid orbitopathy
- Definition: Autoimmune orbital inflammatory condition associated with thyroid dysfunction
- Classic imaging appearance: Enlargement of extraocular muscles (EOMs), particularly **inferior** and **medial recti**
- Most common cause of **proptosis** in adult
- Typical patient is **middle-aged female**

Imaging Findings
General Features
- Best imaging clue: Bilateral enlargement of EOMs
- Symmetric enlargement of EOMs
  - Predilection for **muscle bellies**, sparing of tendons
  - Bilateral in 90%
  - Isolated muscle involvement in 5%
- Order of likelihood of muscle involvement
  - **"I'M SLO"**
  - Inferior, medial, superior, lateral, obliques
- Increased volume of orbital fat
- Enlargement of lacrimal gland
- Straightened ("stretched") optic nerve
- Enlarged superior ophthalmic vein
CT Findings
- Isodense enlargement of EOMs
- Intracranial fat prolapse on CT indicates nerve compression
- Preoperative CT if orbital decompression is planned
MR Findings
- Isointense enlargement of EOMs
- EOM signal correlates with disease activity
- MR shows optic nerve compression better than CT

Thyroid Ophthalmopathy

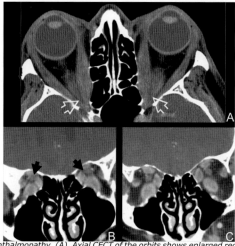

Thyroid ophthalmopathy. (A). Axial CECT of the orbits shows enlarged rectus muscles tightly packing the orbital apices (open arrows). (B-C) Coronal CECT reveals the optic nerves (arrows) compressed by the enlarged extraocular muscles.

Ultrasound Findings
- Enlarged EOMs, enlarged superior ophthalmic vein

Imaging Recommendations
- Imaging not routinely necessary if diagnosis is established clinically
- Non-contrast CT or limited MR adequate for confirmation and follow-up
- Coronal and axial planes are critical for assessing muscle size and relationship to orbital structures

Differential Diagnosis: EOM Enlargement

Infectious Cellulitis-Myositis
- Imaging: Enlarged medial rectus with associated ethmoid sinusitis
- Clinical: Sinusitis

Idiopathic Orbital Pseudotumor (Myositic Type)
- Imaging: Multiple EOMs enlarged
- Clinical: Painful proptosis

Non-Hodgkin Lymphoma or Metastatic Tumor
- Imaging: May mimic any orbital process; invasive mass involving EOM
- Clinical: Systemic NHL or known primary tumor

Pathology

General
- Etiology-Pathogenesis
  - **Autoimmune inflammation** of EOMs, periorbital fat and connective tissues
    - TSH receptor antigen is common to both thyroid and orbit
  - Lymphocyte infiltration leads to fibroblast-mediated glycosaminoglycan deposition and edema
- Epidemiology
  - Most common cause of unilateral and bilateral exophthalmus

Thyroid Ophthalmopathy

- o May precede, follow or coexist with hyperthyroidism or hypothyroidism
- o Incidence: 1 in 2,000
- o Prevalence of orbital disease in patients with Graves
  - ▪ 35% clinically significant orbital disease
  - ▪ ~70% have orbital findings on CT

Gross Pathologic, Surgical Features
- Gross enlargement of EOM bellies
- Increased volume of orbital fat

Microscopic Features
- Lymphocyte infiltration with enlargement of fibroblasts
- Mucopolysaccharide accumulation; increased collagen
- Later stage: Fibrosis and degenerative changes within EOM's

Clinical Issues
Presentation
- Principal presenting symptom: **Bilateral proptosis**
- Other presenting symptoms
  - o Signs and symptoms of thyroid dysfunction
  - o Periorbital edema, chemosis and corneal ulceration
  - o Eyelid retraction and eyelid lag on downgaze
  - o Altered ocular motility due to restrictive myopathy
    - ▪ Strabismus, particularly hypotropia and esotropia
  - o Vision loss in severe cases due to optic nerve compression
- Affects young and middle-aged adults, most 30-50 years old
- 3 to 5 times more common in women

Natural History
- May occur in the setting of hyperthyroidism or hypothyroidism
- Usually has self-limited course over 1 to many years
- More severe cases in older adults
- Other autoimmune diseases have been associated
  - o Myasthenia gravis, Addison disease, pernicious anemia

Treatment
- Treatment of orbital disease is palliative
- Supportive therapy for early and mild cases
  - o Corneal care; close observation for vision impairment
- Medical, radiation or surgical therapy for patients with severe inflammation or optic nerve compression
- Medication: Oral steroids, octreotide, fibroblast cytokine inhibitors
- Radiation: 1500-2000 cGy, fractionated over 10 days
- Surgery: Orbital decompression, correction of strabismus, restore eyelid position and function

Prognosis
- Self-limited condition, favorable outcome
- Vision may be threatened in severe cases

Selected References
1. Mayer E et al: Serial STIR MR imaging correlates with clinical score of activity in thyroid disease. Eye 15:313-8, 2001
2. Jacobson D. Dysthyroid orbitopathy. Semin Neurol 20:43-54, 2000
3. Warwar RE. New insights into pathogenesis and potential therapeutic options for Graves orbitopathy. Curr Opin Ophthalmol 10:358-61, 1999

Optic Nerve Meningioma

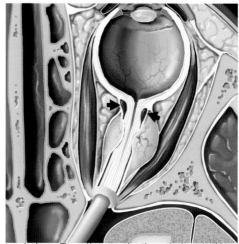

Optic nerve meningioma. The optic nerve sheath meningioma in this axial depiction of the orbit is seen wrapping the optic nerve. Dilatation of the apical subarachnoid space is seen (arrows).

Key Facts
- Synonym: Optic nerve sheath meningioma
- Definition: Benign, slow-growing neoplasm of the intraorbital optic nerve dural sheath
- Imaging appearance: Solid intraconal or orbital apex mass with moderately intense contrast enhancement; **calcification** is a characteristic feature
- 90% of orbital meningiomas are secondary lesions, arising from sites immediately adjacent to the orbit
- Main differential diagnosis is optic nerve glioma (no calcification)

Imaging Findings
General Imaging Features
- Best imaging clue: Enhancing mass along intraorbital optic nerve with tram-track calcifications
- Tubular shape (65%) > pedunculated (25%) > fusiform (10%)
- Encases the nerve in a circumferential pattern, although may show eccentric or pedunculated growth pattern

CT Findings
- Optic nerve meningioma (ONM) appears isodense on non-contrast CT
- When present, linear or punctate calcification within the tumor is characteristic
- **Tram-tracking** may result from tumor enhancement on either side of hypodense optic nerve or from calcification within tumor
- Calcification typically spares the distal-most segment of the optic nerve as it enters the nerve head on the posterior globe

MR Findings
- ONM appears isointense on T1, and variably hypointense on T2 depending on the degree of calcification

Optic Nerve Meningioma

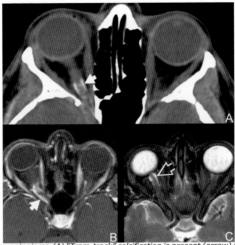

Optic nerve meningioma.(A) "Tram-track" calcification is present (arrow) in this CECT, marking the location of the optic nerve sheath meningioma.(B) T1 C+ MR image shows the enhancing tumor (arrow). (C) Dilated subarachnoid space (open arrow) best seen on T2 axial MR imaging.

- T1 C+ MR shows tumor "tram-tracking" on either side of the hypointense optic nerve
- Increased CSF within the nerve sheath surrounding the distal optic nerve = **perioptic cysts** is a characteristic feature of ONM; best demonstrated on T2 or inversion recovery

Imaging Recommendations
- Contrast-enhanced MR = imaging modality of choice for characterizing the tumor relative to adjacent orbital structures, as well as defining the extent of disease involving the orbital apex, optic canal, and intracranial structures
- CT can provide additional diagnostic information by demonstrating calcification, which is a characteristic feature of ONM
- Be sure to clear the tuberculum sellae and planum sphenoidale of en plaque meningioma as these may extend through optic canal to present as intraorbital ONM; CT will see intracranial origins poorly; if missed, bilateral blindness may result!

Differential Diagnosis: Optic Nerve-Sheath Lesions
Idiopathic Orbital Pseudotumor
- Usually is not isolated to ON sheath
- Painful exophthalmos

Sarcoidosis
- When no systemic disease, can be indistinguishable from ONM on enhanced CT & MR

Optic Neuritis
- Enhancing optic nerve without nerve-sheath enlargement
- Often associated with multiple sclerosis

Optic Nerve Glioma
- No tram-track enhancement or perioptic cysts
- No punctate or linear calcifications

Optic Nerve Meningioma

- Also may be associated with NF-1 (10-50% of cases)

Lymphoma & Metastases
- Systemic symptoms
- Multifocal orbital and extra-orbital lesions

Pathology
General
- Etiology-Pathogenesis
  - Benign tumor arising from arachnoid "cap" cells within the optic nerve sheath
- Epidemiology
  - Of all orbital meningiomas, 10% primary to optic nerve sheath; 90% are secondary lesions, arising from sites immediately adjacent to the orbit

Gross Pathologic, Surgical Features
- Sharply circumscribed, unencapsulated
- Circumferential to optic nerve, tightly adherent to perineural pial microvascular structures

Microscopic Features
- Meningothelial meningiomas most common type encountered in orbit
- Transitional and fibroblastic meningiomas encountered much less frequently

Clinical Issues
Presentation
- Principal presenting symptom: Unilateral loss of vision
- Middle-aged or elderly women or young adults with NF-1
- Other symptoms: Proptosis

Treatment
- Surgical excision first line therapy

Prognosis
- Post-operative visual impairment inevitable because ONM is tightly adherent to ON

Selected References
1. Mafee MF et al: Optic nerve sheath meningiomas. Role of MR imaging. Radiol Clin North Am 37:37-58, 1999
2. Delfini R et al: Primary benign tumors of the orbital cavity: comparative data in a series of patients with optic nerve glioma, sheath meningioma, or neuroma. Surg Neurol 45:147-53, 1996
3. Ortiz O et al: Meningioma of the optic nerve sheath. AJNR 17:901-6 1996

Retinoblastoma

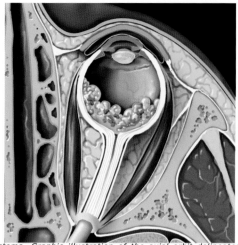

Retinoblastoma. Graphic illustration of the axial orbit delineates a typical retinoblastoma in the posterior globe. A calcified mass in the globe of an infant or young child is a retinoblastoma until proven otherwise.

Key Facts
- Definition: Malignant primary neoplasm of the retina
- Classic imaging appearance: CT shows an intraocular enhancing retinal mass with calcification often with retinal detachment
- Most common intraocular tumor of childhood
- Presents with **leukocoria** (white pupil)
- Retinoblastoma (RB) may involve one (unilateral) or both eyes (bilateral) and rarely may be seen with coexisting PNET in pineal and/or suprasellar area
- When bilateral, follows an autosomal dominant pattern

Imaging Findings
General Imaging Features
- Best imaging clue: Calcified intraocular mass
- Solid intraocular retinal mass, centered posteriorly in the globe
- Moderate or markedly intense contrast enhancement is typical
- Retinal detachment is a commonly associated nonspecific finding
- Extraocular invasion occurs along optic nerve course; tumor may extend into orbit or intracranially through optic canal
- Coexisting tumor in the pineal or suprasellar regions rare
CT Findings
- RB appears as a soft tissue mass with characteristic punctate or finely speckled **calcification** (<90%)
MR Findings
- RB appears moderately hyperintense on T1 and hypointense T2
- T1 C+ images show moderate to marked enhancement
- Extraocular extension best seen by MR
  - Extension along optic nerve into the orbit, optic foramina and intracranial area affect treatment planning and prognosis

Retinoblastoma

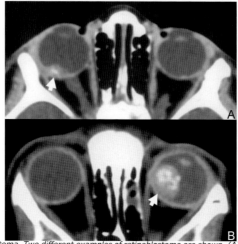

Retinoblastoma. Two different examples of retinoblastoma are shown. (A) Axial CECT shows a small, calcified mass (arrow) in the posterior right globe. (B) A larger example of retinoblastoma is shown in this axial CECT as a calcified, pedunculated mass (arrow).

Imaging Recommendations
- In patients with family history of heritable retinoblastoma (RB), screening eye exam +/- imaging at birth is recommended
- In larger RB as seen by ophthalmic ultrasound, both CT and MR play an important role
  - CT is used for verification of diagnostic calcification
  - MR shows extraocular spread and intracranial lesions

Differential Diagnosis: Lesions Causing Leukocoria
Persistent Hyperplastic Primary Vitreous
- Small globe with increased vitreous density without calcification; tissue band may extend from lens to posterior retina
Coats' Disease
- Increased density in all or part of vitreous in normal-sized globe without calcification
Congenital Cataract
- Vitreous is normal; lens is dense
Toxocariasis
- Ambulating child (2-8 years of age) with dense vitreous without discrete mass or calcification
Retinal Detachment
- Dense vitreous without discrete mass or calcification

Pathology
General
- Genetics
  - Heritable or non-heritable (sporadic) forms
  - Heritable form: Autosomal dominant with complete penetrance

Retinoblastoma

- o Chromosome 13 (q14 band) mutation: Seen in all patients with bilateral disease and 15% with unilateral disease
- Etiology-Pathogenesis
  - o Highly malignant primary neoplasm that arises from neuroectodermal cells of the retina
- Epidemiology
  - o Incidence of 1:20,000 births

Gross Pathologic, Surgical Features
- White to pink retinal mass
- Three growth patterns have been described:
  - o Endophytic form: Protrudes into the vitreous
  - o Exophytic form: Grows subretinal causing retinal detachment
  - o Diffuse form: Grows along the retina in a plaque-like fashion, simulating other inflammatory or nonneoplastic conditions

Microscopic Features
- Differentiated tumor shows Flexner-Wintersteiner rosettes
- Small round cells with scant cytoplasm and large nuclei
- Pineal and/or suprasellar tumors: PNET = Primitive neuroectodermal tumor

Retinoblastoma Types: Based on location
- Unilateral = One eye (70%)
- Bilateral = Both eyes (30%)
- Trilateral = Bilateral and pineal or suprasellar tumor (< 1%)
- Tetralateral = Bilateral plus pineal and suprasellar mass (< .1%)

Clinical Issues
Presentation
- Principal presenting symptom: Unilateral blindness
- Primary physical sign = **leukocoria** (loss of normal retinal red reflex)
- Most common intraocular tumor of childhood
- Over 90% diagnosed before age 5
- Less common symptom = strabismus secondary to glaucoma

Natural History
- RB is a congenital lesion that is present but not usually apparent at birth; average age of diagnosis is 13 months
- If intracranial tumor is present, usually not diagnosed for 2.5 years after initial RB is treated

Treatment
- Focal conservative treatment trend has come from early diagnosis
- Large RB +/- local extension: Enucleation + external beam XRT
- Medium RB with diffuse vitreous seeding: External beam XRT
- Small to medium tumors size: Plaque radiotherapy
- Chemotherapy for "chemoreduction" allowing more conservative therapies such as cryotherapy and photocoagulation

Prognosis
- Unilateral tumor without invasion has excellent prognosis
- Trilateral or tetralateral RB dismal prognosis (<24 mo. survival)

Selected References
1. Shields CL et al: Recent developments in the management of retinoblastoma. J Pediatr Ophthalmol 36:8-18, 1999
2. Provenzale JM et al: Radiologic-pathologic correlation: bilateral retinoblastoma with coexistent pinealoblastoma (trilateral retinoblastoma). AJNR 16:157-65, 1995
3. Stahl A et al: The genetics of retinoblastoma. Ann Genet 37:172-8, 1994

Optic Nerve Glioma

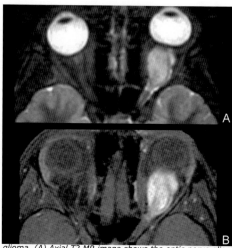

Optic nerve glioma. (A) Axial T2 MR image shows the optic nerve glioma as a high-signal bulbous enlargement of the intraorbital optic nerve. (B) With enhancement the axial T1 fat sat MR image reveals avid tumor enhancement from the immediate retroocular nerve to the orbital apex.

Key Facts
- Synonyms: Grade I astrocytomas of optic nerve; juvenile pilocytic astrocytomas
- Definition: Benign tumor of anterior optic pathway composed of neuroglial tissue
- Classic imaging appearance: Fusiform optic nerve mass with variable enhancement; may involve proximal optic pathway
- Tumor of childhood; 33-50% associated with NF-1
- Optic nerve glioma (ONG) is 4 times more optic sheath meningioma

Imaging Findings
General Imaging Features
- Best imaging clue: Sausage-shaped enlargement of intraorbital ON
- Diffuse **fusiform enlargement** of optic nerve
  - Characteristic **kinking or buckling of optic nerve** course
  - May extend proximally to chiasm, optic tracts, and radiations
- Areas of internal cystic or mucinous change possible
- Moderate enhancement with areas of patchy inhomogeneity
  - Irregular enhancement from ischemia of small nutrient arteries
- Associated CNS findings if patient has NF-1
CT Findings
- Isodense enlargement of optic nerve
- Calcification is rare (cf. optic nerve sheath meningioma)
- Enlargement of bony optic canal if proximal extension of tumor
MR Findings
- T1 signal is iso- to hypointense
- T2 signal is variable but typically hyperintense
- The optic nerve cannot be identified on T1 C+ images as discrete from the ONG

Optic Nerve Glioma

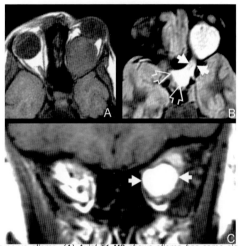

Large optic nerve glioma. (A) Axial T1 MR shows glioma has same signal as gray matter. (B) Avid enhancement of glioma is seen on axial T1 C+ MR. Enlarged optic nerve canal (arrows) transmits tumor intracranially to optic chiasm (open arrows). (C) Coronal T1 C+: Glioma in cross-section (arrows).

- o   In ON meningioma, optic nerve is usually visible passing through the tumor

Imaging Recommendations

- •   MR is preferred imaging tool because it helps with
  - o   Defining involvement of proximal optic pathways
  - o   Correlating degree of vision loss
  - o   Allowing assessment of NF-1 related findings (if present)
- •   CECT adequate for intraorbital ONG assessment without sedation
- •   Does not do as well as MR with proximal disease

Differential Diagnosis: Cystic CPA Mass

Optic Nerve-Sheath Lesion

- •   CECT shows enhancing mass along optic nerve and sheath
- •   Tram-track calcifications is a classic appearance on CT
- •   T1 C+ MR shows enhancing mass wrapping a visible optic nerve

Optic Neuritis (Ischemic, Viral, MS)

- •   T1 C+ fat saturated images show enhancing optic nerve without significant enlargement
- •   T2 whole brain MR shows cerebral plaques in 50% of MS cases

Idiopathic Orbital Inflammatory Disease (Pseudotumor)

- •   Isolated optic nerve involvement rare

Pathology

General

- •   Etiology-Pathogenesis
  - o   Tumor caused by hyperplasia of adjacent glial connective tissue and meninges, not by cell division (mitotic activity)
  - o   This hyperplastic event produces intracellular and extracellular mucopolysaccharides (mucinous substance)

Optic Nerve Glioma

- Epidemiology
  - 3% of orbital tumors
  - 4 times more common than optic sheath meningioma
  - 33-50% of those with ONG have NF-1
  - 15% of patients with NF-1 have optic pathway glioma

<u>Gross Pathologic, Surgical Features</u>
- Diffuse enlargement of the optic nerve with tan-white tumor
- Cystic changes related to mucinous material and/or infarction

<u>Microscopic Features</u>
- Histological appearance of juvenile pilocytic astrocytoma
- Round, spindle-shaped cells similar in appearance to those in the normal optic nerve

Clinical Issues

<u>Presentation</u>
- Childhood ONG
  - Principal presenting symptom: Progressive unilateral vision loss
    - Proptosis with globe motility preserved
    - If proximal pathway involved: Nystagmus, seizures, hydrocephalus possible
  - Funduscopic exam: Optic atrophy
  - Median age at presentation = 5 years
  - 90% show symptoms by age 20 years
- Adult malignant optic glioma (MOG)
  - Distinct lesion that affects middle-aged adults

<u>Natural History</u>
- Childhood ONG: Indolent benign-acting tumor
  - Progression rare after 6 years of age
  - Spontaneous regression reported with or without NF-1
- Adult MOG: Aggressive, fatal glioma with rapid progression

<u>Treatment</u>
- Childhood ONG
  - Difficult to evaluate treatment given natural history
  - Expectant management in patients with indolent course
  - Radiation therapy and surgery in those with bulky tumor
  - Chemotherapy slows tumor progression
- Adult ONG
  - Multimodality therapy

<u>Prognosis</u>
- Childhood ONG
  - With NF-1: Usually stabilizes before 6 years of age
  - Without NF-1: Often continues to grow after age 6 years
- Adult ONG: Very poor prognosis; highly fatal disease

Selected References
1. Grill J et al: When do children with optic pathway tumours need treatment? An oncological perspective in 106 patients treated in a single centre. Eur J Pediatr 159:692-6, 2000
2. Delfini R et al: Primary benign tumors of the orbital cavity: comparative data in a series of patients with optic nerve glioma, sheath meningioma, or neurinoma. Surg Neurol 45: 147-53, 1996
3. Azar-Kia B et al: Optic nerve tumors: role of magnetic resonance imaging and CT. Radiol Clin North Am 25:561-81, 1987

NOSE AND SINUS

Non-Invasive Fungal Sinusitis

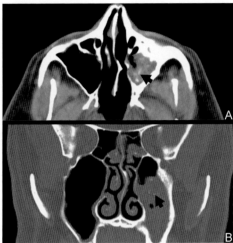

Fungal mycetoma. (A) Axial CT through maxillary sinus shows partial opacification of left maxillary sinus with high-density calcifications evident (arrow). (B) Coronal sinus CT again shows the intrasinus mycetoma with multiple punctate calcifications (arrow).

Key Facts
- Synonyms: **Mycetoma**, fungus ball and aspergilloma
- Definition: Chronic, noninvasive form of fungal sinus infection found in immunocompetent, non-atopic patients
- Classic imaging appearance:
  - Plain CT: Well-defined high-density mass within the involved sinus often with calcified foci
  - MR: Hypointense mass within the affected sinus
  - Single sinus affected; most commonly the maxillary sinus
- Patient profile: Immunocompetent, non-atopic, otherwise healthy patient, minimally symptomatic
- Excision of the mycetoma is the treatment of choice

Imaging Findings
General Features
- Best imaging clue: Single paranasal sinus contains mass with **fine round and linear calcifications** within its matrix
- Most common sinus affected = maxillary sinus
CT Findings
- Plain CT shows a focal mass within the sinus lumen with areas of high density within the mass parenchyma
- Round or linear high density is the result of calcium phosphate and calcium sulfate deposits within necrotic mycetoma
- Thick sinus wall and thickened inflamed sinus mucosa may be seen
MR Findings
- MR shows a low-signal mass in the affected sinus
- Hypointensity on T1 images from the absence of free water in this thick, solid, mycetomatous mass
- T2 MR image hypointensity is from associated macromolecular protein binding creating ultra-short T2 relaxation times

Non-Invasive Fungal Sinusitis

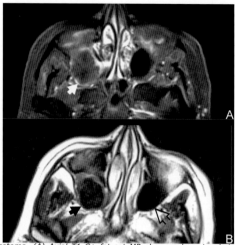

Fungal mycetoma. (A) Axial T1 C+ fat sat MR shows a low signal rim enhancing lesion (arrow) in right maxillary sinus. (B) On a T2 MR image at the same level as (A) the mycetoma (arrow) is seen as low-signal comparable to air in the opposite normal maxillary sinus (open arrow).

- Beware! Non-invasive fungal sinusitis (NIF) hypointensity may be mistaken for air in the sinus; usually not hypointense on all sequences

<u>Imaging Recommendations</u>
- If NIFS is suspected, unenhanced coronal sinus CT is best imaging tool

Differential Diagnosis
<u>Allergic Fungal Sinusitis</u>
- Atopic patient with multiple unilateral or pansinus involvement
- CT shows high-density material within expanded sinuses
- MR may show low signal on both T1 and T2 images

<u>Acute Invasive Fungal Sinusitis</u>
- Immunocompromised patient
- Soft tissue invasion in deep face, orbit, skull base and dura
- Bone destruction is evident on CT

<u>Chronic Invasive Fungal Sinusitis</u>
- Diabetic patient
- Soft tissue invasion in immediate area of affected sinuses

<u>Inverted papilloma</u>
- Mass is in middle meatus, involves sinuses secondarily
- Usually non-calcified with bone remodeling

<u>Ossifying fibroma</u>
- Benign tumor which ossifies, starting at the periphery
- Expansile mass with ossific rim and fibrous center

Pathology
<u>General</u>
- Etiology-Pathogenesis
  - Symbiotic fungal growth within a paranasal sinus
- Epidemiology

    ○   Mycetoma and allergic fungal sinusitis are most common forms of fungal sinusitis

<u>Gross Pathologic, Surgical Features</u>
- Mycetoma physical consistency: Thick, cheesy, semisolid lesion
- Tightly packed hyphae within the mycetoma give the feeling to the surgeon of "shoveling clay"

<u>Microscopic Features</u>
- Tightly packed **fungal hyphae** with no allergic mucin
- The absence of allergic mucin differentiates mycetoma from allergic fungal sinusitis
- No tissue invasion (cf. acute invasive fungal sinusitis)

Clinical Issues
<u>Presentation</u>
- Principal presenting symptom: Asymptomatic or mild sensation of pressure overlying the sinuses
- Immunocompetent, non-atopic, otherwise healthy patients

<u>Natural History</u>
- Indolent course
- May be asymptomatic for years

<u>Treatment</u>
- Resection of the fungus ball is curative
- No systemic treatment is needed

<u>Prognosis</u>
- Excellent response to surgical resection expected

Selected References
1. Fatterpekar G et al: Fungal diseases of the paranasal sinuses. Semin Ultrasound CT MRI 20:391-401, 1999
2. Som PM et al: Hypointense paranasal sinus foci: Differential diagnosis with MR imaging and relation to CT findings. Radiology 176:777-81, 1990
3. Zinreich SJ et al: Fungal sinusitis: Diagnosis with CT and MR imaging. Radiology 169:439-44, 1988

Antrochoanal Polyp

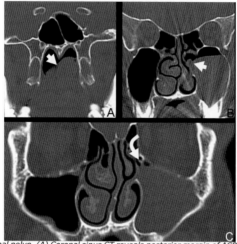

Antrochoanal polyp. (A) Coronal sinus CT reveals posterior margin of ACP in posterior nares (arrow). (B) More anterior coronal image shows ACP emerging from maxillary sinus through accessory ostium (arrow). (C) Coronal image through maxillary infundibulum: ACP does not pass this way (arrow).

Key Facts

- Definition: Antrochoanal polyp (ACP) is a sinonasal inflammatory polyp that arises from the maxillary sinus antrum and herniates through the major or accessory ostium into the nasal cavity
- Classic appearance: Dumbbell cystic mass fills maxillary antrum and ipsilateral nasal cavity; may protrude into nasopharyngeal airway
- **Sphenochoanal** and **ethmochoanal polyps** are less common

Imaging Findings

General Features

- Best diagnostic clue: **Dumbbell shape** with a narrow stalk within the maxillary infundibulum or accessory ostium connecting the two globular ends in the nose and maxillary antrum
- Solitary polypoid mass fills the maxillary antrum, spills through an enlarged maxillary ostium and infundibulum into an enlarged middle meatus and nasal cavity
- Large ACP has bulbous projection posteriorly into the posterior nasal cavity and nasopharyngeal airway
- CT and MR appearances are characteristic of ACP

CT Findings

- CECT shows a dumbbell-shaped mass filling the maxillary antrum and ipsilateral nasal cavity
- Strikingly low mucoid-density polyp; same density is seen in maxillary antrum and in the nose
- Connection between antrum and nasal cavity may be through the maxillary infundibulum or the accessory ostium
  - The stalk or midportion of the dumbbell may be difficult to see on coronal sinus CT

MR Findings

- T2 images show ACP as high, almost water-intensity

Antrochoanal Polyp

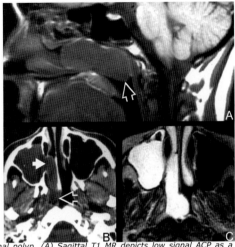

Antrochoanal polyp. (A) Sagittal T1 MR depicts low signal ACP as a nasal mass projecting posteriorly into nasopharynx (open arrow). (B) Axial CECT shows ACP passing through accessory ostium (arrow) into nose and nasopharynx (open arrow). (C) T2 MR shows high signal ACP.

- T1 C+ MR images show no evidence for enhancement of the mass
  - Polyp is low signal on T1 images

Imaging Recommendations
- Nasal mass is best imaged by CECT in axial and coronal plane
- If endoscopic examination clearly reveals ACP, unenhanced coronal sinus CT alone may be sufficient

Differential Diagnosis: Nasal Mass in Teenager

Nasal Glioma
- Anterior nasal septum or bridge of nose mass
- Maxillary sinus and nasal cavity uninvolved

Nasal Encephalocele
- Polypoid mass in nose
- Intracranial origin usually obvious on imaging
- Defect in cribriform plate

Juvenile Angiofibroma
- Males with enhancing mass centered in posterior choanae on the margin of sphenopalatine foramen
- Often herniates into pterygopalatine fossa
- May obstruct maxillary sinus but generally not in this sinus

Nasopharyngeal Carcinoma
- Invasive mass of the nasopharyngeal mucosal space
- Associated adenopathy common
- Maxillary sinus and nose usually spared

Pathology

General
- Embryology-Anatomy
  - Passage of the antral polyp into the nose can occur via two different routes

- Through the maxillary infundibulum
- Through the accessory ostium of the maxillary sinus
- Etiology-Pathogenesis
  - ○ Inflammatory polyp without significant allergic pathophysiology
  - ○ **Intramural cyst** (retention cyst) of the maxillary sinus first fills the maxillary antrum, then passes into nasal cavity
- Epidemiology
  - ○ 3-6% of all sinonasal polyps
  - ○ Antrochoanal >> Sphenochoanal > Ethmochoanal polyp

Gross Pathologic, Surgical Features
- Looks like any other nasal polyp except careful inspection reveals a stalk leading laterally through the maxillary sinus primary or accessory ostium

Microscopic Features
- Edematous hypertrophy of respiratory epithelium of the maxillary antrum rather than distention of the mucous glands of the sinus
- Reactive atypical stromal cells may be seen

Clinical Issues

Presentation
- Principal presenting symptoms: Unilateral nasal obstruction
  - ○ Other symptoms include nasal drainage, cheek pain, headaches and snoring with obstructive sleep apnea
  - ○ When large, protrude into nasopharyngeal airway and mimic nasopharyngeal tumors
- Age on onset: Teenagers and young adults
- Sex predilection: Male > Female
- Rhinoscopic examination: Polyp occludes nasal airway

Natural History
- Herniation of the ACP into the nasal cavity may take years to occur

Treatment
- Complete surgical removal is the treatment of choice
- Traditional Caldwell-Luc antrostomy has been replaced by endoscopic removal through the middle meatus

Prognosis
- If surgical removal of the nasal portion of the ACP is completed without removal of the antral base, recurrence can be expected
- Removal of both components creates a surgical cure

Selected References
1. Aktas D et al: Antrochoanal polyps: analysis of 16 cases. Rhinol 36:81-5, 1998
2. Woolley AL et al: Antrochoanal polyps in children. Am J Otolaryngol 17:368-73, 1996
3. Towbin R et al: Antrochoanal polyps. AJR 132:27-31, 1979

Paranasal Sinuses Mucocele

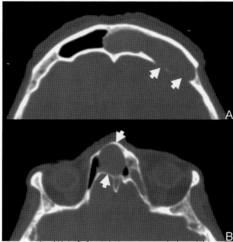

Frontal sinus mucocele. (A) Left frontal sinus mucocele has dehisced the posterior wall (arrows). (B) Axial CT inferior to (A) reveals the enlarged nasofrontal duct (arrows). An expansile mass in a sinus with remodeled bony walls is a mucocele until proven otherwise.

Key Facts
- Definition: Mucous-containing expansile sinus lesion, lined by respiratory epithelium, resulting from major ostial obstruction
- Derivations: From the Latin muco- = mucus + Greek -kele = tumor or "mucous tumor"
- Classic imaging appearance: Expansile, non-enhancing sinus mass
- Mucocele growth stays subclinical until the sinus wall is violated with normal adjacent structure impingement

Imaging Findings
General Features
- Best imaging clue: **Smooth-walled expansion** of a sinus
- **Frontal mucocele**: Expands anteriorly into the skin of the forehead or posteriorly into the anterior cranial fossa
- **Ethmoid mucocele**: Thins and remodels the lamina papyracea (lateral ethmoid air cell wall), bowing it into the orbit
- **Maxillary mucocele**: Expands into the ipsilateral nasal cavity, usually in the area of the secondary ostium of the maxillary sinus
- **Sphenoid sinus mucocele**: Expands anterolaterally into the posterior ethmoids and orbital apex

CT Findings
- Nonenhancing, low-density, expansile mass filling the sinus
- Bony sinus walls remodeled
  - May be thinned, focally absent or normal thickness

MR Findings
- High water content of mucous interior yields low T1, high T2 signal
- When protein content high, may have high T1 signal
- When areas of inspissated mucus exist, may be very low signal
- T1 C+ images sort mucocele from slow-growing tumor
  - Mucocele: No enhancement

Paranasal Sinuses Mucocele

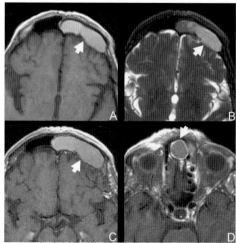

Frontal sinus mucocele. Axial T1 (A), T2 (B), T1 C+ (C) show frontal sinus mucocele with the black line representing the posterior bony wall gone laterally (arrow). High signal on T1 is secondary to high protein content. (D) T1 C+ inferiorly shows enhancing wall of enlarged nasofrontal duct (arrow).

    o   Sinus tumor: Partial or complete enhancement

<u>Plain Film Findings</u>
- "Clouding" of expanded sinus with loss of the normal **mucoperiosteal line** of the sinus wall
- Frontal and maxillary sinus mucocele can be suggested from plain film findings; ethmoid and sphenoid mucocele may be missed

<u>Imaging Recommendations</u>
- Small mucocele may require only unenhanced coronal sinus CT
- Larger mucocele with significant regional compression may benefit from enhanced MR with bone-only CT in the axial and coronal plane
- When MR suggests a low-signal mucocele with inspissated mucus, CT may be helpful in confirming this diagnosis

Differential Diagnosis: Expansile Sinus Mass
<u>Sinonasal Polyposis</u>
- Involves all sinuses; may have multiple small mucoceles associated

<u>Antrochoanal Polyp</u>
- Dumbbell cystic mass that fills the maxillary antrum, herniates through a sinus ostium into the adjacent nasal cavity

<u>Slow Growing Benign or Malignant Tumor</u>
- May mimic mucocele when seen on coronal sinus CT
- Tumors contrast enhance, mucoceles do not

Pathology
<u>General</u>
- General Path Comments
  - Frontal (65%), ethmoid (25%), maxillary (8%), sphenoid (2%)
- Etiology-Pathogenesis
  - Results from obstruction of the main ostium of the affected sinus

- Obstruction from inflammation, trauma, functional endoscopic sinus surgery or any space-occupying, sinonasal mass lesion
  o Secretion of mucus into obstructed sinus creates mucocele
  o Sinus expansion is from pressure necrosis with slow erosion of the inner surface of the bony sinus wall matched by new bone formation on the outer periosteal surface

Gross Pathologic, Surgical Features
- Mucocele lumen filled with mucous secretions

Microscopic Features
- Wall: Flattened, pseudostratified, ciliated columnar epithelium = mucous-secreting respiratory epithelium = normal wall of sinus

Clinical Issues

Presentation
- Principal presenting symptoms
  o Frontal mucocele: Forehead bossing, proptosis and mass in the superomedial orbit
  o Ethmoid mucocele: Proptosis, blurred vision and/or visual loss
  o Maxillary mucocele: Nasal obstruction from medial projection with cheek pressure
  o Sphenoid mucocele: Visual loss, oculomotor palsy, headache
  o If pain present, consider **mucopyocele**

Natural History
- Gradual, clinically silent enlargement over months to years until mucocele interacts with surrounding normal structures and becomes symptomatic

Treatment
- Uncomplicated maxillary or ethmoid mucocele can be surgically cured in most cases by endoscopic sinus surgery
- Deeper posterior ethmoid or sphenoid mucocele requires transfacial surgical approaches to avoid unwanted surgical complications
- Transcranial surgical approach is reserved for mucoceles with intracranial extension or causing compression of the bone structures with optic pathway neurological symptoms

Prognosis
- Surgical cure is the expected result when mucocele is present
- Cranial neuropathy (II, III-VI) may not recover following surgery if chronic at the time of presentation

Selected References
1. Iannetti G et al: Paranasal sinus mucocele: diagnosis and treatment. J Craniofac Surg 8:391-8, 1997
2. Van Tassel P et al: Mucoceles of the paranasal sinuses: MR imaging with CT correlation. AJNR 10:607-12, 1989
3. Hesselink JR et al: Evaluation of mucoceles of the paranasal sinuses with computed tomography. Radiology 133:397-400, 1979

Sinonasal Polyposis

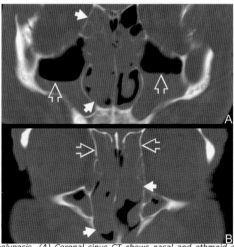

Sinonasal polyposis. (A) Coronal sinus CT shows nasal and ethmoid sinus polyps (arrows) with associated air-fluid levels (open arrows). (B) More anteriorly coronal CT reveals ethmoid sinus polyps (open arrows) and nasal polyps (arrows). Ethmoid trabeculae are deossified by polyp presence.

Key Facts
- Synonym: Polyposis nasi
  - Severe sinonasal polyposis (SNP) = Giant hypertrophic polypoid rhinosinusitis
- Definition: Non-neoplastic inflammatory swelling of the sinonasal mucosa that buckles to form "polyps"
- Classic imaging appearance: Diffuse sinonasal polypoid masses mixed with chronic inflammatory secretions of the sinuses
- SNP has been associated with allergy, asthma, aspirin sensitivity and cystic fibrosis

Imaging Findings
General Features
- Best imaging clue: **Pansinonasal polypoid masses**
- Polyps are usually multiple and bilateral but may be solitary
- Remodeling of the sinonasal bones common in severe cases
CT Findings
- Coronal sinus CT shows pansinonasal polypoid masses
- Other coronal sinus CT findings reported
  - Ethmoid sinus remodeling with trabecular loss and convexed lateral walls bulging into orbits
  - Maxillary infundibular enlargement
  - Air-fluid levels; may signal superinfection or merely trapped fluid
  - Truncation of bulbous bony inferior portion of middle turbinates
- More severe cases have enough aggressive bony distortion for the radiologist to consider a malignant process rather than SNP
- CECT: Polyps maintain "mucoid attenuation" (10-20 HU) with mucosal enhancement surrounding the polyps

Sinonasal Polyposis

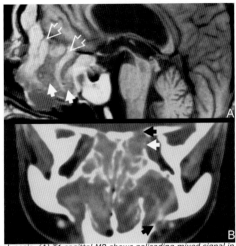

Sinonasal polyposis. (A) T1 sagittal MR shows palisading mixed signal in sinuses and nose. Low signal areas are polyps (arrows) while high signal areas are mucus (open arrows). (B) Areas of focal dehiscent sinus walls (arrows) suggest malignancy but CT shows palisading mixed density of SNP.

- o The characteristic CECT appearance of SNP as **layered high- and low-density tissue** within the nose and sinuses helps differentiate SNP from tumor

MR Findings
- Bizarre mixture of layered signals seen in sinuses and nose as result of polyps mixed with various ages of mucus
- Fresh mucus is close to fluid signal
- Old inspissated mucus can appear low signal on T1 and T2

Imaging Recommendations
- Coronal sinus CT is adequate for most cases
- If concern for tumor is generated, CECT may help diagnose SNP
- If orbital or intracranial extension is suspected based on dehiscent bone on CT, enhanced MR imaging is done to assess extrasinus extent

Differential Diagnosis: Multiple Sinonasal Masses

Retention Cysts
- Within sinuses with relative sparing of nasal cavity
- Fluid density/signal on CT/MR; no enhancement

Allergic Fungal Sinusitis
- Atopic patient with multiple unilateral or pansinus involvement
- CT shows high-density material within expanded sinuses
- MR may show low signal on both T1 and T2 images
- May mimic SNP

Wegener's Granulomatosis
- Bony destruction is mostly nasal walls; septal perforation
- Chronic inflammatory changes of paranasal sinuses

Pathology

General
- Etiology-Pathogenesis

137

Sinonasal Polyposis

- o   Formal pathogenesis of SNP has not been clarified
- o   Multiple factors linked to SNP etiology including allergies, aspirin intolerance, cystic fibrosis and chronic infections
- o   Non-neoplastic hyperplasia of inflamed mucous membranes
- • Epidemiology
  - o   5% of population affected by some form of chronic sinusitis
  - o   1% of population has some degree of SNP
  - o   20% of cystic fibrosis patients have SNP
  - o   30% of intrinsic bronchial asthma patients have SNP
  - o   50% of aspirin intolerant patients have SNP

Gross Pathologic, Surgical Features
- • Pinkish, fleshy, polypoid masses with glistening mucoid surface

Microscopic Features
- • Intact surface respiratory epithelium
- • Underlying stroma is edematous with inflammatory cellular infiltrate and variable vascularity
- • Seromucinous glands usually absent

Clinical Issues

Presentation
- • Principal presenting symptoms: Progressive nasal stuffiness
- • Other symptoms: Rhinorrhea, facial pain, headaches and anosmia
- • Typical patient profile
  - o   Allergic patient with progressive nasal stuffiness
  - o   30% of bronchial asthmatic patients have SNP
  - o   50% of aspirin triad patients have SNP (triad = intolerance to aspirin, nasal polyps and bronchial asthma)

Natural History
- • Often a waxing and waning, chronic, relentless disease
- • Left unattended, may become highly deforming, eventually disrupting the central facial region

Treatment
- • Nasal steroids
- • Antibiotics when superinfected
- • Endoscopic removal for symptomatic relief
  - o   Usually only temporary relief

Prognosis
- • Although not life threatening, chronic SNP unresponsive to therapy can be a chronic, debilitating disease

Selected References
1. Liang EY et al: Another CT sign of sinonasal polyposis: truncation of the bony middle turbinate. Eur Radiol 6:553-6, 1996
2. Hosemann W et al: Epidemiology, pathophysiology of nasal polyposis and spectrum of endonasal sinus surgery. Am J Otolaryngol 15:85-98, 1994
3. Drutman J et al: Sinonasal polyposis: investigation by direct coronal CT. Neuroradiology 36:469-72, 1994

Wegener's Granulomatosis

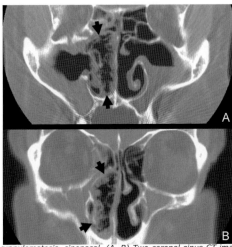

Wegener's granulomatosis, sinonasal. (A, B) Two coronal sinus CT images through the level of the ostiomeatal unit show mucosal crusting (arrows) in the right nasal cavity, a finding consistent with the diagnosis of mild nasal Wegener's granulomatosis. Chronic inflammatory sinus changes also support this diagnosis.

Key Facts
- Synonym: Midline non-healing granuloma
- Definition: Idiopathic, aseptic, necrotizing disease that preferentially involves the upper and lower respiratory tracts and kidneys
- Classic imaging appearance: Soft-tissue mass in nose with septal and non-septal bone destruction
- Other important facts
  - **Classic clinical triad**
    - Necrotizing granulomas of upper and lower respiratory tracts
    - Necrotizing vasculitis of both arteries and veins
    - Glomerulonephritis
  - Elevated antineotrophil cytoplasmic antibodies (ANCA) combined with biopsy showing **noncaseating,** multinucleated, giant cell granulomas makes diagnosis

Imaging Findings
General Features
- Best imaging clue: Septal and non-septal bone destruction
- Soft-tissue mass associated with bone destruction
- Sites of occurrence in sinonasal region
  - Nasal cavity > maxillary > ethmoid > frontal > sphenoid
- Paranasal sinus inflammatory changes
- Orbital soft-tissue from invasion or in absence of nasal disease
  - Orbital Wegener's = late finding
CT Findings
- Nasal septum perforation
- Lateral nasal wall destruction
  - Turbinates, uncinate bone & medial wall maxillary sinus
MR Findings
- Sinonasal findings

Wegener's Granulomatosis

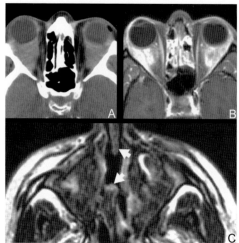

Wegener's granulomatosis. (A) Axial CECT reveals bilateral intraconal, conal and extraconal granulomatous masses. (B) Axial T1 C+ MR, masses seen in (A) are enhancing. (C) Axial T2 MR shows granulomatous material in maxillary sinuses is inhomogeneous low signal. Arrows: Perforated septum.

- T1 and T2 images show mass to be **low signal**
- T1 C+ MR reveals homogenous enhancement
- Intracranial findings
  - Meningeal thickening with enhancement < 5% (late finding)
  - Stroke

Imaging Recommendations
- Bone-only coronal sinus CT is best tool for initial evaluation
- If orbital, deep facial, skull base or meningeal involvement suspected from CT or clinical symptoms, enhanced MR used

Differential Diagnosis: Destructive Midline Nasal Lesions
Cocaine Nose
- History of cocaine abuse
- Septal perforation with nasal inflammatory changes

Invasive Fungal Sinusitis
- Immunocompromised patient
- Rapidly progressive sinonasal destructive process

Non-Hodgkin T-cell Lymphoma
- Midline soft-tissue mass with septal and non-septal bone dehiscence or frank destruction
- May exactly mimic Wegener's on imaging
- Lacks tracheobronchial or renal lesions seen in Wegener's

Pathology
General
- Etiology-Pathogenesis
  - Etiology is not known
- Epidemiology
  - Rare disease
  - Head and neck sites

Wegener's Granulomatosis

- Nose most common, followed by sinuses
- Orbit > larynx/ trachea > T-bone
- Oral cavity, nasopharynx and salivary glands least common
  o Systemic involvement: Lung, kidney & skin

Gross Pathologic, Surgical Features
- Initial appearance: Diffuse mucosal ulcerations with crusting
- Advanced disease: Septal perforation leads eventually to "saddle nose" deformity from underlying bony collapse

Microscopic Features
- **Noncaseating**, multinucleated, giant cell granulomas
- Vasculitis with ischemic necrosis

Clinical Issues

Presentation
- Principal presenting symptom: Nasal obstruction and epistaxis
- Other sinonasal symptoms: Pain, anosmia & purulent rhinorrhea
- Other head and neck symptoms: Hoarseness (larynx); stridor (trachea); hearing loss and ear pain (T-bone)
- 3 year lag in diagnosis common because thought to be sinusitis
- Age at presentation: 40-60
- Laboratory findings
  o Elevated ANCA; titers followed for disease response to therapy
  o Elevated erythrocyte sedimentation rate = ESR
  o Elevated serum creatinine signals presence of renal Wegener's

Natural History
- Generally an indolent disease
- May transition to fulminating fatal disease

Treatment
- Steroids or cyclophosphamide for limited disease
- Fulminant disease treated with high-dose prednisone followed by cyclophosphamide when acute process subsides

Prognosis
- "Limited disease" associated with good to excellent prognosis
- Spontaneous remissions have been reported
- More aggressive disease can be fatal secondary to renal failure or sepsis

Selected References
1. Borges A et al: Midline destructive lesions of the sinonasal tract: simplified terminology base on histopathologic criteria. AJNR 21:331-6, 2000
2. Drake-Lee AB et al: A review of the role of radiology in non-healing granulomas of nose and nasal sinuses. Rhinology 27:231-6, 1989
3. Paling MR et al: Paranasal sinus obliteration in Wegener granulomatosis. Radiology 144:539-43, 1982

Ossifying Fibroma

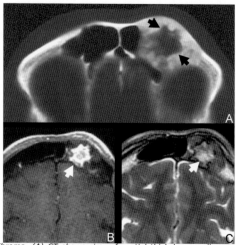

Ossifying fibroma. (A) CT shows circumferential thick bony wall surrounding low-density center (arrows). (B) Axial T1 C+ MR shows enhancing center (arrow) of lesion. (C) T2 axial MR reveals low-signal wall encircling the high-signal center (arrow) of the ossifying fibroma.

Key Facts

- Synonyms: Osteofibroma; fibrous osteoma
- Subtypes described: Juvenile, aggressive, active, psammomatoid and cementifying ossifying fibroma
  - Terms do not have radiologic application
  - Using generic term **ossifying fibroma (OsFi)** recommended
- Definition: Benign fibro-osseous tumor composed of **encapsulated** mixture of fibrous tissue and mature bone
- Classic imaging appearance: Well-demarcated, expansile mass with a **thick bony rim** and unilocular or multilocular low density (CT) or intensity (MR) center located in ethmoid or sphenoid sinuses

Imaging Findings

General Features
- Best imaging clue: Mature bone **surrounds** fibrous center
- Radiologic appearance depends on age of OsFi
  - As tumor grows, **fills in from periphery** with mature bone
- Early stage: OsFi primarily fibrous
- Late stage: OsFi fills in with mature bone
- Characteristically monostotic

CT Findings
- Well-circumscribed lesion of the paranasal sinuses
- Thick bony wall surrounds low attenuation fibrous center

MR Findings
- T1 signal low throughout tumor
- T2 signal mixed low and high
- T1 C+ shows inhomogeneous enhancement of tumor matrix

Imaging Recommendations
- Fibro-osseous lesions of the craniofacial area best studied with enhanced MR followed by bone-only unenhanced CT

Ossifying Fibroma

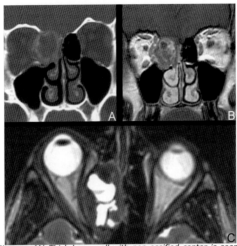

Ossifying fibroma. (A) Thick bony wall with non-ossified center is seen on coronal sinus CT. (B) Coronal T1 C+ shows inhomogeneous enhancement of lesion center. (C) Ossifying fibroma viewed on axial T2 MR reveals low signal in the wall and multiple high-signal foci in the lesion center.

- Since OsFi is treated with surgery, a complete presurgical roadmap of soft tissues at risk as well as bones involved is critical

Differential Diagnosis: Sinonasal Fibro-osseous Lesions

Fibrous Dysplasia
- Poorly-defined expansile lesion of the maxilla
- Mixed pattern of less active ground glass and more active cystic areas
- May be monostotic (70%) or polyostotic (30%)

Osteoma
- Mass of lamellar bone
- Frontal sinus common location

Osteosarcoma
- Destructive lesion of the craniofacial bones
- Often long term sequelae of XRT to the area
- Tumor "new bone" in mass matrix

Pathology

General
- General Path Comments
  - Mandible >> ethmoid or sphenoid > maxillary sinus
  - OsFi may be histologically indistinguishable from the active form of fibrous dysplasia
    - Correct diagnosis may only be achieved when clinical-imaging-pathology cross-correlation is completed
- Epidemiology
  - 75% OsFi found in mandible

Gross Pathologic, Surgical Features
- Gritty, gray to white, hard lesion

Ossifying Fibroma

Microscopic Features
- Encapsulated tumor with matrix of lamellar bone spicules and fibrous stroma mixture
- Central OsFi contains immature (woven) bone while periphery has mature (lamellar) bone

Clinical Issues
Presentation
- Principal presenting symptoms: Exophthalmia
- Other symptoms: Asymptomatic incidental finding
- Large lesions: Visual acuity loss, nasal obstruction
- Mandibular location: Hard jaw mass
- Female to male ratio is 5:1
- First appears in young adult; 20-40 year olds

Natural History
- Slow growing but locally aggressive

Treatment
- Complete surgical excision as lesion permits
- Marked tendency to recur even from ossific wall

Prognosis
- Excellent after complete resection
- When OsFi involves critical anatomical areas, complete surgical removal may be obviated

Selected References
1. Commins DJ et al: Fibrous dysplasia and ossifying fibroma of the paranasal sinuses. J Laryngol Otol 112:964-8, 1998
2. Han MH et al: Sinonasal psammomatoid ossifying fibroma: CT and MR manifestations. AJNR 12:25-30, 1991
3. Morris MR et al: Aggressive paranasal sinus ossifying fibroma. Ear Nose Throat J 68:260-4, 1989

Juvenile Angiofibroma

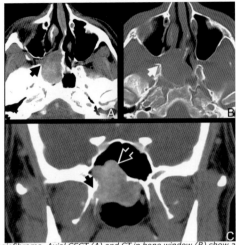

Juvenile angiofibroma. Axial CECT (A) and CT in bone window (B) show an enhancing mass in posterior nose. Lesion does not traverse sphenopalatine foramen (arrows). (C) Coronal CECT through posterior nose reveals tumor entering sphenoid sinus (open arrow). Pterygoid plate invasion: arrow.

Key Facts
- Synonyms: Juvenile nasopharyngeal angiofibroma (JNA); fibromatous or angiofibromatous hamartoma
  - JNA commonly used term but tumor begins in nose, (not in nasopharynx) and spreads secondarily into nasopharyngeal airway
  - JAF of the nasal cavity is a more correct terminology
- Definition: Vascular, non-encapsulated benign nasal cavity mass that is found exclusively in **adolescent males**
- Classic imaging appearance: Heterogeneous, intensely enhancing nasal cavity, nasopharyngeal, maxillary and ethmoid sinus mass extending into pterygopalatine fossa, masticator space and orbit

Imaging Findings
General Features
- Best imaging clue: Posterior nasal mass in a young male
- Benign, vascular, locally aggressive nasal cavity mass
- Centered in posterior wall of nasal cavity, **at margin of sphenopalatine foramen**
- Penetrates the pterygopalatine fossa (PPF) early
- Early involvement of upper medial pterygoid lamina
CT Findings
- Bone remodeling ± destruction
- Ipsilateral nasal cavity and PPF enlarged
- Posterior wall maxillary sinus bowed anteriorly
- If large, penetration of vidian canal ± foramen rotundum conveys tumor into pterygoid plate and medial middle cranial fossa respectively
MR Findings
- Heterogeneous on both T1 and T2 MR images
- Multiple flow voids on T1 C- MR
- T1 C+ MR shows intense enhancement

Juvenile Angiofibroma

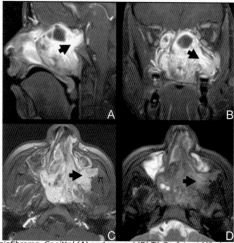

Juvenile angiofibroma. Sagittal (A) and coronal (B) T1 C+ fat sat MR shows enhancing nasal mass spreading into sphenoid sinus (arrow, A) and maxillary sinus (arrow, B). Axial T1 C+ fat sat (C) and T2 (D) reveals lateral spread of tumor into pterygopalatine fossa (arrows).

- Coronal T1 C+ MR images necessary to show cavernous sinus, sphenoid sinus, or skull base extension

Plain Film Findings
- Lateral plain film of face shows anterior displacement of posterior wall of maxillary antrum associated with nasal opacification

Catheter Angiography
- Intense capillary blush is fed by enlarged feeding vessels from ECA
- **Internal maxillary**, ascending pharyngeal arteries from ECA are most common feeding vessels
  - Supply may be from contralateral ECA branches as well
- If skull base/cavernous sinus extension, ICA supply is common

Imaging Recommendations
- Ideal workup to stage and characterize JAF includes
  - Maxillofacial MR with T1 C+ in axial and coronal planes
  - Bone-only non-contrasted CT in axial and coronal planes
  - Catheter angiography of both ECA and ICA
    - Helps plan surgery
    - Embolization of JAF decreases intra-operative blood loss

Differential Diagnosis: Mass in Nasal Cavity of Young Male
Nasal Polyp
- Does not have aggressive bone destruction
- Enhances only peripherally

Antrochoanal Polyp
- Maxillary antrum is full; PPF not involved
- Lesion herniates into anterior nasal cavity, then nasopharynx
- Peripheral enhancement only

Rhabdomyosarcoma
- Homogeneous mass with bone destruction
- Not centered in posterolateral nasal cavity

Juvenile Angiofibroma

- Does not usually penetrate the sphenopalatine foramen into PPF

Pathology
General
- General Path Comments
  - Angiomatous tissue in a fibrous stroma
- Etiology-Pathogenesis
  - Source of fibrovascular tissue of JAF is not known
  - Best current hypothesis: Primitive mesenchyme of sphenopalatine foramen is the source of JAF
- Epidemiology
  - 5-20% extend to skull base, and may have skull base erosion

Gross Pathologic, Surgical Features
- Reddish-purple, compressible, mucosa-covered, nodular mass
- Cut surface has a "spongy appearance"

Microscopic Features
- Vascular and fibrous tissue
  - **Myofibroblast** is cell of origin
  - Fibrovascular stroma, with fine neovascularity
  - May be purely fibrous, with reduced vascularity
- Estrogen, testosterone or progesterone receptors may be present

Clinical Issues
Presentation
- Principal presenting symptom: Unilateral nasal obstruction
- Other symptoms
  - Epistaxis
  - Pain or swelling in the cheek
- Adolescent male with average age at onset = 15 years
- 10-25 yrs reported age range

Natural History
- May rarely spontaneously regress

Treatment
- Complete surgical resection using pre-operative embolization to decrease blood loss
- Radiation therapy
  - Adjuvant to surgery
  - Recommended for intracranial extension, incomplete resection or local recurrence
- Hormonal therapy
  - Not routine, as complete tumor regression does not occur
  - Feminization side-effects undesirable in adolescent male

Prognosis
- Local recurrence rate with surgery 6-24%
- Local recurrence higher with large lesions, intracranial spread

Selected References
1. Gullane PJ et al: Juvenile angiofibroma: A review of the literature and a case series report. Laryngoscope 102:928-33, 1992
2. Harrison DF: The natural history, pathogenesis, and treatment of juvenile angiofibroma. Arch Otolaryngol Head Neck Surg 113:936-42, 1987
3. Lloyd GA et al: Juvenile angiofibroma: Imaging by magnetic resonance, CT and conventional techniques. Clin Otolaryngol 11:247-59, 1986

Inverted Papilloma

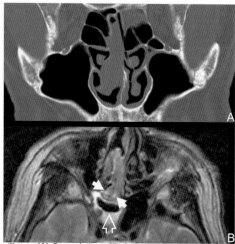

Inverted papilloma. (A) Coronal sinus CT shows a polypoid mass in the right nasal cavity. (B) Axial T2 MR image reveals the inverted papilloma has plugged the sphenoid foramen (arrows), obstructing the right sphenoid sinus. Open arrow: air-fluid level.

Key Facts
- Definition: Epithelial tumor of the nasal mucosa with characteristic histology showing epithelium proliferating into the underlying stroma
- Classic imaging appearance: Focal mass centered in middle meatus causes local bone remodeling and an ostiomeatal unit obstructive pattern of sinus opacification
- Inverted papilloma (IPap) morphology described as **convoluted cerebriform pattern**

Imaging Findings
General Features
- Best imaging clue: Enhancing mass centered in middle meatus with ostiomeatal unit obstructive pattern associated
- Small IPap: Polypoid mass centered in the middle meatal region of the lateral wall of the nose with infundibular obstruction
- Large IPap: Large nasal mass that has completely remodeled the nasal cavity, invaded or obstructed the ipsilateral sinuses
- Unilateral obstruction yields an **ostiomeatal unit pattern** (frontal, anterior ethmoid and maxillary sinuses opacified)
CT Findings
- Coronal sinus CT: Reveals sinus opacification secondary to middle meatal obstruction
  - Small IPap shows no bone changes, making identification of the tumor difficult in the early stages of the disease
  - Larger IPap shows bone remodeling and mass effect in the middle meatal region suggesting the presence of the tumor
- CECT: Shows a characteristic **lobulated tumor surface**
- 10% show tumorous calcification while 40% show "entrapped bone"

Inverted Papilloma

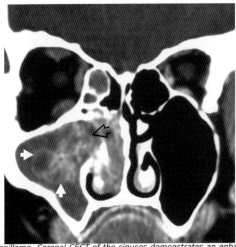

Inverted papilloma. Coronal CECT of the sinuses demonstrates an enhancing mass filling the nasal cavity and entering the maxillary sinus (open arrow) through an enlarged accessory ostium. The "cerebriform" mixed enhancement (arrows) within the maxillary sinus lumen is characteristic.

MR Findings
- T1 C+ MR shows an enhancing mass in the middle meatus with extension into the maxillary ± ethmoid sinus
- Obstructed, mucous-containing sinuses do not enhance and are high signal on T2 images
- "Convoluted cerebriform pattern" is distinctive in the maxillary sinus component primarily

Imaging Recommendations
- Commonly presenting as "sinusitis" with coronal sinus CT ordered
- When a mass is found on CT, do T2 and enhanced MR for pre-operative tumor mapping
- High recurrence rate and propensity for metachronous **associated SCCa** makes radiologic follow-up imperative

Differential Diagnosis: Nasal Mass

Antrochoanal Polyp
- Dumbbell lesion involving maxillary antrum and ipsilateral nose
- Cystic, non-enhancing mass

Sinonasal Polyposis
- Pansinus polyposis
- Bone remodeling

Juvenile Angiofibroma
- Young males
- Mass centered on margin of sphenopalatine foramen in posterolateral nasal cavity

SCCa and Other Nasal Malignancy
- Destroys rather than remodels bones in most cases

Inverted Papilloma

Pathology
General
- General Path Comments
  - Two papilloma types arise from the nasal mucosa, **inverted** and **fungiform**
    - Fungiform papilloma occurs on the nasal septum in young males and is rarely imaged prior to surgical treatment
    - IPap is a benign nasal tumor of older males occurring on the **lateral nasal wall**
- Embryology-Anatomy
  - Usually begins in lateral wall of nose, especially in the mucosa of the middle meatus
- Etiology-Pathogenesis
  - Viral origin postulated
- Epidemiology
  - 1-4% of all tumors of the nasal cavity
  - 10-27% either degenerate into or coexist with SCCa either as a synchronous or metachronous event

Gross Pathologic, Surgical Features
- Bulky, opaque, polypoid mass with red-gray color

Microscopic Features
- Tumor epithelium **inverts** into the underlying stroma of the lateral nasal wall giving it an **endophytic growth pattern**
- Surrounding nasal mucosa often shows squamous metaplasia suggesting incipient IPap

Clinical Issues
Presentation
- Principal presenting symptom: Sinusitis
- Less common symptoms: Nasal discharge, epistaxis, nasal obstruction
- Males (4:1) older than 50; can occur in children and adolescents
- Nasal endoscopy underestimates the extent of mass

Natural History
- High local recurrence rate

Treatment
- Lateral rhinotomy with medial maxillectomy

Prognosis
- High recurrence rates in the 20% range require repeat surgery
- When SCCa is associated, prognosis changes to survival rates associated with nasal SCCa

Selected References
1. Ojiri H et al: Potentially distinctive features of sinonasal inverted papilloma on MR imaging. AJR 175:465-8, 2000
2. Dammann F et al: Inverted papilloma of the nasal cavity and the paranasal sinuses: using CT for primary diagnosis and follow-up. AJR 172:543-8, 1999
3. Yousem DM et al: Inverted papilloma: evaluation with MR imaging. Radiology 185:501-5, 1992

Paranasal Sinus Osteoma

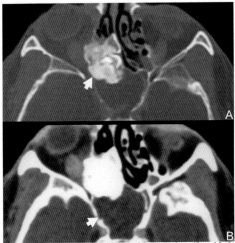

Ethmoid osteoma. (A) Axial bone CT shows the posterior ethmoid sinus osteoma (arrow) obstructing the sphenoethmoidal recess, causing complete opacification of right sphenoid sinus. (B) With soft tissue window the CT image shows the sphenoid sinus is mucus-filled (arrow).

Key Facts
- Definition: Benign, slowly-growing tumor that is bone-forming
- Classic imaging appearance: CT shows osteoma as a well-marginated bone-density lesion arising in the wall of the paranasal sinus that protrudes into the sinus lumen
- Other key facts
  - Usually asymptomatic observation on CT
  - Some experts believe that osteoma is actually the end-stage of a fibro-osseous lesion, not a true benign neoplasm

Imaging Findings
General Features
- Best imaging clue: Bone-based high-density foci on CT
- Traditionally named for the sinus lumen invaded by the osteoma, not the sinus they originate in
CT Findings
- Usually **sessile**, projecting off wall of frontal or ethmoid sinus
- Homogeneous dense bony texture
- Larger osteoma is associated with following findings
  - Sinus opacification from ostial obstruction
  - Mucocele
  - Pneumocephalus
  - Brain abscess
MR Findings
- Low signal on all sequences; often not seen
Plain Film Findings
- Well-defined bony density within a sinus lumen with or without associated inflammatory opacification of remaining sinus

Paranasal Sinus Osteoma

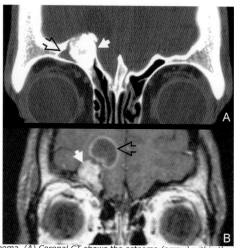

Frontal osteoma. (A) Coronal CT shows the osteoma (arrow) within the frontal sinus lumen. Lateral opacification is obstructed secretions (open arrow). (B) T1 C+ MR at same level as A. reveals enhancing osteoma marrow space (arrows) and a pedunculated intracranial mucocele (open arrow).

Imaging Recommendations
- Coronal bone-only sinus CT easily diagnoses osteoma
- When larger osteoma involves a dural surface, MR may be warranted before surgery to assess adjacent intracranial structures

Differential Diagnosis: High Density Lesions of the Sinus
Bony Exostosis
- Localized overgrowth of bone
- "Bubble on bone" with cortical covering and extension of parent bone medullary cavity into lesion

Fibrous Dysplasia
- Expansile lesion of bone most typically with ground-glass matrix

Ossifying Fibroma
- Thick, mature bony wall transitioning to immature woven bone centrally
- Most of center of lesion is low density on CT (fibro-osseous)

Osteosarcoma
- Bone-forming invasive malignant tumor of bone
- Periosteal elevation, permeative margins present

Pathology
General
- General Path Comments
  - Growth rate of average osteoma = 1.6 mm per year
- Etiology-Pathogenesis
  - Osteoma development has been linked to trauma and infection
  - Have been called "hamartomas of bone"
  - Also called fibro-osteodysplastic lesions
- Epidemiology
  - Very common lesion in general population (= 3% incidence)
  - Almost all osteomas in craniofacial skeleton

Paranasal Sinus Osteoma

- o **80%** of osteomas are in **frontal sinus**
- o **20%** of osteomas are in **ethmoid sinus**
- o Other areas of reported involvement: T-bone (especially the bony external auditory canal), skull, maxilla, and mandible

<u>Gross Pathologic, Surgical Features</u>
- Rock-hard mass protruding into sinus lumen

<u>Microscopic Features</u>
- 4 histological types described
  - o Ivory (eburnated): Hard, dense, mature bone with total absence of Haversian canals
  - o Compact: Compact lamellar bone with small Haversian canals
  - o Spongiose: Periphery of compact bone with radial septa and intervening marrow spaces
  - o Mixed: Bone and fibrous tissue

Clinical Issues

<u>Presentation</u>
- Principal presenting symptom: Asymptomatic
  - o < 5% of all osteomas are symptomatic
- Other symptoms
  - o Related to obstruction of sinus ostium
  - o Headache, facial pain, sinusitis
  - o Rarely, meningitis from intracranial extension
- Age of presentation: Broad; reported in all ages > 20 years old
  - o > 50% between 50-70 years
- If multiple osteomas are discovered, consider **Gardner's syndrome** = autosomal dominant trait
  - o **Multiple craniofacial osteomas**
  - o Intestinal colorectal polyposis may progress to adenocarcinoma
  - o Lesions of the soft tissues: Fibromatosis, cutaneous epidermoid cysts, lipomas, and leiomyomas

<u>Natural History</u>
- Slow-growing benign tumor that remains asymptomatic until large
- Degeneration into osteosarcoma has not been reported

<u>Treatment</u>
- If asymptomatic, can treat with watchful waiting
- Complete surgical removal for cure if:
  - o Unrelenting symptoms
  - o Located near frontal sinus ostium
  - o Greater than 50% of volume of frontal sinus filled by osteoma
  - o Extends intra-orbitally or intracranially
  - o CT evidence of significant enlargement
- Endoscopic resection possible when small and frontoethmoidal

<u>Prognosis</u>
- Excellent; often does not need treatment

Selected References
1. Namdar I et al: Management of osteomas of the paranasal sinuses. Am J Rhinol 12:393-8, 1998
2. Earwaker J: Paranasal sinus osteomas: a review of 46 cases. Skeletal Radiol 22:417-23, 1993
3. Savic DL et al: Indications for the surgical treatment of osteomas of the frontal and ethmoid sinuses. Clin Otolaryngol 15:397-404, 1990

Esthesioneuroblastoma

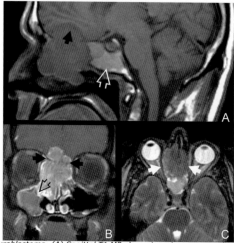

Esthesioneuroblastoma. (A) Sagittal T1 MR shows invasive mass eroding the floor of anterior cranial fossa (arrow). Open arrow: High protein mucus in sphenoid sinus. (B) Coronal T1 C+ shows cribriform plate destruction (arrows). Open arrow: Obstructed maxillary sinus. (C) T2 axial MR shows ethmoid tumor (arrows).

Key Facts
- Synonym: **Olfactory neuroblastoma**
- Definition: Uncommon neuroendocrine malignancy of neural crest origin that arises from the olfactory epithelium of the olfactory rim of the superior nasal cavity
- Classic imaging appearance: Dumbbell mass with upper portion in intracranial fossa and lower portion in nasal cavity; "waist" is at level of cribriform plate
- Imaging approach: Enhanced MR with bone-only CT best maps esthesioneuroblastoma (ENB) for en bloc craniofacial surgery

Imaging Findings
General Features
- Best imaging clue: **Dumbbell mass** in anterior cranial fossa and nose with "waist" at the cribriform plate
- Smaller ENB: Unilateral nasal mass centered on superior nasal wall
- Large ENB: Tumor in anterior cranial fossa, ipsilateral ethmoid and maxillary sinuses; orbital involvement is late

CT Findings
- CECT shows a homogeneously-enhancing mass
- Bone remodeling causing enlargement of the nasal cavity mixed with bone destruction, especially of the cribriform plate area
- Speckled pattern of calcification within the tumor matrix unusual

MR Findings
- Intermediate signal mass on most sequences
- T1 C+ MR shows homogeneous tumor enhancement
- **Peripheral tumor cysts** at the intracranial tumor margin is highly suggestive of the diagnosis of ENB

Imaging Recommendations
- Enhanced MR best imaging tool

Esthesioneuroblastoma

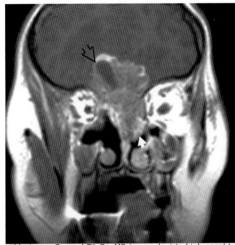

Esthesioneuroblastoma. Coronal T1 C+ MR image depicts high nasal tumor (arrow) invading the anterior cranial fossa with displacement of the frontal lobes of the brain. Along the cephalad margin of the tumor is a cystic component (open arrow), characteristic of esthesioneuroblastoma.

- o   T2 sequences best differentiate tumor from sinus secretions
- Plain bone-only CT shows precise extent of bone destruction and may alter extent of craniofacial resection
- Anterior cranial fossa, sinonasal area and the cervical neck should all be scanned when ENB is suspected
- Follow-up imaging: Long-term follow-up (5-10 years) necessary given the documented tendency of this tumor to recur late

Differential Diagnosis: Nasal Mass
Antrochoanal Polyp
- Dumbbell lesion involving maxillary antrum and ipsilateral nose
- Cystic, non-enhancing mass with benign, expansile bone changes
Inverting Papilloma
- Mass centered in middle meatus
- Benign, expansile bony changes
Squamous Cell Carcinoma & Other Nasal Malignancy
- If the malignancy begins high in nasal vault, may be indistinguishable from ENB

Pathology
General
- Embryology-Anatomy
  - o   **Olfactory mucosa** lines the roof of nasal cavity
- Etiology-Pathogenesis
  - o   Tumor of neural crest origin begins in olfactory mucosa
- Epidemiology
  - o   2% of all malignant nasal tumors
Gross Pathologic, Surgical Features
- Lobulated, soft, red-gray mass that frequently contains areas of necrosis and calcification

Esthesioneuroblastoma

Microscopic Features
- Nests of small cells separated by fibrovascular septa with **neurofibrillary intercellular matrix** and **rosette** formations
- When only sheets of small round cells are identified, an incorrect histopathologic diagnosis of anaplastic carcinoma, large cell lymphoma, melanoma or other nasal malignancy may occur
- Electron microscopy showing **neurosecretory granules** can help make the correct diagnosis when light microscopy is inconclusive

Staging Criteria: Kadish Classification
- **Group A**: Localized to the nasal cavity
- **Group B**: Localized to the nasal cavity and sinuses
- **Group C**: Extends beyond the nasal cavity and sinuses to skull base, anterior cranial fossa, orbit, neck nodes ± distant metastases
  - Most common group since late presentation is norm

Clinical Issues

Presentation
- Principal presenting symptom: Unilateral nasal mass
- Larger ENB: Nasal obstruction, repeated epistaxis, rhinorrhea, sinus pain and headache
- Age at presentation
  - Bimodal distribution clustered around 20 and 50
  - Age range 3-88 years
- Rhinoscopy: Nasal mass may be indistinguishable from polyposis, chronic sinusitis or other nasal malignancies

Treatment
- Combined therapy using radical craniofacial surgery (en bloc resection) with radiotherapy is treatment of choice
- Chemotherapy reserved for larger, high-grade ENB

Prognosis
- 8-year disease-free survival is approximately 80%
- 35% of patients have one or more episodes of metastatic disease
- Negative prognostic indicators
  - Female sex, age less than 20 or over 50 years at presentation, tumor grade, extensive intracranial spread, cervical or distant metastasis and tumor recurrence
  - Tumor grade is most significant
    - 5-year survival rate of 80% for low-grade tumors
    - 5-year survival 40% for high-grade tumors

Selected References
1. Som PM et al: Sinonasal esthesioneuroblastoma with intracranial extension: marginal tumor cysts as a diagnostic MR finding. AJNR 15:1259-62, 1994
2. Schuster JJ et al: MR of esthesioneuroblastoma (olfactory neuroblastoma) and appearance after craniofacial resection. AJNR 15:1169-77, 1994
3. Morita A et al: Esthesioneuroblastoma: prognosis and management. Neurosurg 32:706-15, 1993

Paranasal Sinus SCCa

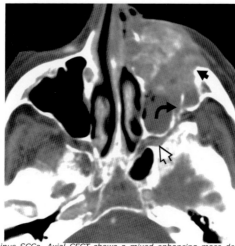

Maxillary sinus SCCa. Axial CECT shows a mixed enhancing mass destroying the anterior maxillary sinus wall (arrow). Perineural tumor follows the canal of the infraorbital nerve (curved arrow) into the pterygopalatine fossa (open arrow).

Key Facts
- Synonyms: Epidermoid carcinoma; transitional carcinoma
- Definition: Malignant epithelial tumor growing from sinus surface epithelium into sinus lumen
- Classic imaging appearance: Enhancing mass in the sinus lumen with invasion and destruction of sinus wall
- Other important facts
  - Most common malignancy of the sinonasal area
  - Maxillary >> nasal > ethmoid > frontal or sphenoid sinuses

Imaging Findings
General Features
- Best imaging clue: **Destroyed** sinus **bony wall**
- Unilateral sinonasal mass involving the nasal vault, maxillary antrum and ethmoid sinuses
- The radiologist creates pre-surgical tumor map of spread
  - Anterior: Subcutaneous tissues of the cheek
  - Posterior: Retroantral fat pad and pterygopalatine fossa (PPF)
  - Cephalad: PPF => inferior orbital fissure => orbit
  - Lateral: Malar eminence and subcutaneous tissues
  - Superior: Through the orbital floor into orbit proper
  - Inferior: Maxillary alveolar ridge, buccal space & hard palate
  - **Perineural spread**: Inferior orbital nerve or PPF => V2 (foramen rotundum) => cavernous sinus

CT Findings
- Solid, moderately-enhancing mass with aggressive bone destruction

MR Findings
- Intermediate signal mass on T1 and T2 sequences
- T2 differentiates high signal obstructed sinus secretions from tumor
- T1 C+ fat saturated images great for perineural tumor spread

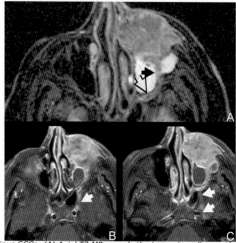

Maxillary sinus SCCa. (A) Axial T2 MR reveals the tumor traveling on the infraorbital nerve (arrow) into the pterygopalatine fossa (open arrow). (B-C) Two axial T1 C+ MR, (B) just above (C), shows deep perineural spread of SCCa along V2 through the foramen rotundum (arrows).

Imaging Recommendations
- Lead with enhanced MR from sellar floor to hyoid bone
- Follow with bone-only axial and coronal CT

Differential Diagnosis: Destructive Sinonasal Lesion
Invasive Fungal Sinusitis
- Rapidly progressive destructive lesion
- ICA invasion and thrombosis may be associated
- Immunocompromised patient
Wegener's Granulomatosis
- Septal and non-septal bone destruction in nose
- Chronic sinusitis associated
- Sinonasal disease associated with tracheobronchial and renal disease
T-Cell Non-Hodgkin Lymphoma (Midline Granuloma)
- Tendency to cause nasal bone dehiscence
- Midline nasal mass is typical
- May exactly mimic Wegener's granulomatosis
Minor Salivary Gland Malignancy
- Suggested when the T2 signal of the mass is high
- If not present, may exactly mimic SCCa

Pathology
General
- Etiology-Pathogenesis
  - No direct link to smoking
- Epidemiology
  - SCCa is 80% of malignant tumors of the sinonasal area
  - Maxillary (85%), ethmoid (10%), frontal/sphenoid (< 5%)
  - 15% with maxillary sinus SCCa have malignant adenopathy
    - Retropharyngeal or jugulodigastric lymph nodes

Gross Pathologic, Surgical Features
- Friable polypoid or fungating growth with a tan-to-white or red-to-pink color

Microscopic Features
- Two subtypes: Keratinizing (80%) and non-keratinizing (20%)

Primary Tumor (T) Staging Criteria
- T staging criteria based on a plane joining the medial canthus of the eye with the angle of the mandible (**Ohngren's line**)
  - Anteroinferior = maxillary **infrastructure**
  - Posterosuperior = maxillary **suprastructure**
- **T1**: Limited to antral mucosal without bone destruction
- **T2**: Confined to suprastructure mucosa without bone destruction, or infrastructure with inferior or medial bony wall destruction
- **T3**: Invades skin of cheek, posterior wall maxillary sinus, floor or medial wall orbit, masticator space, pterygoid plates or ethmoid sinus
- **T4**: Invades orbit or cribriform plate, posterior ethmoid or sphenoid sinuses, nasopharynx, soft palate or skull base

Clinical Issues

Presentation
- Principal presenting symptoms: **Chronic sinusitis** symptoms overshadows tumor presence
  - Tumor presents in advanced stage as a result
- Older males: 50-70 year old
- Larger maxillary tumors: Unilateral nasal obstruction, epistaxis, nasal discharge and cheek numbness
- Regional invasion: Tooth pain or loosening, proptosis and diplopia, trismus and headache

Treatment
- Combined treatment with en bloc surgery and XRT
- Relapse occurs at primary site > regional lymph nodes
- If tumor recurs, 90% < 1 year
- Prophylactic XRT of ipsilateral neck or neck dissection also done

Prognosis
- Overall 5 year survival rate = 75%
- Survival statistics heavily influenced by tumor stage
  - T1 SCCa treated aggressively have 100% survival
  - 5-year survival rates with T4 SCCa drop to 60%
- Better prognosis: Ethmoid sinus SCCa, low tumor stage, treatment with both surgery and XRT and history of inverted papilloma

Selected References
1. Nishino H et al: Combined therapy with conservative surgery, radiotherapy, and regional chemotherapy for maxillary sinus carcinoma. Cancer 89:1925-32, 2000
2. Hermans R et al: Squamous cell carcinoma of sinonasal cavities. Semin Ultrasound CT MRI 20:150-61, 1999
3. Som PM et al: Sinonasal tumors and inflammatory tissues: differentiation with MR imaging. Radiology 167:803-8, 1988

PHARYNGEAL
MUCOSAL SPACE

Nasopharyngeal Carcinoma

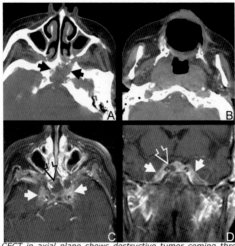

NPCa. (A) CECT in axial plane shows destructive tumor coming through roof of nasopharynx into floor of sella (arrows). (B) Inferior CECT reveals NPCa filling pharyngeal mucosal space of nasopharynx. Axial (C) and coronal (D) T1 C+ MR. Arrows: Cavernous sinus invasion: Open arrows: sellar invasion.

Key Facts
- Definition: SCCa arising from the nasopharyngeal (NP) mucosal space, with **3 histoclinical subtypes** including 1) keratinizing SCCa (WHO Type 1), 2) nonkeratinizing carcinoma (WHO Type 2) and 3) undifferentiated carcinoma (WHO Type 3)
- High risk patient profile = Southern Chinese and Eskimos
- Strong relationship to Epstein-Barr virus, diet and genetic factors

Imaging Findings
General Features
- Best imaging clue: Mass centered in the lateral pharyngeal recess of NP
- Early spread is submucosal causing infiltration of the palate
  - Levator veli palatini infiltration leads to eustachian tube dysfunction and serous otitis media
- Nasopharyngeal carcinoma (**NPCa**) spread patterns include
  - Anterior: Into nasal vault, then into pterygopalatine fossa
  - Lateral: Into parapharyngeal space (PPS)
  - Posterior: Through RPS into prevertebral musculature
  - Inferior: Into oropharyngeal soft palate and faucial tonsils
  - Superior: Into anterior clivus, sphenoid sinus, foramen lacerum-ICA (perivascular) and V3-foramen ovale (perineural)
- Nodal metastases present in 90% of cases at presentation
  - RPS nodes, deep cervical and spinal accessory chains
- Distant metastases are present at presentation < 10% time
  - Bone > lung > liver

CT Findings
- NP mucosal space mass pushes posterolaterally into the PPS
- CECT shows mild enhancement of mass with invasive margins

MR Findings
- T1 images show tumor is hypo- to isointense to muscle

Nasopharyngeal Carcinoma

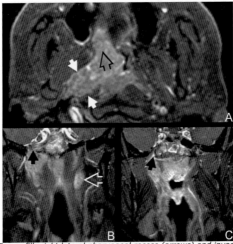

NPCa. (A) Tumor fills right lateral pharyngeal recess (arrows) and invades posterior nasal cavity (open arrow) on this T1 C+ fat sat MR image. (B-C) Two coronal T1 C+ fat sat MR images shows invasion into foramen lacerum (arrows) of skull base. Open arrow: malignant lateral retropharyngeal node.

- T2 images reveal moderate hyperintensity compared to muscle
- Fat saturated C+ T1 images demonstrate mild enhancement; fat saturation greatly assists in recognition of tumor margins

Nuclear Medicine Studies
- FDG-SPECT or FDG-PET may locate tumor when it is entirely submucosal (unknown primary search)

Imaging Recommendations
- Enhanced MR imaging best tool for evaluating intracranial extent via direct, perivascular and/or perineural routes
- Bone only CT in axial and coronal planes with slice thickness of 1-3 mm helps assess bone invasion
- MR imaging is recommended for 1) staging of known NPC, 2) SCCa in neck nodes without a mucosal primary seen and 3) unilateral middle ear fluid in an adult without a cause

Differential Diagnosis: NP Mucosal Space Mass
Lymphoid Hyperplasia of the Adenoids
- Patients under 20 years old (SCCa usually older)
- Symmetric enlargement of adenoidal tissue; internal enhancing **septa** seen on T1 C+

Non-Hodgkin Lymphoma, NP Adenoids
- Systemic illness may be present; submucosal mass evident
- Diffusely involves the adenoids with no enhancing septa on T1 C+

Minor Salivary Gland Malignancy, PMS of NP
- May be indistinguishable from head and neck SCCa
- Associated nodal metastases rare

Pathology
General
- Genetics

Nasopharyngeal Carcinoma

- o Marker for Chinese (undifferentiated) NPCa susceptibility is the human leukocyte antigen (HLA) locus, on the short arm on chromosome 6
- Etiology-Pathogenesis
  - o Etiology based on interaction between environmental factors (carcinogens), genetics and Epstein-Barr virus (EBV)
- Epidemiology
  - o Epidemic incidence in Southern Chinese: 40 per 100,000

Microscopic Features
- NPCa is defined as mostly squamous differentiation with intracellular bridges or keratinization (and/or keratin pearls)
- Histologic subtypes include keratinizing SCCa, non-keratinizing carcinoma and undifferentiated carcinoma
  - o Within the undifferentiated subtype, lymphoepitheliomas are the most common variety and show a favorable response to XRT
- Further classified as well, moderate and poorly differentiated by amount of differentiation identified

T Staging Criteria for NPCa
- **T1** = Tumor in one subsite or entirely submucosal
- **T2** = Tumor invades more than one subsite in NP
- **T3** = Tumor invades nasal cavity and/or oropharynx
- **T4** = Tumor involves skull base, cranial nerves, or both

N Staging Criteria
- **N1** = Single positive node, ≤ 3cm
- **N2** = Single or multiple node(s), >3 cm but not > 6cm
- **N3** = Ipsilateral nodes > 6cm, bilateral or contralateral nodes

Clinical Issues

Presentation
- Principal presenting symptom: Nodal neck mass
- Depends on tumor site and route of spread
- T4 tumors usually have multiple cranial neuropathy (9-12)
- Clinical Epidemiology
  - o Children–adolescents–middle aged, maximum 40-49 years
  - o Male:Female ratio is 2.5:1

Treatment & Prognosis
- External beam radiotherapy is mainstay treatment
  - o Imaging is vital for tumor mapping and recurrence assessment

Prognosis
- Superficial mucosal recurrences may be best detected with direct endoscopy
- Treatment complications: Temporal lobe necrosis, encephalopathy, cranial nerve palsies, hypothalamic-pituitary dysfunction

Selected References
1. Wenig BM: Nasopharyngeal carcinoma. Ann Diagn Pathol 3:374-85, 1999
2. Chong VFH et al: Carcinoma of the nasopharynx. Semin Ultrasound CT MR 19:449-62, 1998
3. Chong VFH et al: Detection of recurrent nasopharyngeal carcinoma: MR imaging versus CT. Radiology 202:463-470, 1997

Oropharyngeal SCCa

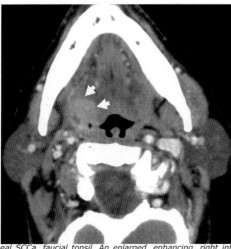

Oropharyngeal SCCa, faucial tonsil. An enlarged, enhancing, right inferior faucial tonsil (arrows) seen on this axial CECT is a Stage T2 (2-4 cm in maximum diameter) primary SCCa. Oropharynx SCCa stage is determined by size until mandibular or soft-tissue invasion is present (Stage T4).

Key Facts
- Definition: Epithelial tumors of epidermoid lineage arising in the oropharyngeal (OP) mucosal space
- Classic imaging appearance: Enhancing mass in the oropharyngeal mucosal space with invasive deep margins and malignant nodes
- Increased incidence in patients with tobacco or alcohol use/abuse

Imaging Findings
General Features
- Best imaging clue: Referring clinician localization of primary tumor mucosal extent for radiologist
- 60% have cervical lymphadenopathy at presentation; 15% bilateral
- OP SCCa spread patterns by primary tumor site
  - Soft palate: Greater palatine nerve to pterygopalatine fossa
  - Tonsillar pillars: Masticator space (MS), V3 intracranially
  - Posterior OP wall: Posterior into RPS directly or to RPS node
  - Lingual tonsil (tongue base): Posteriorly to tonsillar pillar, anteriorly into sublingual space or inferiorly into supraglottic larynx
CT Findings
- All SCCa lesions enhance moderately, invade locally
- Small lesions may demonstrate mild asymmetry only
- Larger lesions reveal heterogeneity due to central necrosis
MR Findings
- Low T1 and high T2 signal; T1 C+ reveals avid enhancement
Imaging Recommendations
- CECT or MR can be used to stage primary and nodal extent
- MR preferred in OP area because
  - Not as affected by dental amalgam artifact as CT
  - Multiplanar capabilities and improved tumor contrast
- Dental CT may be helpful in evaluating mandibular invasion

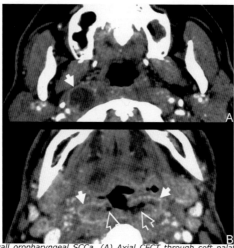

Posterior wall oropharyngeal SCCa. (A) Axial CECT through soft palate reveals a malignant retropharyngeal SCCa node (arrow). (B) CT image in mid-oropharynx shows posterior wall primary tumor outlined by an enhancing line (arrows) with areas of ulceration marked by air (open arrows).

- When imaging primary OP SCCa look for
  - ○ Possible perineural invasion
    - ▪ Palate => greater palatine nerve to pterygopalatine fossa
    - ▪ Retromolar trigone/faucial tonsil => MS => V3 to foramen ovale => Meckel's cave => preganglionic segment of V
  - ○ Possible multifocal disease
    - ▪ 15% second primary SCCa in neck and chest
  - ○ Nodal stage

Differential Diagnosis: Lingual or Faucial Tonsil Mass
Lingual or Faucial Tonsillar Hyperplasia
- No discrete mass seen within enlarged tonsil on CT or MR
- Deep invasion not present
Benign Mixed Tumor of Minor Salivary Gland
- Sharply-marginated mass: Pedunculated into airway when large
Non-Hodgkin Lymphoma in Lingual or Faucial Tonsil
- Submucosal mass enlarges tonsil ± deep invasion
- May have systemic illness ± large, non-necrotic neck nodes
Minor Salivary Gland Malignancy
- May be indistinguishable from OP SCCa
- Nodal metastases are rare

Pathology
General
- Etiology-Pathogenesis
  - ○ Smoke/alcohol cause metaplasia => neoplasia of OP mucosa
- Embryology-Anatomy
  - ○ OP defined as soft palate, faucial tonsil, lingual tonsil (tongue base) and pharyngeal wall between the hard palate above and the pharyngoepiglottic fold below

Oropharyngeal SCCa

- Epidemiology
  - 2% of all malignant tumors in United States

Gross Pathologic, Surgical Features
- Ill-defined, ulcerative, indurated mucosal lesion
- Tan or white in color; exophytic or infiltrative

Microscopic Features
- OP SCCa is defined as having squamous differentiation with intracellular bridges or keratinization (and/or keratin pearls)
- Further classified per amount of differentiation seen
  - Well, moderately, poorly differentiated

Primary Tumor (T) Staging Criteria
- T1 = Tumor $\leq$ 2 cm in greatest dimension
- T2 = Tumor 2-4 cm in greatest dimension
- T3 = Tumor > 4 cm in greatest dimension
- T4 = Tumor invades adjacent structures

Clinical Issues

Presentation
- Principal presenting symptom: Ulcerative mucosal lesion
- Men >> Women; > 40 years old
- Usually presents with painless, non-healing mucosal ulcer
- Larger lesions: Otalgia, induration and cervical lymphadenopathy
- Location specific symptoms
  - Masticator space invasion: Trismus, V3 numbness
  - Mandibular invasion: Inferior alveolar nerve => chin numbness
  - SLS invasion: Tongue dysfunction from 12th nerve injury

Natural History
- Metastatic disease: Lungs > skeletal > hepatic

Treatment
- Surgical resection with XRT is mainstay of treatment, often with ipsilateral selective or modified radical neck dissection
- Tumor volume considered more important than T-stage for therapy
  - Small volume tumors treated with XRT alone
  - Large volume tumors treated with combinations of XRT, chemotherapy and surgical resection
- Lingual tonsil SCCa most commonly treated with partial glossectomy (when tumor unilateral)
- Small SCCa lesions of the palate and tonsillar pillars
  - Treated with transoral wide local excision

Prognosis
- Nodes important indicator of survival (if present, 50% ↓ survival)

Selected References
1. Mukherji SK et al: Squamous cell carcinoma of the oropharynx and oral cavity: how imaging makes a difference. Semin Ultrasound CT MRI. 19:463-75, 1998
2. Sigal R et al: CT and MR imaging of squamous cell carcinoma of the tongue and floor of the mouth. RadioGraphics 16:787-810, 1996
3. Muraki AS et al: CT of the oropharynx, tongue base, and floor of the mouth: normal anatomy and range of variations, and applications in staging carcinoma. Radiology 148:725-31, 1983

Tornwaldt's Cyst

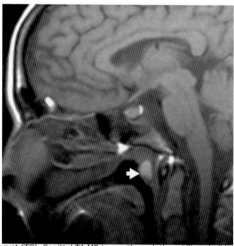

Tornwaldt's cyst (TC). Sagittal T1 MR image through the midline skull base shows an ovoid, high-signal mass (arrow) nestled in the submucosal posterior nasopharyngeal wall. The high signal is due to high protein concentration in the fluid of the cyst lumen.

Key Facts
- Synonyms: Nasopharyngeal bursa, pharyngeal bursa, Thornwaldt's cyst
- Definition: Benign developmental nasopharyngeal (NP) midline cyst covered by mucosa anteriorly and bounded by the longus muscles posteriorly
- Classic imaging appearance: High T1 and T2 signal lesion in midline of posterior nasopharyngeal mucosal space is characteristic
- Most common congenital lesion of the nasopharynx
- Incidental finding on 1-5% of brain MR; rarely becomes infected

Imaging Findings
General Features
- Best imaging clue: Midline NP cyst
- Cystic mass found in the midline on the posterior wall of the nasopharynx nestled between the prevertebral muscles
- Size: TC ranges from a few mm to 2-3 cm in diameter
CT Findings
- Density: Ranges from hypodense to muscle attenuation
- On CECT images may rim enhance but lesion itself remains relatively low attenuation
- Can be indistinguishable from normal lymphoid tissue when small on non-contrasted CT studies
MR Findings
- T1 MR lesion signal usually intermediate to high depending on protein concentration of luminal fluid
- T2 and IR sequences show lesion as homogeneously high signal
- On T1 C+ MR TC usually does not enhance
  - Slight enhancement of cyst wall on T1 C+ images may be seen
Imaging Recommendations
- Easily seen and diagnosed on T2 MR images

Tornwaldt's Cyst

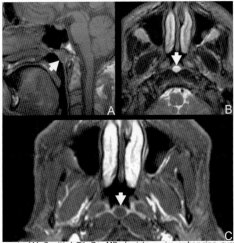

Tornwaldt's cyst. (A) Sagittal T1 C+ MR depicts a rim-enhancing cyst (arrow) in posterior wall of nasopharynx. (B) The high-signal cyst (arrow) is nestled in the notch between the longus muscles on axial T2 image. (C) The cyst rim-enhancement (arrow) is best seen on axial T1 C+ MR.

Differential Diagnosis: Cystic Masses of PMS of Nasopharynx

Cephalocele
- Sphenoid cephalocele may project inferiorly into nasopharynx but stalk connecting lesion from above is obvious on MR imaging

Rathke's Cleft Cyst
- When low, nestled in posterior sphenoid bone
- Does not reach PMS of nasopharynx

Adenoidal Retention Cyst
- Often multiple; T1 signal low
- Off midline or lateral pharyngeal recess location distinctive
- Pear-shaped morphology when in lateral location is characteristic

Adenoidal Hyperplasia
- Diffuse adenoidal hyperplasia that may be low density/intensity without central midline cyst
- Enhancing septa traverse the hyperplastic tissue

Suppurative Pharyngitis
- Multifocal areas of pus within adenoids, paramedian or lateral

Antrochoanal Polyp
- Cystic mass projects from maxillary antrum through nose into nasopharyngeal airway

Pathology

General
- Embryology
  - Tornwaldt's cyst = notochordal remnant
  - In the early embryo, the notochord contacts the endoderm of the primitive pharynx
  - If an adhesion occurs at point of contact, a small midline diverticulum lined by pharyngeal mucosa is formed as the notochord ascends into the clivus

Tornwaldt's Cyst

- Etiology-Pathogenesis
  - If pharyngitis closes the opening to the midline diverticulum, a Tornwaldt's cyst is formed
- Epidemiology
  - Most common lesion of the nasopharyngeal mucosal space

Gross Pathologic, Surgical Features
- Smooth, translucent cyst if uninfected; may be thick walled with adhesions to adjacent adenoidal tissue if infected

Microscopic Features
- Cyst lining: Respiratory epithelium, little or no lymphoid tissue is seen in the cyst wall
- Cyst fluid: Usually with high protein concentration

Clinical Issues

Presentation
- Incidence: 4% autopsy specimens, 1–5% MRI studies
- Principal presenting symptom: Asymptomatic
- > 99% both incidentally found and asymptomatic
- Age range: 39-78yo, peak 15-60
- More common in Caucasians
- **Tornwaldt's syndrome** (rare)
  - Chronically-infected cyst usually seen in large lesions (> 2 cm)
  - Periodic halitosis with unpleasant taste in the mouth
  - Intermittent nasopharyngeal drainage
  - Cervical musculoskeletal tenderness, especially with motion
  - Occipital headache

Natural History
- Most exist in harmony with patient
- Rarely they may release anaerobic bacteria into nasopharynx, leading to periodic halitosis and rarely forming a nasopharyngeal abscess
  - Other potential complications include
    - Eustachian tube dysfunction
    - Constant or periodic nasal speech
    - Chronic pharyngeal discomfort

Treatment
- Asymptomatic cysts require no treatment = benign neglect
- Chronically-infected, painful lesions treated with excision or marsupialization via a trans-oral route
- Rarely, palatal split required for large, symptomatic cysts

Prognosis
- The observation of a Tornwaldt's cyst on routine brain MR is of no clinical significance

Selected References
1. Ikushima I et al: MR imaging of Tornwaldt's cysts. AJR 172:1663-1665, 1999
2. Kwok P et al: Tornwaldt's cyst: clinical and radiological aspects. J Otolaryngol 16:104-107, 1987
3. Miller RH et al: Tornwaldt's bursa. Clin Otolaryngol 10:21-25, 1985

Tonsillar Abscess

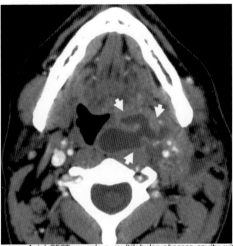

Tonsillar abscess. Axial CECT reveals a multilobular abscess cavity within the left enlarged faucial tonsil (arrows). The abscess has so enlarged the tonsil that the oropharyngeal airway has been seriously compromised.

Key Facts
- Synonym: Intratonsillar abscess
- Definitions
  - **Tonsillar abscess**: Faucial (palatine) tonsil suppurates, with abscess forming within the tonsil itself
  - **Peritonsillar abscess**: When tonsillar abscess spreads to the adjacent parapharyngeal (PPS) +/- submandibular (SMS) spaces
- Classic imaging appearance: Rim-enhancing fluid collection within the faucial tonsil of the oropharynx +/- PPS and SMS involvement

Imaging Findings
General Features
- A cystic oropharyngeal mucosal space mass is seen within an enlarged facial tonsil with effacement of medial wall of PPS
- Tonsillar abscess: Pus within an enlarged faucial tonsil
- Peritonsillar abscess: Extension of infection from tonsil to peritonsillar structures, including masticator space, PPS and SMS

CT Findings
- CECT shows swollen tonsil with intratonsillar fluid density mass with enhancing rim
- Surrounding tissues are poorly defined, swollen with enhancing cellulitis
- May see asymmetric obliteration of ipsilateral oral airway
- Reactive bilateral cervical adenopathy is common

Ultrasound Findings
- Hypoechoic foci within tonsil suggests abscess

Imaging Recommendations
- CECT best differentiates tonsillar abscess from cellulitis
- CECT also best delineates deeper peritonsillar inflammatory changes or abscess formation

Tonsillar Abscess

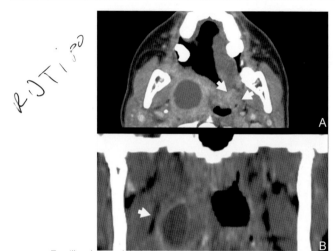

Tonsillar abscess. (A) Thick enhancing wall surrounds this right intratonsillar abscess on axial CECT through the oropharynx. Arrows mark reactive left faucial tonsil. (B) Coronal reconstructed CECT shows ovoid fluid density mass in right faucial tonsil. Arrow: Parapharyngeal space.

Differential Diagnosis: Tonsillar Mass

Tonsillar Retention Cyst
- Discrete area of focal faucial tonsillar fluid without surrounding soft tissue enhancement or edema

Lymphoid Hyperplasia of Tonsils
- No discrete mass is seen within the enlarged tonsil on CT or MR
- Tonsillar prominence is bilateral and symmetric
- Enhancing septa are visible on T1 C+ MR and CECT

Benign Mixed Tumor of Minor Salivary Gland
- Sharply-marginated mass; pedunculated when large

Tonsillar SCCa
- Faucial tonsil mucosal surface with obvious erosive lesion
- Poorly-circumscribed faucial tonsil mass +/- invasive margins
- Associated malignant adenopathy common in ipsilateral Level II

Non-Hodgkin Lymphoma in Faucial Tonsil
- Systemic illness may be present; submucosal mass evident
- Unilateral faucial tonsil mass +/- invasive margins
- No enhancing septa are seen on T1 C+ MR or CECT
- Associated large, non-necrotic nodes (50%)

Minor Salivary Gland Malignancy
- May be indistinguishable from faucial tonsillar SCCa
- Associated nodal malignancy rare

Pathology

General
- Embryology-Anatomy
  - The middle layer of deep cervical fascia surrounds the non-airway side of the pharyngeal mucosal space
  - When tonsillar infection occurs, this fascia tends to confine the early infection in the tonsillar fossa

Tonsillar Abscess

- Etiology-Pathogenesis
  - Acute exudative tonsillitis undergoes internal cavitation and suppuration creating **tonsillar abscess**
  - Rupture of tonsillar abscess into the deeper PPS, masticator and/or SMS creates **peritonsillar abscess**
- Epidemiology
  - Tonsillar-peritonsillar abscess is the most common deep neck infection in children and young adults

Gross Pathologic, Surgical Features
- Putrid yellow-green fluid drains from abscess cavity

Microscopic Features
- Abscess wall = granulation tissue (capillaries, fibroblasts) and fibrous connective tissue (fibroblasts, collagen fibers)

Microscopic Features
- Beta-hemolytic streptococcus, staphylococcus, pneumococcus and hemophilus are most common organisms
- Pus = necrotic debris, polymorphonuclear leukocytes, lymphocytes and macrophages

Clinical Issues

Presentation
- Begins as acute tonsillitis in the adolescent or young adult
- Progression to severe sore throat with tonsillar area edema despite antibiotic treatment suggests the diagnosis of tonsillar abscess
- Physical exam
  - Edema and erythema of affected tonsil with associated uvular edema and contralateral displacement
  - "Bulging" tonsil

Natural History
- Left untreated, tonsillar abscess may rupture into the pharyngeal airway (autodrainage) or deep into the PPS, masticator and SMS (transpatial abscess formation)

Treatment
- Needle aspiration, incision and drainage and antibiotics or abscess tonsillectomy
- Tonsillectomy usually performed after acute infection has resolved, usually at least 6 weeks later
- **Abscess** tonsillectomy is definitive, avoiding follow-up aspirations and post-abscess tonsillectomy
  - Carries higher risk of complications

Prognosis
- Excellent if treated with incision, drainage and intravenous antibiotics
- Both aspiration and incision and drainage techniques may require repeat drainage

Selected References
1. Schraff S et al: Peritonsillar abscess in children: a 10-year review of diagnosis and management. Int J Pediatr Otorhinolaryngol 57:213-8, 2001
2. Herzon FS: Peritonsillar abscess: incidence, current management practices and a proposal for treatment guidelines. Laryngoscope 105:1-17, 1995
3. Patel KS et al: The role of computed tomography in the management of peritonsillar abscess. Otolaryngol Head Neck Surg 107:727-32, 1992

Minor Salivary Gland Ca

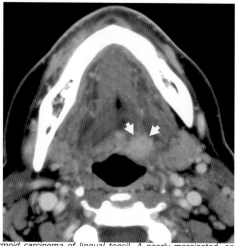

Mucoepidermoid carcinoma of lingual tonsil. A poorly-marginated, enhancing left lingual tonsillar mass (arrows) is seen on this axial CECT image. There is no mucosal lesion present on endoscopic examination of the lingual tonsil.

Key Facts
- Minor salivary gland malignancies (MSGM) are rare, pernicious, aggressive tumors of the pharynx
- The 3 principal MSGM are adenoid cystic carcinoma (ACCa), adenocarcinoma (ADCa) and mucoepidermoid carcinoma (MECa)
- The imaging appearance of these 3 cell types is indistinguishable
- Treatment success must be judged by long-term survival rates as these tumors tend to grow slowly and recur late

Imaging Findings
General Features
- Infiltrating mass of the pharyngeal mucosal space (PMS)
- Locations of MSGM: Palate > sinonasal region > tongue > faucial, lingual or adenoidal tonsils
- When in PMS unilateral mass invading parapharyngeal and other deeper spaces from medial to lateral is seen

CT Findings
- Enhancing, infiltrating mass centered at the pharyngeal surface

MR Findings
- Pharyngeal surface mass with T2 signal spectrum from low (more cellular, poorer prognosis) to high (less cellular, better prognosis)
- Enhancing mass on T1 C+ MR images with infiltrating margins

Imaging Recommendations
- These tumors, especially ACCa, have a tendency to spread via **perineural** and perivascular routes
  - Radiologist must check perineural and perivascular "way stations" deep to primary tumor site on imaging study
    - Palatal MSGM: Greater palatine foramen/nerve => pterygopalatine fossa => foramen rotundum/V2
    - Faucial tonsillar MSGM: Masticator space => V3 => foramen ovale => Meckel's cave

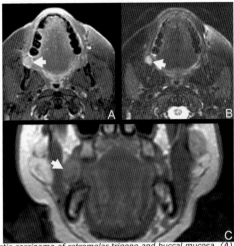

Adenoid cystic carcinoma of retromolar trigone and buccal mucosa. (A) Axial T1 C+ MR shows a nodular enhancing tumor (arrow) in retromolar trigone. (B) T2 fat sat axial image shows tumor as high signal (arrow). (C) Coronal T1 MR demonstrates tumor (arrow) centered in buccal mucosa.

- NP adenoidal tonsil: Carotid space => ICA => vertical and horizontal segments of petrous ICA
- **Fat saturation** recommended as part of the T1 C+ MR sequence
  o Helps define deep tissue extent of the tumor & perineural spread
- Long-term (5-10 year) imaging follow-up recommended given the tendency of these tumors to recur late

Differential Diagnosis: Pharyngeal Mucosal Space Mass
Lymphoid Hyperplasia of Tonsils
- No discrete mass is seen within the enlarged tonsil on CT or MR
- Enhancing septa are visible on T1 C+ MR
Benign Mixed Tumor of Minor Salivary Gland
- Sharply-marginated mass; pedunculated when large
Squamous Cell Carcinoma
- Mucosal surface with obvious erosive lesion
- Poorly-circumscribed mass in PMS with invasive deep margins
- Associated malignant adenopathy common
Non-Hodgkin Lymphoma
- Systemic illness may be present; submucosal mass evident
- Diffusely involves the adenoids while a unilateral mass is seen when faucial or lingual tonsil is affected
- No enhancing septa are seen on T1 C+ MR
- Associated large, non-necrotic nodes (50%)

Pathology
General
- General Path Comments
  o MSG are mucous or seromucous secreting tubuloalveolar glands
  o Three principal MSGM seen: ACCa, ADCa and MECa

- o ACCa specific comments
  - Most common MSGM; classic tumor with perineural spread
  - Arises from peripheral segments of salivary duct system (intercalated ducts and acini)
- Embryology
  - o MSG occur normally along the mucosal surfaces of the sinuses, nose, nasopharynx, oropharynx, oral cavity, hypopharynx, larynx and tracheobronchial tree
  - o MSG are most commonly found in posterior hard and soft palate
- Etiology-Pathogenesis
  - o Spectrum of malignant tumors arising from minor salivary glands that normally line the surfaces of the upper aerodigestive tract
- Epidemiology
  - o Rare, cf. to major salivary gland malignancy (1/10 as common)
  - o Frequency of occurrence: ACCa > ADCa > MECa

Gross Pathologic, Surgical Features
- Tan-white mass

Microscopic Features
- ACCa
  - o Unencapsulated neoplasm with varied growth patterns consisting of cribriform, tubular and solid; individual tumors most commonly are composed of multiple growth patterns
- ADCa
  - o Encapsulated tumor with a variety of growth patterns including solid, microcystic, papillary-cystic and follicular
- MECa
  - o Malignant epithelial minor or major salivary gland tumor composed of a variable admixture of epidermoid, intermediate and mucous-secreting cells

Clinical Issues
Presentation
- **Submucosal**, often painful mass in the pharyngeal wall
- Larger, more invasive lesions can have cranial neuropathy (V2, V3)
- ACCa: Usually no lymph nodes at presentation
- MECa: Higher grade lesions usually have associated nodes

Natural History
- Begin as slow-growing tumors that tend to recur late
- **80%** 5-year survival is in stark contrast to **20%** 20-year survival

Treatment
- Wide surgical removal is treatment of choice
- Post-operative radiotherapy is used routinely

Prognosis
- Late stage MSGM and the presence of neck node metastases predict both early recurrence and high eventual mortality
- Survival is favored by histological type (MECa > ACCa > ADCa) and site of primary (OC and OP > NP > sinus-nose)

Selected References
1. Jones AS et al: Tumors of the minor salivary glands. Clin Otolaryngol 23:27-33, 1998
2. Sigal R et al: Adenoid cystic carcinoma of the head and neck: evaluation with MR imaging and clinical-pathologic correlation in 27 patients. Radiology 184:95-101, 1992
3. Parker GD et al: Clinical-radiologic issues in perineural tumor spread of malignant diseases of the extracranial head and neck. RadioGraphics 11:383-99, 1991

Non-Hodgkin Lymphoma, Tonsils

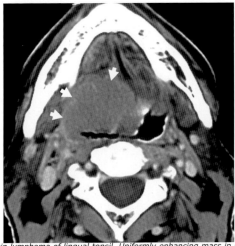

Non-Hodgkin lymphoma of lingual tonsil. Uniformly enhancing mass in right lingual tonsil (arrows) is seen in this axial CECT. For its size, the absence of necrosis would suggest NHL. However, only biopsy can differentiate this NHL mass from SCCa.

Key Facts
- Definition: Pharyngeal mucosal space (PMS) contains Waldeyer's lymphatic ring
  - Nasopharyngeal PMS holds the adenoids
  - Oropharyngeal PMS holds the faucial and lingual tonsils
- PMS NHL key differential diagnosis is **lymphoid hyperplasia**
- Imaging shows PMS NHL diffusely involves NP adenoids but is unilateral-asymmetric in the facial and lingual tonsil areas
- Associated large, non-necrotic nodes present 50% of time

Imaging Findings
General Features
- PMS foci = **extranodal, lymphatic** NHL deposit
  - PMS tonsils aka **MALT** = **M**ucosa-**A**ssociated **L**ymphoid **T**issue
  - PMS most common sites of occurrence: Faucial (palatine) tonsil > nasopharyngeal adenoids > lingual tonsil
  - NP adenoidal involvement is usually diffuse
  - Faucial and lingual tonsillar involvement is usually unilateral
- Nodal NHL is associated (50%)
  - Large (> 2cm), non-necrotic nodes most common
  - Nodes may be necrotic in more invasive NHL (esp. AIDS NHL)
- Non-nodal, non-tonsillar NHL rarely associated = **extranodal, extralymphatic** (ENEL) NHL deposit
  - ENEL sites: Sinonasal, orbit, parotid, larynx, thyroid
CT Findings
- Enhancing tonsillar mass without bone invasion
MR Findings
- Enhancing tonsillar mass on T1 C+ MR images
  - **No** internal enhancing septa present (cf. lymphoid hyperplasia)
- T2 MR shows markedly nonhomogeneous high-signal intensity

Non-Hodgkin Lymphoma, Tonsils

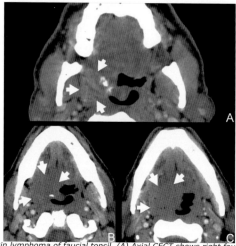

Non-Hodgkin lymphoma of faucial tonsil. (A) Axial CECT shows right faucial tonsillar mass (arrows). Calcifications are from previous inflammation. (B-C) Inferior CECT reveals enlarging faucial tonsillar NHL (arrows). It is not possible to differentiate NHL from SCCa by CT imaging.

Imaging Recommendations
- Imaging (CT or MR) should cover the entire extracranial head and neck from the sellar floor above to the clavicles below
- Enhanced MR imaging can differentiate PMS NHL from lymphoid hyperplasia by the absence of **internal hypervascular septa**

Differential Diagnosis: Tonsillar Mass
Lymphoid Hyperplasia of Waldeyer's Lymphatic Ring
- Patients under 20 years old (NHL usually > 40 years old)
- Symmetric enlargement of tonsillar tissue; internal enhancing **septa** seen on T1 C+ MR images

Squamous Cell Carcinoma, PMS of NP or OP
- Older, smoking patient
- Erosive mucosal lesion; unless tumor began in crypts of a tonsil
- Poorly-circumscribed mass in the PMS with invasive deep margin
- Associated malignant adenopathy common (often with necrosis)

Minor Salivary Gland Malignancy, PMS of NP or OP
- May be indistinguishable from head and neck SCCa
- Associated nodal metastases rare

Pathology
General
- General Path Comments
  - PMS (MALT) NHL tend to remain localized, grow slowly
  - PMS NHL tend to be of the B-cell type
- Etiology-Pathogenesis
  - Primary malignancy of the lymphatic system
- Epidemiology
  - PMS (Waldeyer's ring) is most common extranodal site in H & N
  - 35% of extranodal NHL in H & N is in the PMS

- o   When PMS NHL present, 20% have GI NHL involvement
- o   50% of PMS NHL have malignant lymph nodes at presentation

Microscopic Features
- Any of the NHL patterns and cell types can be seen
- Most common histologic pattern = diffuse with immunoblastic or large cell (B cell) cytologic features
  - o   Immunochemistry differentiates NPCa from NHL
    - NHL, immunoblastic or large cell type: LCA positive, cytokeratin negative
    - NPCa, undifferentiated: LCA negative, cytokeratin positive
- PMS NHL usually derived from follicular center cells
  - o   Positive reactivity, B-cell markers

Clinical Staging (I-IV)
- **I**: One lymph node region or one extralymphatic organ/site
  - o   Treatment: Radiotherapy; Prognosis: 50% 5 yr. survival
- **II**: 2 or more nodal regions or involvement of an extralymphatic site and > 1 nodal region on same side of diaphragm
  - o   Treatment: Radiotherapy; Prognosis: 25% 5 yr. survival
- **III**: Nodal involvement on both sides of the diaphragm with or without splenic and extralymphatic organ involvement
  - o   Treatment: Total lymphoid radiotherapy, chemotherapy if spleen is involved; Prognosis: 17% 5 yr. survival
- **IV:** Diffuse or disseminated involvement of one or more extralymphatic organs with or without lymph node involvement
  - o   Treatment: Chemotherapy alone; Prognosis: <10% 5 yr. survival

Clinical Issues

Presentation
- NP adenoidal NHL: Nasal obstruction; serous otitis media
- Faucial or lingual tonsil NHL: Sore throat, otalgia, tonsillar mass
- Can occur at any age but more common with advancing age
- Predisposing conditions: AIDS, Sjogren's syndrome

Natural History
- 2/3 of patients have remission after initial therapy
  - o   Of these, 2/3 are cured and have no further relapse
- 75% of those who relapse after achieving remission die

Treatment & Prognosis
- Based on clinical stage at presentation (see Clinical Staging above)
- High histopathologic grade and recurrent disseminated disease have the poorest prognosis
- Overall survival rate for head and neck PMS NHL is 60%

Selected References
1.   Hanna E et al: Extranodal lymphomas of the head and neck. A 20-year experience. Arch Otolaryngol Head Neck Surg 123:1318-23, 1997
2.   Harnsberger HR et al: Non-Hodgkin's lymphoma of the head and neck: CT evaluation of nodal and extranodal sites. AJR 149:785-91, 1987
3.   Isaacson PG et al: Malignant lymphoma of mucosa-associated lymphoid tissue (MALT). Histopathology 11:445-62, 1987

Benign Mixed Tumor, Pharynx

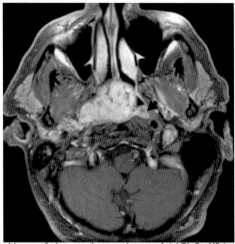

Benign mixed tumor of pharyngeal mucosal space. Axial T1 C+ MR image shows a pear-shaped, mixed-enhancing mass arising from the right lateral pharyngeal recess of the nasopharyngeal mucosal space. The BMT originated in a minor salivary gland. Arrow: opposite lateral pharyngeal recess.

Key Facts
- Synonym: Pleomorphic adenoma
- Definition: Benign, heterogeneous tumor of minor salivary gland origin made up of an admixture of epithelial, myoepithelial and stromal components
- Classic imaging appearance: Well-circumscribed, submucosal, pharyngeal mass that becomes pedunculated when large

Imaging Findings
General Features
- Best imaging clue: sharply-marginated, submucosal mass
- Locations affected: Soft palate >> oropharyngeal mucosal space (lingual or faucial tonsil) > nasopharyngeal mucosal space
- Oval to round, well-circumscribed mass without invasive margins
- Small, benign, mixed tumor of minor salivary gland (BMT-MSG) appear as a marble in the mucosal "rug"
- Large BMT-MSG is exophytic, projecting into pharyngeal airway
CT Findings
- If tumor is adjacent to bone (e.g., hard palate), benign-appearing remodeling is seen as a concavity in this bone
MR Findings
- Sharply-marginated mass with low-intermediate T1, high T2 signal
- Enhancement pattern: Variable; homogeneous enhancement
- Deep margins show no evidence for deep tissue invasion

Differential Diagnosis: Pharyngeal Mucosal Space Mass
Lymphoid Hyperplasia of Tonsils
- No discrete mass is seen within the enlarged tonsil on CT or MR
- Enhancing septa are seen on T1 C+ MR

Benign Mixed Tumor, Pharynx

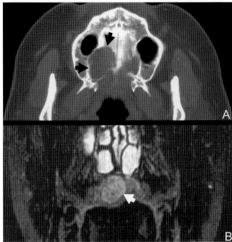

Benign mixed tumor of minor salivary gland. (A) Axial bone-only CT through hard palate reveals an oval area of scalloping (arrows) from BMT remodeling. (B) Coronal T2 fat sat MR image shows the BMT (arrow) in the submucosal area just below the hard palate.

Squamous Cell Carcinoma
- Mucosal surface will have obvious erosive lesion unless tumor began in crypts of a tonsil
- Poorly-circumscribed mass in the pharyngeal mucosal space with CT or MR evidence of invasion on its deep margin
- Associated malignant adenopathy common

Non-Hodgkin Lymphoma
- Systemic illness may present; submucosal mass evident
- Usually diffusely involves the adenoids while faucial or lingual tonsil is asymmetrically affected
- No enhancing septa are seen on T1 C+ MR
- Associated large, non-necrotic nodes may be seen

Minor Salivary Gland Malignancy
- May be indistinguishable from head and neck SCCa
- Associated nodal malignancy rare

Pathology

General
- General Path Comments
  - **MSG** occur normally along the mucosal surfaces of the nose, nasopharynx, oropharynx, oral cavity, hypopharynx, larynx and tracheobronchial tree
  - MSG are most commonly found in the posterior hard and soft palate
- Etiology-Pathogenesis
  - Benign tumor arising spontaneously from minor salivary glands that normally line all surfaces of the upper aerodigestive tract
- Epidemiology
  - 6.5% of head and neck BMT arise from MSG
  - 85% in parotid gland

o   8% in submandibular glands
o   0.5% in sublingual glands

<u>Gross Pathologic, Surgical Features</u>
- Exophytic mass projecting into pharyngeal airway; 1-4 cm in size
- Tan-white, either encased in a fibrous capsule or well-demarcated

<u>Microscopic Features</u>
- Interspersed epithelial, myoepithelial and stromal cellular components must be identified to diagnose BMT-MSG
- BMT-MSG are more commonly well-demarcated but not encased in a fibrous capsule
  o   BMT of major salivary glands are usually encapsulated

Clinical Issues

<u>Presentation</u>
- Principal presenting symptom: Submucosal mass of pharynx
- When small, focal submucosal mass is seen; larger lesions present as obvious pedunculated masses within the airway
- Location-dependent symptoms and signs
  o   Nasopharynx: Posterior nasal obstruction
  o   Oropharynx (lingual or faucial tonsil, soft palate): Dysphagia
- Clinical epidemiology
  o   Female: male ratio 2:1
  o   Most common age of presentation: 30-60 years

<u>Natural History</u>
- Slow-growing, painless, benign tumor that is usually treated early in patients unless denial is a part of the clinical presentation

<u>Treatment</u>
- Complete surgical resection of mass without spillage

<u>Prognosis</u>
- Excellent if no spillage occurs during surgery
- Recurrent tumor tends to be **multifocal**

Selected References
1.   Lopes MA et al: A clinicopathologic study of 196 intraoral minor salivary gland tumours. J Oral Pathol Med 28:264-7, 1999
2.   Waldron CA et al: Tumors of the intraoral minor salivary glands: a demographic and histologic study of 426 cases. Oral Surg Oral Med Oral Path 66:323-33, 1998
3.   Horky JK et al: True malignant mixed tumor (carcinosarcoma) of tonsillar minor salivary gland origin. AJNR 18:1944-8, 1997

PocketRadiologist™
Head and Neck
100 Top Diagnoses

LYMPH NODES

Nodal Squamous Cell Carcinoma

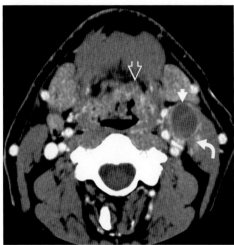

Malignant SCCa node with extranodal tumor. Axial CECT reveals a thick-walled necrotic jugulodigastric lymph node (arrow). Enhancing area of thickened anterior margin of sternomastoid muscle (curved arrow) indicates extranodal spread. Open arrow: submucosal lingual tonsil primary SCCa.

Key Facts
- Synonym: Nodal metastases from head and neck SCCa primary
- Definition: Primary SCCa of H & N spreads to regional lymph nodes to create metastatic intranodal SCCa
- Classic imaging appearance: Enlarged lymph node(s) with round or oval configuration, loss of normal nodal morphology and fatty hilum and central inhomogeneous matrix
- Incidence of nodal disease in H & N SCCa varies by primary site
  - Nasopharynx (90%), oropharynx (60%), oral cavity (50%), hypopharynx (60%), supraglottic (40%) glottic and subglottic (<10%)
  - Warning: Suppurative adenitis can mimic malignant adenopathy

Imaging Findings
General Features
- Best imaging clue: Large node ± central matrix inhomogeneity in regional lymph node drainage of known primary H & N SCCa
- Most masses over 3 cm are nodal conglomerates
- Imaging studies can **NOT** accurately diagnose microscopic nodal neoplastic involvement
- **Nodal neoplastic involvement** is suggested by
  - Loss of normal "kidney-bean" shape & fatty hilum
  - Nodal internal matrix inhomogeneity
- **Extranodal tumor** suggested by indistinct nodal margins with enhancing tissue spreading into adjacent soft tissues
- **Malignant nodal criteria**
  - Deep cervical, spinal accessory, submandibular nodes: ≥ 1.5 cm
  - Retropharyngeal and parotid nodes: ≥ 1.0 cm
  - Any size lymph node with internal matrix inhomogeneity

Nodal Squamous Cell Carcinoma

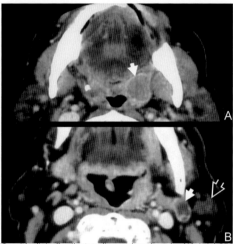

Tonsillar SCCa with clinically silent malignant lymph node. (A) Axial CECT shows the left tonsillar primary SCCa. (B) More inferior axial CECT reveals the non-palpable but clearly malignant jugulodigastric necrotic node (arrow). Open arrow: Overlying parotid tail.

CT Findings
- CECT shows diffuse or rim enhancement of ovoid node(s)

MR Findings
- T1 C+ MR reveals internal matrix inhomogeneous enhancement

FDG-PET Findings
- Focal areas of metabolic activity are seen in larger nodal deposits

Ultrasound Findings
- Loss of normal nodal architecture, echo lucent nodal matrix
- Can be used to needle biopsy suspicious nodes

Imaging Recommendations
- Staging of malignant lymph nodes done concurrently with primary
- CECT or CEMR can be used

Differential Diagnosis: Lateral Cervical Mass

2nd Branchial Cleft Cyst
- No primary SCCa present; usually younger patient
- Single cystic mass with thinner, non-nodular wall

Internal Jugular Vein Thrombosis
- Tubular mass in location of IJV

Non-Hodgkin Lymphoma Nodes
- Large, non-necrotic nodes in absence of primary SCCa
- When tonsil involved and NHL is aggressive (necrotic), may be indistinguishable from SCCa adenopathy

Other Systemic Nodal Malignancy
- Often found in deep cervical and spinal accessory nodes in low neck
- As a single node on imaging, may be indistinguishable from SCCa

Pathology

General
- General Path Comments

Nodal Squamous Cell Carcinoma

- o   Nodal internal inhomogeneity from necrosis or replacement of normal nodal medulla with neoplastic cells
- o   CT (probably MR) nodal staging accuracy 95%
  - ▪   Compared with clinical staging accuracy of 80%
- •   Embryology-Anatomy: AJCC Nodal Level Classification Scheme
  - o   Level **I**: Submandibular and submental
  - o   Level **II**: Upper jugular (deep cervical); above hyoid bone
  - o   Level **III**: Mid-jugular (deep cervical); hyoid to inferior cricoid
  - o   Level **IV**: Lower jugular (deep cervical); below inferior cricoid
  - o   Level **V**: Spinal accessory chain (posterior cervical space)
  - o   Level **VI**: Anterior midline (paratracheal, Delphian chains)
  - o   Level **VII**: Upper mediastinal nodes
- •   Epidemiology
  - o   30-50% of metastatic nodes are < 1 cm

Microscopic Features
- •   Squamous differentiation with intracellular bridges or keratinization

Nodal Staging Criteria
- •   AJCC classification for cervical lymphadenopathy is uniform for mucosal primary SCCa (with exception of thyroid & NPC primaries)
  - o   **N1** = Single positive node, ≤ 3 cm
  - o   **N2** = Single or multiple node(s), 3-6 cm
  - o   **N3** = Ipsilateral nodes > 6 cm, bilateral or contralateral

Clinical Issues

Presentation
- •   Principal presenting symptom: Firm, painless, non-tender mass
- •   10% of malignant nodes clinically occult secondary to deep location

Natural History
- •   Single nodal disease will increase in size, incorporating surrounding nodal groups and finally encasing surrounding structures

Treatment
- •   Surgical excision is classic treatment for nodal disease
  - o   Nodes removed with primary resection
  - o   Radical neck dissection has given way to conservative techniques
- •   Cervical nodal dissections types
  - o   Radical neck dissection: Resection of nodal groups I-V, along with SCM, IJV and spinal accessory nerve
  - o   Modified radical neck dissection: Resection of nodal groups I–V, **without** resection of all three above structures
  - o   Selective neck dissection: Cervical lymphadenectomy in which one or more of groups I–V are preserved
- •   XRT can be used alone for nodes less than 1 cm
- •   If extracapsular spread present, postoperative XRT is required

Prognosis
- •   Nodal tumor associated with **50%** reduction in long-term survival
- •   Extracapsular extension decreases survival rate by **50%**
  - o   Single best prognosticator of local failure of control

Selected References
1.   Som PM et al: Imaging-based nodal classification for evaluation of neck metastatic lymphadenopathy. AJR 174:837-44, 2000
2.   Curtin HD et al: Comparison of CT and MR imaging in staging of neck metastases. Radiology 207:123-30, 1998
3.   Anzai Y et al: Imaging of nodal metastases in the head and neck. JMRI 7:774-83, 1997

Nodal Lymphoma

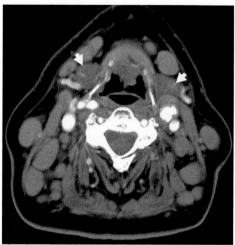

Non-Hodgkin lymphoma (NHL) lymph nodes. CECT shows multiple, large, non-necrotic lymph nodes in the submandibular, deep cervical, parotid and spinal accessory chains bilaterally. Arrows: submandibular glands. NHL nodes are usually non-necrotic unless the NHL is high grade.

Key Facts
- Definition: Cancer that develops in the lymphoreticular system, thought to arise from lymphocytes and their derivatives
- Classic imaging appearance: Multiple, bilateral, homogeneous, enlarged lymph nodes involving all nodal chains in the neck
- Other key facts
  - Cervical lymphadenopathy is one of the most common presentations of **Hodgkin lymphoma** (HL)
  - **Non-Hodgkin lymphoma** (NHL) is second most common neoplasm of the head and neck (5% of head and neck cancers)
  - NHL sites in head and neck
    - **Nodal** (most common site)
    - **Extranodal, lymphatic** (Waldeyer's ring)
    - **Extranodal, extralymphatic** (orbit, sinonasal, etc.)

Imaging Findings
General Features
- Best imaging clue: Multiple, bilateral, **non-necrotic** enlarged nodes involving usual and unusual (RPS, SMS, occipital) nodal chains
- All nodal chains may be involved
  - When RPS, occipital and submandibular nodes appear, think NHL
  - Deep cervical and spinal accessory nodes commonly involved
- If nodes show necrosis ± extranodal spread, aggressive NHL (e.g., AIDS, NHL) is implied
- HL usually spreads up from chest to lower cervical nodes 1st
  - Progression cephalad into neck seen in severe cases

CT Findings
- CECT shows multiple, large (> 2 cm), ovoid masses bilaterally in multiple lymph node chain areas of the neck
  - Nodal density equal or less than muscle

Nodal Lymphoma

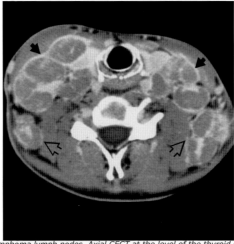

Hodgkin lymphoma lymph nodes. Axial CECT at the level of the thyroid gland shows multiple rim-enhancing lymph nodes bilaterally. Deep cervical nodes: arrows. Spinal accessory nodes: open arrows.

- Calcifications usually seen only post-therapy or from previous neck granulomatous infection
- HL: Tend to have more rim enhancement than NHL nodes

<u>MR Findings</u>
- Isointense to muscle on T1; hyperintense on T2 and STIR

<u>Gallium-67 Nuclear Medicine Imaging</u>
- Useful for lymphoma whole body screening
- Low specificity

<u>Imaging Recommendations</u>
- CECT or MR can adequately stage head and neck lymphoma

Differential Diagnosis

<u>Reactive Adenopathy</u>
- Imaging: Diffuse, non-necrotic adenopathy < 2 cm
- Clinical: < 20 year old with upper respiratory tract infection

<u>Granulomatous Disease (TB)</u>
- Imaging: Diffuse, necrotic adenopathy

<u>Sarcoidosis</u>
- Diffuse cervical lymphadenopathy that may exactly mimic NHL
- Mediastinal nodes commonly associated

Pathology

<u>General</u>
- Epidemiology
  - HL risk factors
    - 2 age ranges: 15-40yo, and >55yo; rare <5yo
    - Increased incidence in siblings of HL cases; EBV association
  - NHL risk factors
    - Incidence increases with age, in immunocompromised patients
    - Increased association with EBV and HTLV-1

- Exposure to chemicals (pesticides, fertilizer, solvents)
  o Incidence
    - HL: 7,000 cases/year, <1% cancer cases in US
    - NHL: 50,000 cases/year, 5% cancer cases in US

<u>Gross Pathologic, Surgical Features</u>
- Nodes can range in size from 1-10cm

<u>Microscopic Features</u>
- B-cells are usually located in the cortex of the follicles and medullary cords, T-cells are usually located in the paracortex
- Neoplastic changes demonstrate large, non-cleaved cells
- HL: Presence of Reed-Sternberg cells (not seen in NHL)

<u>Revised European-American Lymphoma (REAL) Classification</u>
- B-cell neoplasms
  o Precursor B-lymphoblastic leukemia/lymphoma
  o Peripheral B-cell neoplasms
- T-cell and putative NK-cell neoplasms
  o Precursor T-lymphoblastic leukemia/lymphoma
  o Peripheral T-cell and NK-cell neoplasms
- Hodgkin's Disease
  o Lymphocyte predominance; nodular sclerosis; mixed cellularity; lymphocyte depletion

<u>Ann Arbor NHL Staging Criteria</u>
- **Stage I**: Single nodal region or single extralymphatic organ
- **Stage II**: Involvement of ≥ 2 nodal regions, or single extralymphatic organ involvement and adjacent nodes on same side of diaphragm
- **Stage III**: Positive nodal regions on both sides of diaphragm
- **Stage IV**: Multifocal involvement with ≥ 1 extralymphatic organ

Clinical Issues

<u>Presentation</u>
- Principal presenting symptom: Multiple, bilateral, painless masses
- Other symptoms: Night sweats, recurrent fevers, unexplained weight loss/fatigue, itchy skin rash/red skin patches

<u>Natural History</u>
- Not well understood, cases can go into permanent or temporary remission, or continue to progress despite aggressive therapy

<u>Treatment</u>
- Usually treated with XRT and/or chemotherapy
  o Bone marrow transplantation under investigation
- NHL limited to head and neck can be treated with XRT
- Exact treatment of NHL depends on stage, cell type, patient age
- Disseminated NHL treated with chemotherapy

<u>Prognosis</u>
- Prognosis depends on tumor stage and response to therapy
- Estimated cure rates: Stage I and II: 85% with XRT
- Stage II and IV: 50% with combined XRT and chemotherapy

Selected References
1. Kaji AV et al: Imaging of cervical lymphadenopathy. Semin Ultrasound CT MRI 18:220-49, 1997
2. Harnsberger HR et al: Non-Hodgkin lymphoma of the head and neck: CT evaluation of nodal and extranodal sites. AJNR 8:673-9, 1987
3. Lee Y et al: Lymphomas of the head and neck: CT findings at initial presentation. AJNR 8:665-71, 1987

Spinal Accessory Nodal Mets

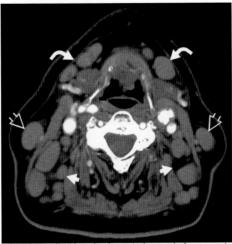

Non-Hodgkin lymphoma (NHL) nodes in posterior cervical space spinal accessory nodes. Axial CECT at the level of the vallecula shows multiple non-necrotic nodes in the spinal accessory chain bilaterally (arrows). NHL nodes in the parotid tail (open arrows) and submandibular chain (curved arrows) also seen.

Key Facts
- Definitions
  - Malignant lymph nodes in spinal accessory chain (SAC) in the posterior cervical space (PCS) of the cervical neck
  - Spinal accessory lymph node chain = posterior cervical chain
- Most common histologies: Squamous cell carcinoma (SCCa), non-Hodgkin lymphoma (NHL), Hodgkin lymphoma (HL) and differentiated thyroid carcinoma (DTCa)
- Classic imaging appearance: Multiple round to oval masses in the fat of the PCS
  - SCCa: > 1.5cm or any size with central nodal necrosis
  - NHL: Large (> 2cm) usually without central nodal necrosis
  - HL: Any size with inhomogeneous enhancement
  - DTCa: Solid nodules of enhancement, cystic change, calcifications, hemorrhage

Imaging Findings
General Features
- Multiple oval to round masses within the fat of the PCS
CECT Findings
- SCCa: > 1.5cm or any size with central nodal low density
- NHL: Large (> 2cm) usually without central nodal necrosis
- HL: Any size node with inhomogeneous enhancement
- DTCa: Bizarre-appearing nodes with solid nodules of enhancement, cystic change and calcifications possible
T1 C+ Fat Saturated MR Findings
- SCCa: > 1.5cm or any size with central low signal
- NHL: Large (> 2cm) usually without central nodal necrosis
- HL: Any size with inhomogeneous enhancement

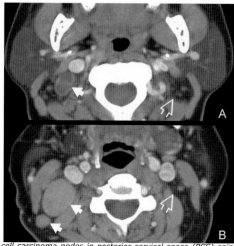

Squamous cell carcinoma nodes in posterior cervical space (PCS) spinal accessory nodes. (A) Axial CECT through mid-oropharynx reveals a malignant necrotic node in spinal accessory chain on right (arrow). Open arrow: PCS. (B) Low oropharynx image shows 2 more malignant nodes (arrows). Open arrow: PCS.

- DTCa: Bizarre-appearing nodes with solid nodules of enhancement, cystic change and hemorrhage (high signal on T1 pre-C+)

Imaging Recommendations
- Enhanced CT or MR can both adequately assess PCS nodal disease

Differential Diagnosis: PCS Mass
Cystic Hygroma of PCS
- Cystic mass fills PCS in younger patient

Reactive Adenopathy, SAC
- Multiple, bilateral, non-necrotic SAC nodes
- Adenoidal and faucial tonsillar hypertrophy may be associated

Suppurative Adenopathy, SAC
- Intranodal abscess seen as single or multiple necrotic SAC nodes
- Patient usually septic with tender neck masses

Brachial Plexus Schwannoma or Neurofibroma
- Single tubular mass emerges from between anterior and middle scalene muscles into the PCS

Pathology
General
- General Path Comments
  - SCCa, NHL, HL or DTCa commonly found in SAC of PCS
  - Any systemic malignancy can go via hematogenous spread to spinal accessory lymph nodes of the neck
- Embryology-Anatomy
  - The PCS = posterior triangle clinically
  - PCS normally contains only the spinal accessory nerve, SAC and fat
- Etiology-Pathogenesis
  - SCCa: Primary tumor (NPCa, OPCa) seeds the SAC
  - NHL: Nodal NHL may affect any nodal chain in the body

- o HL: Nodal HL may affect any nodal chain in the body
- o DTCa: SAC is only seeded if paratracheal and deep cervical chains are already involved
- Epidemiology
  - o SCCa from H & N, > 80% of SAC malignant adenopathy
  - o NHL > NL > PTCa of remaining 20%

Microscopic Features
- Four histologies to consider: SCCa, NHL, HL and DTCa

N Staging Criteria
- For SCCa
  - o **N1** = Single positive node, < or = 3cm
  - o **N2** = Single or multiple node(s), >3cm but not > 6cm
  - o **N3** = Ipsilateral nodes > 6cm, bilateral or contralateral nodes
- For NHL
  - o **Stage I**: One nodal region or one extralymphatic organ/site
  - o **Stage II**: Two or more nodal regions or involvement of an extralymphatic site and > 1 nodal region, same side diaphragm
  - o **Stage III**: Nodal involvement on both sides of the diaphragm with or without splenic and extralymphatic organ involvement
  - o **Stage IV**: Diffuse or disseminated involvement of one or more extralymphatic organs with or without lymph node involvement
- For DTCa
  - o **N0**: No regional metastasis
  - o **N1**: Regional nodal metastasis
    - **N1a**: Nodal metastasis in ipsilateral cervical neck
    - **N1b**: Bilateral, midline or contralateral cervical or mediastinal

Clinical Issues
Presentation
- Principal presenting symptom: Mass or masses palpable along the posterior border of the sternocleidomastoid muscle
- If extranodal tumor present, masses may be "fixed"

Treatment
- Determined by histology
- SCCa
  - o In NPCa primary, radiotherapy and chemotherapy
  - o In OPCa primary, neck dissection and radiotherapy
- NHL or NL
  - o Radiotherapy +/- chemotherapy depending on stage
- DTCa
  - o Surgical resection of tumor with I-131 post-op

Prognosis
- Determined by histology
- SCCa, NHL and NL all stage dependent
- DTCa: Excellent prognosis overall

Selected References
1. Mazzaferri EL: An overview of the management of papillary and follicular thyroid carcinoma. Thyroid 9:421-7, 1999
2. Chong VF et al: Carcinoma of the nasopharynx. Semin Ultrasound CT MR 19:449-62, 1998
3. Harnsberger HR et al: Non-Hodgkin's lymphoma of the head and neck: CT evaluation of nodal and extranodal sites. AJR 149:785-91, 1987

PocketRadiologist™
Head and Neck
100 Top Diagnoses

LARYNX

Supraglottic SCCa

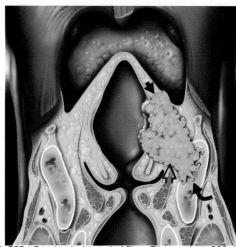

Supraglottic SCCa. Drawing depicts typical Stage T4 supraglottic SCCa involving the aryepiglottic fold (arrow) and paraglottic space (open arrow). At the deep margin of the tumor invasion of the thyroid cartilage can be seen (curved arrow). Cartilage invasion makes this lesion Stage T4.

Key Facts
- Definitions
  - **Supraglottic (SG) SCCa** = Primary SCCa originating on the mucosa of any part of the supraglottic larynx
  - **Supraglottic larynx** = Larynx above true vocal cords including false cords, aryepiglottic (AE) folds and epiglottis as well as the deep pre-epiglottic (PES) and paraglottic (PGS) spaces
- Classic imaging appearance: Moderately-enhancing, infiltrating mass of the epiglottis, AE fold ± false vocal cord often with associated malignant adenopathy
- Other important facts
  - SG larynx lymphatic rich, resulting in frequent metastatic nodes
  - 30% of all endolaryngeal SCCa = supraglottic SCCa

Imaging Findings
General Features
- Best imaging clue: Endoscopic assessment of **mucosal extent** of tumor; rendering your imaging report without this knowledge will lead to large errors in radiologic stage
- Moderately-enhancing mass invades the deep tissues of the larynx including PES ± PGS
- Larger tumors: Laryngeal cartilage destruction ± malignant nodes
CT Findings
- Moderately-enhancing mass seen involving the epiglottis, AE fold or false vocal cord
  - **Epiglottic SCCa**: Side-to-side symmetric enlargement of epiglottis may be missed by those searching for "asymmetry"; PES spread is a clinical blind spot
  - **AE fold SCCa**: May spread posteriorly to involve pyriform sinus or anteriorly to involve false cord

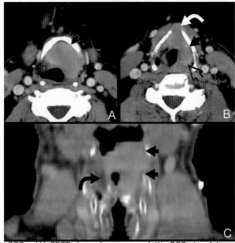

Supraglottic SCCa. (A) CECT shows large supraglottic SCCa involving pre-epiglottic space (arrow). (B) Inferior CECT reveals SCCa in paraglottic space (arrow), aryepiglottic fold (open arrow) & thyroid notch (curved arrow). (C) Coronal CT reformation. Arrows: Supraglottic SCCa. Curved arrow: Normal paraglottic space.

   o   **False cord SCCa**: Deep invasion into PGS should be sought

<u>MR Findings</u>
- Low to intermediate T1, increased PD, bright on T2
- Homogeneous or heterogeneous enhancement on T1 C+ MR

<u>PET/SPECT-FDG</u>
- Most useful in post-laryngectomy patient where CT or MR is suspicious but definite for recurrent tumor

<u>Imaging Recommendations</u>
- Because of motion issues (breathing, coughing, swallowing), CECT is preferred imaging tool in staging SG-SCCa
- MR serves an adjunctive role in questions of cartilage invasion
- CT protocol: **2 pass technique**; stage primary and nodes
  - **1st pass**: Quiet respiration 3 mm axial scans from mandibular fillings to clavicles with maximum intravascular contrast
  - **2nd pass**: Breath-holding axial image set from hyoid to cricoid
    - Multiplanar reconstruction of this set in coronal plane best delineates craniocaudal spread of SG-SCCa

Differential Diagnosis: Endolaryngeal Mass
<u>Rheumatoid Arthritis of the Larynx</u>
- Crico-arytenoid swelling
- History of rheumatoid arthritis

<u>Chondrosarcoma</u>
- Tumor centered in thyroid or cricoid cartilage
- Chondroid calcifications confirm diagnosis

<u>Adenoid Cystic Carcinoma of Minor Salivary Gland</u>
- Very rare
- Indistinguishable on imaging from SG-SCCa

Supraglottic SCCa

Pathology

General
- Genetics
  - Allelic loss on chromosome 8 is an indicator of poor prognosis
- Embryology-Anatomy
  - The larynx is divided embryologically into two distinct parts
    - Supraglottic larynx: Vascular and lymphatic rich
    - Glottic-subglottic larynx: Vascular and lymphatic poor
  - Supraglottic larynx components:
    - PES is deep to epiglottis; PGS is deep to false cords
    - Laryngeal cartilages = thyroid, cricoid & arytenoids
- Epidemiology
  - Laryngeal SCCa = 2.5% of all cancers in men; 0.5% in women
  - > 95% of malignant tumors of the larynx are SCCa
  - 30% of all laryngeal SCCa are supraglottic
  - 35% have nodal metastases at presentation

Gross Pathologic, Surgical Features
- Poorly-marginated, ulcerative and/or indurated mucosal lesion

Microscopic Features
- Usually nonkeratinizing, moderately or poorly differentiated
- Squamous differentiation with intracellular bridges or keratinization

Staging Criteria: SG-SCCa Primary T Stage
- **T1** = Tumor in 1 laryngeal subsite with normal cord mobility
- **T2** = Tumor in > 1 subsite without laryngeal fixation
- **T3** = Endolaryngeal tumor with fixed cord ± post-cricoid or PES
- **T4** = Cartilage invasion ± extralaryngeal soft-tissue extension

Clinical Issues

Presentation
- Principal presenting symptom: Sore throat
- Other symptoms: Hoarseness, aspiration
- Classic patient profile: Male patient over 50 years with history of **alcohol** and **tobacco** use

Natural History
- Presents late with nodal disease because SG itself is clinically silent

Treatment
- Smaller tumors: Laser surgery or XRT only
  - Speech-preserving supraglottic laryngectomy may be used for isolated supraglottic lesions, without cord fixation
- Larger tumors: XRT and partial or total laryngectomy
- For clinically negative neck, some surgeons undertake complete bilateral neck dissections

Prognosis
- 5-year survival rate = 75% for all SG-SCCa
- Prognosis best for inferiorly located tumors (present earlier)

Selected References
1. Hicks WL et al: Patterns of nodal metastasis and surgical management of the neck in supraglottic laryngeal carcinoma. Otolaryngol Head Neck Surg 121:57-61, 1999
2. Mancuso AA et al: Preradiotherapy computed tomography as a predictor of local control in supraglottic carcinoma. J Clin Oncol 17:631-7, 1999
3. Castelijns JA et al: Imaging of laryngeal cancer. Semin Ultrasound CT MR 19:492-504, 1998

Glottic SCCa

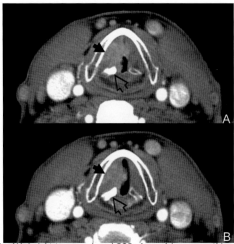

Glottic SCCa. (A) A right true vocal cord SCCa (arrow) is seen on this axial CECT at level of the glottis. Tumor abuts the arytenoid cartilage, causing sclerosis (open arrow). (B) Under surface of true vocal cord image shows right cord irregularity (arrow) and arytenoid cartilage sclerosis (open arrow).

Key Facts
- Definition: SCCa arising on the mucosal surface of the glottic larynx
  - **Glottis** = air space between the true vocal cords (TVC) is the strict definition; for imaging purposes = TVC including the anterior and posterior commissures
- Classic imaging appearance: Enhancing invasive mass of the TVC
- Other important facts
  - Although 60% of laryngeal SCCa are glottic, early glottic (G) SCCa are not imaged but instead are treated based on mucosal extent only
  - Larger G-SCCa are imaged to define submucosal extent and presence or absence of cartilaginous invasion

Imaging Findings
General Features
- Best imaging clue: Endoscopic assessment of mucosal extent of tumor; rendering your imaging report without this knowledge will lead to large errors in radiologic stage
- Moderately-enhancing invasive or exophytic mass centered on TVC
  - If anterior commissure > 1 mm thick, G-SCCa is there
- Glottic SCCa spread patterns
  - Anteromedial to anterior commissure
  - Posterior into arytenoids or cricoid cartilage, cricoarytenoid joint or posterior commissure (often leading to fixed cord)
  - Inferiorly into subglottis
  - Superiorly into supraglottic paraglottic space beneath false vocal cord
- Low incidence (≤ 10%) nodal disease at presentation
  - Secondary to relative lack of lymphatics

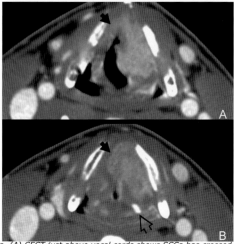

Glottic SCCa. (A) CECT just above vocal cords shows SCCa has crossed the anterior commissure to the anterior margin of the right cord (arrow). (B) CECT through glottis shows left cord SCCa has reached the arytenoid cartilage (open arrow). Right anterior cord invasion is again noted (arrow).

CT Findings
- Contrast-enhancing, soft-tissue, infiltrative or exophytic mass of TVC

MR Findings
- Low to intermediate T1 signal; high signal on T2
- Homogeneous enhancement on T1 C+ MR

Imaging Recommendations
- Because of motion issues (breathing, coughing & swallowing), CECT is preferred imaging tool in G-SCCa
- MR serves an adjunctive role in questions of cartilage invasion
- CECT protocol: **2 pass technique**; stage primary tumor and nodes
  - **1st pass**: Quiet respiration 3 mm axial images from mandibular fillings to clavicles with maximum intravascular contrast
  - **2nd pass**: Breath-holding axial image set from hyoid to cricoid
    - Multiplanar reconstruction of this set in coronal plane best delineates craniocaudal spread of G-SCCa

Differential Diagnosis: Invasive Lesions of Larynx
Wegener's Granulomatosis of Larynx
- Glottic and supraglottic thickening
- Present in association with renal, nasal & other areas of disease

Rheumatoid Arthritis of Larynx
- Crico-arytenoid swelling
- History of rheumatoid arthritis

Chondrosarcoma
- Tumor centered in thyroid or cricoid cartilage
- Chondroid calcifications confirms diagnosis

Pathology
General
- Embryology-Anatomy

Glottic SCCa

- o   TVC is relatively avascular and alymphatic
    - G-SCCa rarely spread to regional nodes
- Epidemiology
    - o   Laryngeal SCCa = 0.5% of all cancers
    - o   Over 95% of malignant tumors of the larynx are SCCa
    - o   60% of laryngeal SCCa are glottic

Gross Pathologic, Surgical Features
- Small tumor: Irregular area of mucosal thickening
- Large tumor: Ulcerating, invasive or exophytic mucosal lesion

Microscopic Features
- Usually keratinizing well-to moderately-differentiated SCCa

Staging Criteria for Primary Glottic SCCa
- **T1** = Limited to cord(s) with normal mobility
- **T2** = Extension (supraglottis ± subglottis) with impaired VC mobility
- **T3** = Limited to larynx with fixed vocal cord
- **T4** = Thyroid-cricoid cartilage invasion ± extralaryngeal soft tissues

Clinical Issues

Presentation
- Principal presenting symptom: Hoarseness
- Other symptoms: Change in the voice, sore throat
- Classic patient profile: > 50-year-old male with history of **tobacco** use; less commonly alcohol abuse
- Physical-endoscopic exam
    - o   Ulcerative mucosal lesion on TVC
    - o   Clinical blind spots for endoscopic examination include paraglottic space and cartilage invasion

Natural History
- G-SCCa spreads to contralateral TVC via anterior commissure
- If untreated, transglottic SCCa will result

Treatment
- Direct endoscopic evaluation preferred for mucosal involvement
- Smaller tumors (T1): Usually not imaged and can be treated with laser surgery or XRT only
- Higher stage, larger tumor: Combination of XRT and partial or radical laryngectomy
    - o   Inferior extension into subglottis necessitates total laryngectomy
    - o   Speech-preserving partial laryngectomy
        - Vertical laryngectomy: TVC lesions without fixation and less than 1/3 contralateral cord involvement

Prognosis
- T1, > 90%
- T4, 25% 5-year survival rate

Selected References
1. Barthel SW et al: Primary radiation therapy for early glottic cancer. Otolaryngol Head Neck Surg 124:35-9, 2001
2. Castelijns JA et al: Imaging of laryngeal cancer. Semin Ultrasound CT MR 19:492-504, 1998
3. Castelijns JA et al: MR imaging of laryngeal cancer. J Comput Assist Tomogr 11:134-40, 1987

Subglottic SCCa

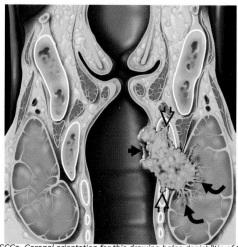

Subglottic SCCa. Coronal orientation for this drawing helps depict "tip of the iceberg" nature of subglottic SCCa. Mucosal lesion (arrow) can be seen at endoscopy but the cricoid cartilage (open arrows) and thyroid gland invasion (curved arrows) is only seen with cross-sectional imaging.

Key Facts
- Definition: SCCa involving mucosal surface of subglottis
  - **Subglottis** = mucosal surface extending from the inferior true vocal cords (TVC) to the lower border of the cricoid cartilage
- Classic imaging appearance: Enhancing, invasive mass centered below the glottis and above the inferior margin on cricoid cartilage
- Other important facts
  - Poor prognosis because lesion becomes large and invasive in this clinically silent area prior to discovery
  - **Alymphatic subglottis** means infrequent associated malignant adenopathy ($\leq$ 20%)

Imaging Findings
General Features
- Best imaging clue: Endoscopic assessment of mucosal extent of lesion provides the clinical stage of the primary tumor
  - Rendering an opinion regarding imaging stage of subglottic SCCa without knowledge of mucosal stage will lead to an incomplete or inaccurate assessment
- Any tissue seen on the airway side of the subglottic larynx should be considered tumor in this setting
- Subglottic SCCa spread patterns
  - Anterior through cricothyroid membrane into thyroid gland
  - Posterior into cricoid cartilage and esophagus
  - Cephalad to invade the TVC and supraglottis
  - Inferior into the tracheal lumen and cartilaginous rings
- Alymphatic subglottis leads to low incidence nodal disease ($\leq$10%)
CT Findings
- Contrast-enhancing mass centered below the TVC which may be invasive or exophytic

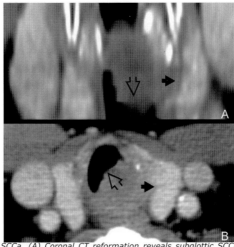

Subglottic SCCa. (A) Coronal CT reformation reveals subglottic SCCa extending inferiorly into trachea (open arrow) and laterally into the thyroid lobe (arrow). (B) Axial CECT through subglottis shows tumor encroachment on the tracheal lumen (open arrow) and invasion into thyroid lobe (arrow).

MR Findings
- Low to intermediate T1 signal; high signal on T2
- Heterogeneous enhancement on T1 C+ MR

Imaging Recommendations
- Inherent motion of the larynx makes CECT a better staging tool than MR for subglottic SCCa
  - Motion comes from breathing, coughing and swallowing
- MR advantages may give MR adjunctive role in complex cases
  - Better at detection cartilage invasion
  - Direct coronal images give craniocaudal extent
- CECT protocol: 2 pass method
  - 1st pass: Quiet respiration 3 mm axial images from mandibular fillings to clavicles with maximum intravascular contrast (node search)
  - 2nd pass: Breath-holding axial image set from hyoid to 2nd tracheal ring
    - Multiplanar reconstruction in the coronal plane gives best sense of craniocaudal extent of subglottic SCCa

Differential Diagnosis: Subglottic Mass
Chondrosarcoma
- Tumor centered in thyroid or cricoid cartilage
- Chondroid calcifications seal diagnosis

Adenoid Cystic Carcinoma of Minor Salivary Gland
- Indistinguishable by imaging from SCCa
- Very rare in this location

Pathology
General
- Embryology-Anatomy

Subglottic SCCa

- o Glottis and subglottis are embyrologically distinct from the supraglottic larynx
- o They are both relatively avascular and alymphatic
- Epidemiology
  - o Least common of laryngeal SCCa
  - o **5%** of laryngeal carcinoma cases are **subglottic**

Gross Pathologic, Surgical Features
- Usually large, exophytic, fungating mass

Microscopic Features
- Predominantly squamous differentiation with intracellular bridges or keratinization (and/or keratin pearls)
- Subglottic SCCa are more likely to be undifferentiated

T Staging Criteria
- **T1** = Tumor limited to the subglottis
- **T2** = Extends to vocal cords with normal or impaired mobility
- **T3** = Tumor limited to larynx with fixed vocal cord
- **T4** = Invasion of cricoid or thyroid ± extension into adjacent tissues

Clinical Issues

Presentation
- Principal presenting symptom: Stridor
- Classic patient profile: > 50 year old male smoker and/or drinker
- Other presenting symptoms: Dyspnea, hoarseness
- Usually patients > 50 years with history of alcohol and/or tobacco abuse
- Male > Female

Natural History
- Subglottic SCCa tend to remain clinically silent
- Invasion of surrounding tissues has occurred when discovered

Treatment
- Large tumors at presentation require total laryngectomy and XRT
- Subglottic stomal recurrences are common

Prognosis
- Overall 5-year survival is < 40% because of advanced disease at time of discovery

Selected References
1. Chiesa F et al: Surgical treatment of laryngeal carcinoma with subglottis involvement. Oncol Rep 8:137-40, 2001
2. Castelijns JA et al: Imaging of laryngeal cancer. Semin Ultrasound CT MR 19:492-504, 1998
3. Dahm JD et al: Primary subglottic cancer. Laryngoscope 108:741-6, 1998

Hypopharynx SCCa

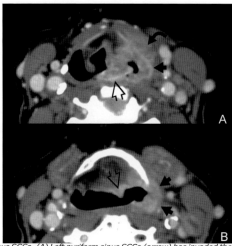

Pyriform sinus SCCa. (A) Left pyriform sinus SCCa (arrow) has invaded the aryepiglottic fold (open arrow) and the strap muscle (curved arrow) on this axial CECT. (B) Image above (A) shows typical posterolateral invasion of neck soft tissues (arrows). Open arrow: Aryepiglottic fold invasion.

Key Facts
- Definitions
  - Hypopharyngeal (HP)-SCCa = Primary SCCa originating on mucosal surface of any part of hypopharynx
  - **Hypopharynx** = Area between the floor of the oropharynx above, the supraglottic larynx anteroinferior and the cervical esophagus directly inferior; HP subsites include
    - **Pyriform sinus**
    - **Post-cricoid** region (pharyngo-esophageal junction)
    - Posterior hypopharyngeal wall
- Classic imaging appearance: Moderately-enhancing, infiltrating mass of subsite(s) of HP often with malignant adenopathy
- Other important facts
  - Like supraglottis, HP is lymphatic rich creating a high rate of malignant adenopathy at presentation (> 50%)
  - Most HP-SCCa found in pyriform sinus subsite (60%)

Imaging Findings
General Features
- Best imaging clue: Knowledge of clinical tumor stage as assessed by endoscopic examination will allow you to focus your imaging assessment to deep tissue beneath mucosal lesion
- Moderately-enhancing, invasive mass in HP with invasive patterns dependent on part of HP originating from
  - **Pyriform sinus SCCa**: Posterolateral spread into cervical soft tissues, eroding ipsilateral thyroid cartilage ala on its way there
  - **Posterior HP wall SCCa**: Infiltrates posteriorly into RPS, then PVS ± laterally into cervical soft tissues; RPS adenopathy common
  - **Post-cricoid HP SCCa**: Infiltrates anteriorly into larynx and inferiorly into cervical esophagus

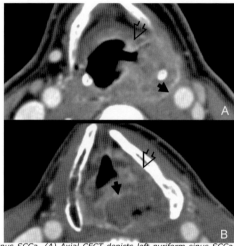

Pyriform sinus SCCa. (A) Axial CECT depicts left pyriform sinus SCCa with typical posterolateral soft tissue neck invasion (arrow) and aryepiglottic fold involvement (open arrow). (B) Paraglottic space (open arrow) and post-cricoid (arrow) invasion is seen on this more inferior CECT image.

- Overall, 50% of HP-SCCa have malignant nodes at presentation

CT Findings
- Moderately-enhancing, invasive mass involving pyriform sinus, posterior HP wall or post-cricoid HP
    - Pyriform sinus SCCa: Look for posterior thyroid cartilage destruction, invasion into neck to involve carotid space
    - Posterior HP wall SCCa: Look for invasion through deep layer of deep cervical fascia into PVS and RPS malignant adenopathy
    - Post-cricoid HP SCCa: Search for invasion into endolarynx with associated cricoid or thyroid cartilage destruction

MR Findings
- HP mass with low to intermediate T1 signal; high signal on T2
- Heterogeneous enhancement on T1 C+ MR

Imaging Recommendations
- Breathing, coughing and swallowing motions make CECT the preferred imaging tool for staging HP-SCCa
- MR serves an adjunctive role in determining cartilage invasion or soft tissue extent
- CT protocol: 2 pass technique; Stage primary and nodes
    - 1st pass: Quiet respiration 3 mm axial scans from mandibular fillings to clavicles with maximum intravascular contrast
    - 2nd pass: Breath-holding axial image set from hyoid to 1st tracheal ring; glottic angle (approximately 10 degrees to feet)
        - Multiplanar reconstruction in coronal plane best demonstrates craniocaudal spread of HP-SCCa

Differential Diagnosis: Hypopharyngeal Mass

Kaposi's Sarcoma
- AIDS-related malignancy
- Hypopharyngeal or oropharyngeal mucosal mass

Hypopharynx SCCa

- SCCa imaging mimic

Adenoid Cystic Carcinoma of Minor Salivary Gland
- Primary tumor indistinguishable from HP-SCCa
- Usually no malignant adenopathy at presentation

Pathology
General
- Embryology-Anatomy
  - HP is embryologically associated with the supraglottic larynx
  - Has same rich vascular-lymphatic architecture
- Epidemiology
  - 95% of HP tumors are SCCa
  - 60% pyriform sinus; 25% post-cricoid; 15% posterior wall

Gross Pathologic, Surgical Features
- Poorly-marginated ulcerative or exophytic mass of the HP

Microscopic Features
- Squamous differentiation with intracellular bridges or keratinization
- More aggressive than laryngeal SCCa; often of anaplastic histology

Staging Criteria: HP-SCCA Primary T Stage
- **T1** = Tumor limited to one subsite of HP and $\leq$ 2 cm
- **T2** = > 1 subsite or >2 cm, <4 cm without hemilarynx fixation
- **T3** = Tumor > 4 cm with hemilarynx fixation
- **T4** = Tumor invading local structures
  - Thyroid/cricoid cartilage, cervical soft tissues

Clinical Issues
Presentation
- Principal presenting symptom: Sore throat
- Other symptoms: Dysphagia, cervical pain
- Classic patient profile: Male smoker and/or drinker over age 50
- **Plummer-Vinson syndrome**: Female with postcricoid carcinoma with dysphagia, iron-deficiency anemia, weight loss and hypopharyngeal and esophageal webs

Treatment
- Surgical resection as possible combined with XRT
- When large, laryngopharyngectomy often necessary
- Posterior HP wall SCCa that violates the deep layer of deep cervical fascia (carpet) generally felt to be unresectable for cure

Prognosis
- Pyriform sinus > posterior HP wall > post-cricoid SCCa prognosis
- Post-cricoid SCCa worst prognosis, with 5 year survival <25%

Selected References
1. Pameijer FA et al: Imaging of squamous cell carcinoma of the hypopharynx. Semin Ultrasound CT MR 19:476-91, 1998
2. Zbaren P et al: Pretherapeutic staging of hypopharyngeal carcinoma. Clinical findings, computed tomography, and magnetic resonance imaging compared with histopathologic evaluation. Arch Otolaryngol Head Neck Surg 123:908-13, 1997
3. Ho CM et al: Squamous cell carcinoma of the hypopharynx: analysis of treatment results. Head Neck 15:405-12, 1993

Laryngocele

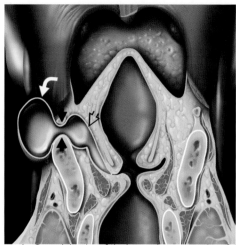

Mixed laryngocele. Coronal drawing of the larynx shows narrowing of the laryngeal ventricle yielding a mixed laryngocele with internal (open arrow) and external (curved arrow) components. Notice the isthmus (arrows) by the passage of the laryngocele through the thyrohyoid membrane.

Key Facts
- Synonym: Lateral saccular cyst, laryngeal mucocele
- Definitions
  - **Internal laryngocele** = Laryngocele confined to supraglottis, deep to the false vocal cord, in the paraglottic space
  - **Mixed (external) laryngocele** = Laryngocele with both internal and external components; lesion has herniated through the thyrohyoid membrane into the soft tissues of the anterior neck
  - **Pyolaryngocele** = Either internal or mixed superinfected laryngocele containing pus
  - **Secondary laryngocele** = Internal or mixed laryngocele resulting from inferior supraglottic or glottic SCCa obstructing the laryngeal ventricle; 15% of laryngoceles
- Classic imaging appearance: Cystic mass in paraglottic (internal) or submandibular (mixed) space

Imaging Findings
General Features
- **Internal (simple) laryngocele**: An air or fluid-filled cystic mass is **identified in the paraglottic space** of the supraglottis deep to the false vocal cord that can be followed down to the ventricle
- **Mixed (external) laryngocele**: An air or fluid-filled cystic mass seen in lower submandibular space directly adjacent to the thyrohyoid membrane; the **isthmus** (or waist) through the perforation in this membrane is usually readily identifiable
- Pyolaryngocele: Laryngocele wall thickening suggest this diagnosis
- Secondary laryngocele: Infiltrating mass in the low supraglottis or glottis is associated with an internal or mixed laryngocele
CT Findings
- Internal laryngocele: Low-density mass in paraglottic space

Laryngocele

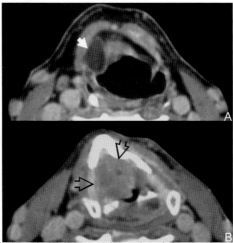

Secondary laryngocele. (A) CECT in axial plane through the supraglottic larynx shows an ovoid cystic mass (arrow) in the right paraglottic space. (B) The internal laryngocele seen in (A) is secondary to the large glottic SCCa (open arrows) seen in this axial CECT at the level of the glottis.

- Mixed laryngocele: Low-density, thin-walled mass seen in low submandibular space that can be followed into larynx
  o Internal component may be collapsed or dilated
- Pyolaryngocele: Thick, enhancing wall surrounds laryngocele

MR Findings
- Low T1, high T2, thin walled, cystic mass seen in the paraglottic space of the supraglottis (internal laryngocele); extends into soft tissues of neck (mixed laryngocele)
- Coronal images best display origin of laryngocele in the laryngeal ventricle; in mixed laryngocele coronal image shows connection between internal and external components

Plain Film
- Air pocket seen in upper neck soft tissues

Imaging Recommendations
- This is an easy radiologic diagnosis; just do not forget to look for the occult SCCa in the low supraglottis or glottic larynx!
- CECT of cervical neck = best imaging tool

Differential Diagnosis: Cystic Neck Mass, Hyoid Bone level

2nd Branchial Cleft Cyst
- Cystic mass posterior to submandibular gland at angle of mandible
- No connection to larynx

Thyroglossal Duct Cyst
- Midline cystic mass adjacent to mid-portion of hyoid bone
- May project in the midline into pre-epiglottic space

Hypopharyngeal Diverticulum
- Air or fluid-filled pseudopod projecting off the lateral hypopharyngeal wall

Laryngocele

Pathology
<u>General</u>
- General Path Comments
  - Laryngocele may be air, fluid or pus filled
  - The appendix of the laryngeal ventricle = saccule is the site of origin of laryngocele
- Etiology-Pathogenesis
  - Rarely congenital, commonly acquired
  - When the laryngeal ventricle or its more distal sacculus (appendix) is functionally obstructed because of increased intraglottic pressure (e.g., from excessive coughing, playing an instrument, or blowing glass), laryngocele develops
  - Obstruction of the proximal saccule by postinflammatory stenosis, trauma or tumor is a less common cause of laryngocele
  - With continued growth the laryngocele penetrates the thyrohyoid membrane to enter the neck in the lower submandibular space
- Epidemiology
  - Bilateral laryngoceles: 30%
  - Internal laryngocele twice as common as mixed laryngocele

<u>Gross Pathologic, Surgical Features</u>
- Smooth-surfaced, sac-like specimen

<u>Microscopic Features</u>
- Lined by respiratory epithelium (ciliated, columnar); fibrous wall

Clinical Issues
<u>Presentation</u>
- Principal presenting symptom
  - Internal laryngocele: Hoarseness
  - Mixed laryngocele: Submandibular mass
- Internal laryngocele: When small, often incidental and asymptomatic; larger lesions present with hoarseness or stridor
- Mixed laryngocele: Present with an anterior neck mass, just below the angle of the mandible which may expand with modified Valsalva
- More common in Caucasians
- Glass blowers, wind instrument players, chronic coughers
- Age at presentation: >50 years old

<u>Natural History</u>
- Gradual enlargement over time with continued ventricular pressure

<u>Treatment & Prognosis</u>
- Isolated internal laryngocele: Endoscopic laser therapy
- Mixed laryngocele: Requires an external surgical procedure

Selected References
1. Thabet MH et al: Lateral saccular cysts of the larynx. Aetiology, diagnosis and management. J Laryngol Otol 115:293-7, 2001
2. Alvi A et al: Computed tomographic and magnetic resonance imaging characteristics of laryngocele and its variants. Am J Otolaryngol 19:251-6, 1998
3. Glazer HS et al: Computed tomography of laryngoceles. AJR 140:549-52, 1983

ORAL CAVITY

Oral Cavity SCCa

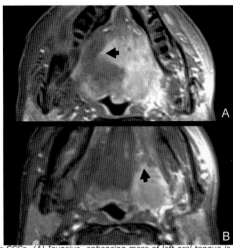

Oral tongue SCCa. (A) Invasive, enhancing mass of left oral tongue is seen on this axial T1 C+ MR image. Arrow: Tumor invasion across lingual septum. (B) Lower axial image shows the tumor primarily involving the lateral lingual tonsil, but spreading anteriorly into the posterior sublingual space (arrow) of the oral tongue.

Key Facts
- Definitions: Oral cavity (OC)-SCCa includes all epithelial tumors of epidermoid lineage arising in the oral cavity
  - **Oral cavity** = region anterior to the lingual tonsil of oropharynx
- Lip most common oral cavity primary site, followed by oral tongue
- SCCa accounts for 90% of neoplasms in oral cavity and oropharynx & 5% of malignant neoplasms in US
- Increased incidence in patients with tobacco and alcohol use/abuse

Imaging Findings
General Features
- Best imaging clue: Enhancing, invasive mass of mucosal surface
- Principal locations of primary where imaging is employed
  - Oral tongue: Floor of mouth invaded? Thick mylohyoid muscle?
  - Gingivobuccal sulcus: Is mandible invaded?
  - Retromolar trigone: Mandible ± masticator space/V3 invasion?
  - Hard palate: Maxillary sinus invasion? Perineural V2?
CT Findings
- Small lesions: Show mild asymmetry of mucosal surface
- Larger lesions: Show heterogeneity due to central necrosis
MR Findings
- SCCa usually shows low T1 and high T2 signal
- Avid enhancement on T1 C+ MR is expected
SPECT-FDG or FDG-PET
- Locate tumor when entirely submucosal (unknown primary search)
Imaging Recommendations
- MRI preferred imaging modality
  - Less affected by dental amalgam artifact than CT
  - Multiplanar capabilities + better contrast for primary evaluation
  - Mandibular marrow invasion assessment

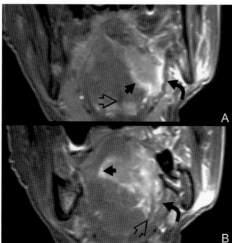

Oral tongue SCCa. (A) Coronal T1 C+ MR through posterior tongue reveals invasive tumor (arrow) spreading laterally to mylohyoid muscle (curved arrow). Open arrow: lingual septum. (B) More anterior image shows tumor crosses midline (arrow). Open arrow: hyoglossus muscle; curved arrow: mylohyoid muscle.

- CECT is excellent when dental amalgam artifact is not present
  - Preferred for evaluation of cortical bone invasion
  - Always attempt to angle sections around dental amalgam
- Radiologist interpretation affected by following important issues
  - Primary tumor (T) stage (see below)
    - Measure tumor and assess for deep invasion
  - Nodal (N) stage
    - Are metastatic nodes present?
  - Hard palate-maxillary alveolar ridge SCCa
    - Maxillary antrum invasion?
  - Retromolar trigone-faucial tonsil SCCa
    - Pterygoid musculature invasion, V3 perineural tumor?
  - Oral tongue SCCa
    - Extension into tongue root = floor of mouth?
    - Has the tumor crossed the lingual septum to involve the contralateral neurovascular bundle?

Differential Diagnosis: Oral Cavity Mass
Minor Salivary Gland Malignancy
- Invasive mass mimics OC-SCCa
- May require biopsy to differentiate

Pathology
General
- Genetics
  - Possible association with aberrations of chromosome 17
- Embryology-Anatomy
  - Oral cavity mucosal surface is defined as
    - Junction of the skin and vermilion border, anteriorly
    - Upper and lower gingival and buccal mucosa

- Mucosa overlying hard palate and alveolar ridges
- Oral (mobile) tongue (anterior 2/3 of the tongue)
  - Three potential spaces are defined in the OC
    - **Oral mucosal space** (all of above)
    - **Sublingual space** = superomedial to mylohyoid muscle, deep to the mucosal surface of the oral tongue
    - **Submandibular space** = inferolateral to mylohyoid muscle, deep to platysma muscle; only real fascia-defined space of OC
- Epidemiology
  - SCCa accounts for 90% of neoplasms in oral cavity and oropharynx
  - 5% of malignant neoplasms in US
  - 30-60% of cases have malignant nodes at presentation

Gross Pathologic, Surgical Features
- Usually presents as an ill-defined, ulcerative, mucosal lesion
- May be tan or white in color; exophytic and/or infiltrative

Microscopic Features
- OC-SCCa is defined as having squamous differentiation with intracellular bridges or keratinization (and/or keratin pearls)
- Further classified per amount of differentiation seen
  - Well, moderately or poorly differentiated

Primary Tumor (T) Staging Criteria in Oral Cavity
- **T1**: Tumor ≤ 2 cm in greatest dimension
- **T2**: Tumor 2-4 cm
- **T3**: Tumor > 4 cm
- **T4**: Tumor invading **adjacent structures**
  - Mandible, maxillary sinus, floor of mouth and skin

Clinical Issues
Presentation
- Principal presenting symptoms: Non-healing ulcer of oral mucosa
- Male > Female, usually > 40 yo

Treatment
- Most cases treated with surgery and/or XRT; chemotherapy alone has not been demonstrated to be effective
  - If oral tongue tumor has crossed lingual septum, usually means hemiglossectomy no longer a treatment option
  - Mandibular invasion requires cortical resection, partial or complete mandibulectomy depending on depth of invasion
  - Nodal involvement dictates extent of nodal dissection
    - Suprahyoid, conservative or radical neck dissection

Prognosis
- Most important prognostic factor = nodal stage
- Estimated over all 5-year survival of 50%

Selected References
1. Mukherji SK et al: Squamous cell carcinoma of the oropharynx and oral cavity: how imaging makes a difference. Seminars Ultrasound CT MR. 19:463-75, 1998
2. Sigal R et al: CT and MR imaging of squamous cell carcinoma of tongue and floor of the mouth. RadioGraphics 16:787-810, 1996
3. Muraki AS et al: CT of the oropharynx, tongue base, and floor of the mouth: normal anatomy and range of variations, and applications in staging carcinoma. Radiology 148:725-31, 1983

Sublingual Space Abscess

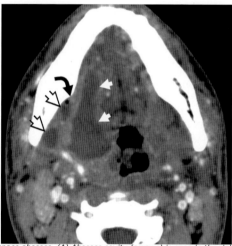

Sublingual space abscess. (A) Abscess cavity (arrows) is seen in the right sublingual space on this axial CECT through the oropharynx. The mylohyoid muscle (curved arrow) can be seen separating this abscess cavity from the more inferolateral submandibular space abscess (open arrows).

Key Facts
- SLS abscess the same as **Ludwig's angina**
  - Ludwig's angina is defined as diffuse, rapidly spreading, phlegmonous **cellulitis** of the soft tissues of the tongue, sublingual space (SLS) and submandibular space secondary to posterior molar infection
  - No abscess is seen with imaging in Ludwig's angina
- Primary cause is dental decay of premolar, canine or incisor with root abscess leading to mandibular osteomyelitis; rupture of root abscess above the mylohyoid line pours pus down the cephalad surface of the mylohyoid muscle into the sublingual space
- Sublingual space abscess when unilateral is a rim-enhancing pus collection superomedial to the mylohyoid muscle; when bilateral, SLS abscess has a "horseshoe" appearance

Imaging Findings
General Features
- Best imaging clue: Fluid in SLS
- Ipsilateral medial cortex of mandible may be dehiscent secondary to pus draining from an infected premolar, canine or incisor tooth
CT Findings
- Bone-only CT of oral cavity will show mandibular dental infection if present; root abscess, cortical dehiscence
- Enhanced CT shows a rim-enhancing cystic mass in the SLS often with extensive adjacent tongue and soft tissue cellulitis-edema
- If SLS abscess has spread to contralateral side, a "horseshoe" shaped cystic mass is seen
- Submandibular chain reactive adenopathy associated

Sublingual Space Abscess

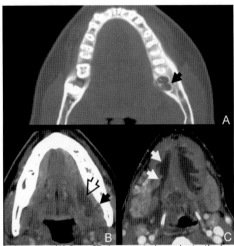

Bilateral SLS abscesses. (A) Bone CT shows posterior molar tooth absence (arrow). Medial wall of tooth socket is dehisced. (B) Axial CECT just inferior to (A) reveals a tract of pus (arrow) projecting into a SLS abscess (open arrow). (C) Abscess spreads to contralateral SLS (arrows).

MR Findings
- T1 C+ fat saturated coronal MR images reveal rim-enhancing low-signal mass superomedial to mylohyoid muscle in the SLS
- T2 MR images show lesion to be high signal (water intensity)
- Marrow of adjacent mandible will be abnormal if dental infection is source of abscess; MR misses submandibular duct calculus if small

Imaging Recommendations
- Contrast-enhanced CT reviewed in both soft tissue and bone algorithm-window is superior to MR in head and neck region
- Special dental CT algorithm that allows "Panorex-like" and 1 mm axial images enhances understanding of dental source of infection

Differential Diagnosis: Cystic Mass SLS

Epidermoid Cyst of SLS
- Unilateral low density/signal mass in SLS with thin, non-enhancing wall; no associated cellulitis-edema
- By imaging looks identical to simple ranula

Dermoid Cyst of SLS
- Unilateral mass in SLS with evidence of soft tissue and fat within its matrix; low density (CT) or high signal (T1 MR) is characteristic

Ludwig's Angina
- Cellulitis-edema seen in tongue, SLS and submandibular space without evidence for drainable pus
- 2nd or 3rd molar root abscess is causal in 90%

Simple Ranula
- Unilateral low density/signal mass in SLS with thin, non-enhancing wall (unless superinfected)
- By imaging looks identical to epidermoid cyst of SLS
- No associated cellulitis-edema in tongue or adjacent soft tissues

Sublingual Space Abscess

Sialocele of Submandibular Duct
- Enlarged proximal submandibular duct +/- obstructing calculus
- Fluid collection adjacent to duct in SLS without enhancing wall

Pathology
General
- Etiology-Pathogenesis
  o Premolar, canine or incisor tooth root abscess breaks out above the mylohyoid line of the medial mandible with pus then walled off in the SLS = SLS abscess
  o Suppurative sublingual sialadenitis with secondary abscess of SLS is a less common cause of SLS abscess
Gross Pathologic, Surgical Features
- Putrid-smelling abscess pocket is entered with a surgical drain
Microscopic Features
- Oral flora predominate: Streptococcus, Staphylococcus
- The abscess is usually a mixed culture of these with anaerobes

Clinical Issues
Presentation
- Principal presenting symptom: Sublingual swelling
- Older patients with bad dentition
- Painful tongue with dysphagia, dysphonia
- Elevation and backward displacement of the tongue may compromise the patient's airway
- History of recent oral antibiotic treatment common
Treatment
- Surgical drainage of abscess cavity with removal of infected tooth
- Intravenous antibiotics
Prognosis
- Prognosis for full recovery excellent

Selected References
1. Sumi M et al: Sublingual gland: MR features of normal and diseased states. AJR 172:717-22, 1999
2. Holliday RA et al: Imaging inflammatory processes of the oral cavity and suprahyoid neck. Oral Maxillofac Surg Clin N Am 4:215-40, 1992
3. Nguyen VD et al: MR: Ludwig angina: an uncommon and potentially lethal neck infection. AJNR 13:215-9, 1992

Submandibular Sialadenitis

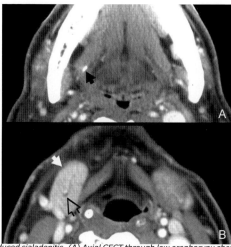

Calculus-induced sialadenitis. (A) Axial CECT through low oropharynx shows a calcified calculus (arrow) in the proximal right submandibular duct. (B) More inferiorly, right submandibular gland is enlarged and enhancing (arrow) indicating submandibular sialadenitis. Open arrow: Enlarged ductal hilum.

Key Facts
- Sialadenitis is 90% secondary to ductal calculus or stenosis
- Unrelenting submandibular gland (SMG) sialadenitis is treated with gland removal

Imaging Findings
General Features
- Acute or subacute sialadenitis: Unilateral enlarged SMG with associated ductal dilatation and ductal calculus or stenosis
- Chronic sialadenitis: Unilateral atrophic SMG with associated ductal dilatation with ductal calculus or stenosis

CT Findings
- Acute or subacute sialadenitis secondary to calculus: Unilateral enhancing enlarged SMG with large duct obstructed by stone
  - Sublingual space (SLS) cellulitis and myositis often present
- When no stone is visible but the duct has a transition zone from large to small, a search for anterior floor of mouth tumor is undertaken
  - In the absence of tumor, previous suppurative sialadenitis with ductal **stricture** is implicated

MR Findings
- Acute or subacute sialadenitis secondary to calculus: T1 C+ MR images with fat saturation shows unilateral enhancing SMG with large duct
  - SLS cellulitis and myositis often present
  - Stone may be missed if small

Imaging Recommendations
- Contrast-enhanced CT reviewed in both soft tissue and bone algorithm-window is superior to MR in head and neck infection
  - MR sialography can be used in this setting but CT is quicker
- Axial CT must be 3 mm or less not to miss small ductal calculi

Submandibular Sialadenitis

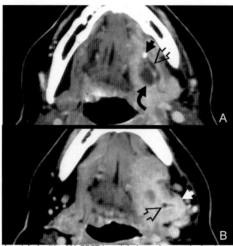

Submandibular sialadenitis. (A) CECT in axial plane shows calculus in submandibular duct (arrow) with proximal duct enlargement (open arrow) and SLS abscess (curved arrow). (B) Axial image below (A) reveals enhancing left submandibular gland (arrow) and enlarged ductal hilum (open arrow).

- Pre-contrast plain CT images are not required as density of ductal stones is different from small arteries in area
- Submandibular sialography no longer used
- **Radiologist questions** to answer at time of image interpretation
  - If stone is present, is it in the anterior or posterior SMG duct?
    - Anterior stones are removed per oral route
    - Posterior stones require removal of gland and ductal system
  - Is ductal stenosis present without calculus present?
    - Is either post-suppurative sialadenitis ductal stenosis vs. obstructing anterior floor of mouth tumor
  - Is the gland affected without ductal pathology?
    - Consider Sjogren's syndrome, AIDS or primary SMG infection

Differential Diagnosis: Submandibular Gland Mass
Reactive Submandibular Lymph Node
- SMS mass distinct from SMG with enhancing septa

Suppurative Submandibular Lymph Node
- SMS mass distinct from SMG with a fluid center

Ludwig's Angina
- Cellulitis-edema seen in tongue, SLS and submandibular space enveloping the SMG without evidence for drainable pus
- 2nd or 3rd molar root abscess is causal in 90%

BMT, Submandibular Gland
- Well-circumscribed mass projecting into SMS from within the SMG
- No fat plane can be seen between the SMG and the mass

Submandibular Gland Malignancy (ACCa or MECa)
- Infiltrating mass emanating from the SMG

Submandibular Nodal Metastases (SCCa or NHL)
- SCCa nodes: Primary SCCa is in oral cavity; central nodal necrosis is present in mass or masses distinct from SMG

- NHL nodes: Large, usually non-necrotic nodes in SMS; no enhancing septa within nodes seen

Pathology
General
- General Path Comments
  - SMG sialadenitis result from ductal obstruction from calculus, stenosis or anterior floor of mouth tumor
  - Primary glandular inflammation can be seen in Sjogren's syndrome, AIDS and bacterial or viral infection
- Etiology-Pathogenesis
  - Most common etiology: Calculus obstructs SMG duct with secondary sialadenitis that may become suppurative sialadenitis
  - Less common etiology: Suppurative sialadenitis causes SMG duct stenosis leading to chronic sialadenitis
  - Rare etiology: Primary glandular inflammation in Sjogren's syndrome, AIDS or bacterial or viral infection
- Epidemiology
  - Major salivary ductal calculi
    - 85% occur in SMG duct; 15% occur in parotid ductal system
  - 90% of all inflammatory disease of the SMG is sialadenitis

Gross Pathologic, Surgical Features
- At the time of SMG extirpation, acutely or subacutely inflamed gland is enlarged and annealed to surrounding soft tissue structures

Microscopic Features
- Acute and subacute SMG sialadenitis shows mostly parenchymal inflammation and lymphoid germinal centers
- Chronic SMG sialadenitis reveals predominantly atrophy and fibrosis

Clinical Issues
Presentation
- Unilateral, painful SMG swelling associated with eating or psychological gustatory stimulation = **salivary colic**
- Physical examination: If calculus is present in anterior SMG duct, may be palpable to bimanual examination

Treatment & Prognosis
- Standard surgical technique in unrelenting obstructive SMG sialadenitis is extirpation of submandibular gland
  - If offending calculus is in anterior duct, may be removed per oral without necessity of SMG removal
- When gland is inflamed in absence of ductal dilatation, antibiotics may preclude need for surgical therapy

Selected References
1. Ellies M et al: Surgical management of nonneoplastic diseases of the submandibular gland. A follow-up study. Int J Oral Maxillofac Surg 25:285-9, 1996
2. Holliday RA et al: Imaging inflammatory processes of the oral cavity and suprahyoid neck. Oral Maxillofac Surg Clin N Am 4:215-40, 1992
3. Aasen S et al: CT appearances of normal and obstructed submandibular gland duct. Acta Radiologica 33:414-9, 1992

Ranula

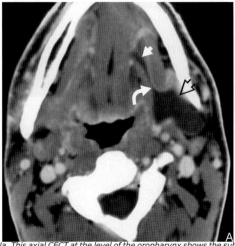

Diving ranula. This axial CECT at the level of the oropharynx shows the submandibular space aspect of the diving ranula (open arrow). The "tail" of the ranula (arrow) is seen within the sublingual space. Connection between the two areas (curved arrows) is at posterior margin of mylohyoid muscle.

Key Facts
- Definitions
  - **Simple ranula (SR)** = Postinflammatory retention cyst of the sublingual glands or the minor salivary glands of the SLS with an epithelial lining
  - **Diving ranula (DR)** = Plunging ranula = Extravasation pseudocyst; term used when a simple ranula becomes large and ruptures out the back of the SLS into the SMS to become a **pseudocyst** that lacks an epithelial lining
- Term ranula derives from the Latin **rana** for frog; the sublingual blebs in the frog's mouth resemble a simple ranula

Imaging Findings
General Features
- SR: Oval-lenticular **unilocular** mass confined to the SLS
- DR: Comet-shaped unilocular mass with its tail in the collapsed SLS and its head in the posterior submandibular space
  - **"Tail sign"** = collapsed SLS portion of DR
  - When large will involve the inferior parapharyngeal space
  - If plunges through mylohyoid muscle defect, may end up anterior to the submandibular gland

CT Findings
- SR: Low-density unilocular mass within the SLS with enhancing wall
- DR: Low-density unilocular multilobular mass emanating from the SLS and extending into the adjacent SMS and/or inferior PPS

MR Findings
- Well-defined, homogeneous masses with low signal on T1 C- and markedly high-signal on T2 MR images
- Even if uninfected, wall is enhancing on T1 C+ MR

Ranula

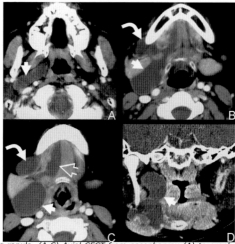

Giant diving ranula. (A-C) Axial CECT from nasopharynx (A) to oropharynx (B, C) shows a giant diving ranula in the parapharyngeal space (arrows), submandibular space (curved arrows) and sublingual space (open arrow). (D) Coronal CECT reveals parapharyngeal space cephalad extension (arrow).

Imaging Recommendations
- Enhanced CT is quickest and cheapest way to define the margins of a ranula; dental amalgam may degrade

Differential Diagnosis: Cystic Masses of SLS and/or SMS
Epidermoid of SLS
- Unilocular mass in SLS is radiologic mimic of simple ranula
Dermoid of SLS or SMS
- Mixed density/intensity mass with fatty component
2nd Branchial Cleft Cyst
- Round to oval unilocular mass in posterior SMS without SLS tail
Cystic Hygroma
- Multilocular transpatial mass filling space available
Suppurative Submandibular Lymph Node
- Multiple SMS nodes with intranodal fluid in clinical setting of infection
Ludwig's Angina
- Cellulitis-edema seen in tongue, SLS and submandibular space enveloping the Submandibular gland without evidence for drainable pus
- 2nd or 3rd molar root abscess is causal in 90%
Submandibular Gland Retention Cyst (Mucocele)
- Fluid bubble off margin of submandibular gland; no SLS tail

Pathology
General
- Etiology-Pathogenesis-Pathophysiology
  - Post-inflammatory or post-traumatic obstruction of sublingual or minor salivary glands of the SLS causes retention cyst formation
  - Rupture of the retention cyst (mucus escape reaction) into the subjacent SMS and low PPS creates a pseudocyst called a DR

Ranula

<u>Gross Pathologic, Surgical Features</u>
- SR: Fluctuant sublingual mass, often with a bluish color

<u>Microscopic Features</u>
- SR: Unilocular cystic lesion with an epithelial lining (squamous, cuboidal or columnar); cyst contains mucus-saliva
- DR: Pools of mucus surrounded by fibrous tissue, chronic inflammatory cells; **no** epithelial lining is present

Clinical Issues
<u>Presentation</u>
- Principal presenting symptom: Painless swelling of the SLS (SR) or of the SMS (DR).
- Median age at presentation is 30 years
- 50% have history of preceding trauma to the neck or oral cavity

<u>Natural History</u>
- If SR is left unattended, will continue to grow in SLS, then rupture into the subjacent SMS to become a DR

<u>Treatment</u>
- SR: Removal of the sublingual gland via an oral route
- DR: Removal of sublingual gland via a cervical approach
- Excision of the pseudocyst is unnecessary and places surrounding structures at risk of damage, but a biopsy of the pseudocyst wall is important to confirm the diagnosis

<u>Prognosis</u>
- Surgical excision yields permanent cure
- Transient lingual nerve damage during surgery

Selected References
1. Kurabayashi T et al: MRI of ranulas. Neuroradiology 42:917-22, 2000
2. Davison MJ et al: Plunging ranula: clinical observations. Head Neck 20:63-8, 1998
3. Coit WE et al: Ranulas and their mimics: CT evaluation. Radiology 163:211-6, 1987

Submandibular Gland BMT

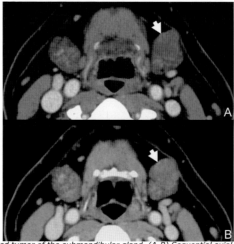

Benign mixed tumor of the submandibular gland. (A-B) Sequential axial CECT in low oropharynx shows a well-circumscribed mass (arrows) projecting from the anterior margin of the left submandibular gland. Notice the absence of a fat plane between the mass and the gland.

Key Facts
- Synonym: Pleomorphic adenoma
- Definition: Benign heterogeneous tumor of submandibular gland origin made up of an admixture of epithelial, myoepithelial and stromal components
- BMT is the most common tumor of the submandibular gland (SMG)
- Imaging shows a well-circumscribed intraglandular mass that pedunculates off the margin of the gland into the SMS when large
- BMT must be removed in total with the parent SMG and a collar of normal tissue to prevent tumor spillage
- If rupture of BMT capsule occurs at time of surgery, it may be years before the multifocal recurrent tumors are detected clinically

Imaging Findings
General Features
- Best imaging clue: Submandibular space mass
- Smaller BMT is solitary, ovoid, well-demarcated mass
- Larger BMT are multilobular with foci of necrosis, hemorrhage or focal calcification

CT Findings
- Smaller BMT: Smoothly marginated, homogenous, spherical mass that is higher density than the gland pre-contrast with mild to moderate enhancement when contrast is administered
- Larger BMT: Nonhomogeneous, lobulated, mixed-density mass with areas of lower attenuation representing foci of degenerative necrosis and old hemorrhage

MR Findings
- Smaller BMT: Sharply-marginated mass with low T1, high T2 signal
- Larger BMT: Inhomogeneous mixed T1 and T2 signal; multilobular
- Enhancement pattern: Variable; homogeneous enhancement

Submandibular Gland BMT

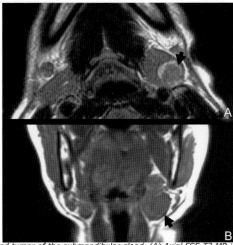

Benign mixed tumor of the submandibular gland. (A) Axial FSE-T2 MR image shows a well-demarcated mixed-intensity mass (arrow) projecting from the posterior margin of the left submandibular gland. (B) Coronal T1 MR reveals the mass (arrow) as lower signal than its associated submandibular gland.

Imaging Recommendations
- CECT or CEMR adequate for SMS mass evaluation
- Differentiation of submandibular space masses
  - In masses of the submandibular space, first decide if the mass is intrinsic to the submandibular gland (mucocele, **BMT**, ACCa or MECa) or is extrinsic to the gland (nodal)
  - If intrinsic to the gland, smaller BMT is easily recognized by its well-demarcated, homogeneous tissue appearance
  - Larger BMT may be difficult to tell from SMG malignancy because of its multilobular, inhomogeneous appearance on CT and MR imaging

Differential Diagnosis: Submandibular Gland Masses
Submandibular Gland Sialadenitis
- Acute or subacute: Enlarged gland that completely enhances, often with associated submandibular duct stone
- Chronic: Shrunken gland with little or no enhancement usually with associated submandibular duct stone
Mucocele of Submandibular Gland
- Well-circumscribed cystic mass emanating from the submandibular gland; may look like a bleb on the side of the gland
Malignant Tumor of Submandibular Gland (ACCa or MECa)
- Enhancing, invasive mass emanating from the submandibular gland
- Adjacent malignant adenopathy may be present

Pathology
General
- General Path Comments
  - 3 types of malignancies are associated with BMT
    - Carcinoma ex-pleomorphic adenoma (malignant mixed tumor)
    - Carcinosarcoma

- Metastasizing benign mixed tumor
  o If left untreated, 25% of BMT will undergo malignant transformation
    - Hence the surgical adage, "all salivary gland tumors must come out"
- Etiology-Pathogenesis
  o Benign tumor arising from intercalated duct-myoepithelial cell unit
- Epidemiology
  o 55% of tumors of the SMG are benign; 45% malignant
  o Distribution of BMT in major and minor salivary glands
    - **8%** of head and neck BMT arise in submandibular glands
    - 0.5% in sublingual glands
    - 85% in parotid glands
    - 6.5% in minor salivary glands on surface of nose, pharynx and tracheobronchial tree

Gross Pathologic, Surgical Features
- 1-4 cm mass growing out of the submandibular gland
- Tan-white, either encased in a fibrous capsule or well demarcated

Microscopic Features
- Interspersed epithelial, myoepithelial and stromal cellular components must be identified to diagnose BMT of SMG
- Epithelial elements may be glandular, ductal or solid
- SMG-BMT is more commonly encased in a **fibrous capsule**

Clinical Issues

Presentation
- Slowly-growing, painless mass in the SMS
- Clinical epidemiology
  o 2:1, female:male ratio
  o Most common age of presentation: > 40

Treatment
- Complete surgical resection of mass without spillage

Prognosis
- Recurrent tumor tends to be **multifocal**
- Recurrence will take years to develop because of slow growth rate

Selected References
1. Weissman JL et al: Anterior facial vein and submandibular gland together: predicting the histology of submandibular masses with CT or MR imaging. Radiology 208:441-6, 1998
2. Kaneda T et al: MR of the submandibular gland: normal and pathologic states. AJNR 17:1575-81, 1996
3. Weber RS et al: Submandibular gland tumors: adverse histologic factors and therapeutic implications. Arch Otolaryngol Head Neck Surg 116:1055-60, 1990

Submandibular Gland Carcinoma

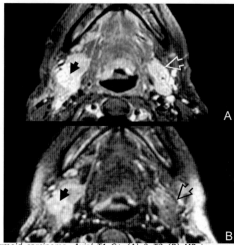

Mucoepidermoid carcinoma. Axial T1 C+ (A) & T2 (B) MR images through low oropharynx reveal an invasive mass projecting off posterior margin of the right submandibular gland (arrow). In absence of infectious symptoms, this mass is malignant until proven otherwise. Open arrows: Normal left submandibular gland.

Key Facts
- Definition: Two major carcinomas of the submandibular gland (SMG) are adenoid cystic carcinoma (ACCa) and mucoepidermoid Ca (MECa)
- Classic imaging appearance: Invasive mass arising from the submandibular gland (SMG) is carcinoma until proven otherwise
- Treatment: Wide surgical removal of tumor with post-operative radiation therapy is treatment of choice

Imaging Findings
General Features
- Best imaging clue: **Invasive mass** emanating from SMG
- Adjacent malignant adenopathy may be present (esp. with MECa)

CT Findings
- Enhancing mass with irregular borders arising from SMG
- Necrotic malignant adenopathy may be present

MR Findings
- Inhomogeneous signal intensity on T1 and T2 sequences
- Mass arising in the SMG with aggressive margins
- Inhomogeneous enhancement also expected

Imaging Recommendations
- CECT is recommended in the setting of submandibular mass since SMG sialadenitis with obstructing calculus is part of the differential diagnosis
- Long term (5-10 year) imaging follow-up recommended given the tendency of these tumors to recur late
- The radiologist and SMS masses
  - In masses of the SMS, first decide if the mass is **intrinsic** to the submandibular gland (mucocele, BMT, **ACCa** or **MECa**) or **extrinsic** to the gland (submandibular node)
  - If intrinsic to the gland, smaller carcinoma is recognized by its glandular invasion and its irregular surface anatomy

Submandibular Gland Carcinoma

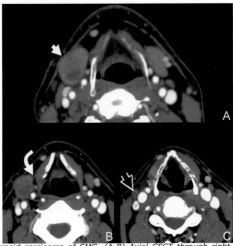

Mucoepidermoid carcinoma of SMG. (A-B) Axial CECT through right SMG shows enlargement of gland. Posteroinferior gland has an inhomogeneous mass (arrows) with irregular margins (curved arrow). (C) More inferior CECT reveals a small but necrotic malignant lymph node (open arrow) clinching malignant nature of mass.

- o Larger SMG carcinoma reveals ragged, irregular margins as it invades the fat of the SMS; malignant SMS nodes may be present

Differential Diagnosis: Submandibular Gland Masses
Submandibular Gland Sialadenitis
- Acute or subacute: Enlarged gland that completely enhances often with associated submandibular duct stone
- Chronic: Shrunken gland with little or no enhancement usually with associated submandibular duct stone

Mucocele (Retention Cyst) of Submandibular Gland
- Well-circumscribed, cystic mass emanating from the submandibular gland; may look like a bleb on the side of the gland

BMT of SMG
- Well-demarcated, solid, homogeneous, ovoid mass arising in the submandibular gland
- When large, lobulation occurs

Pathology
General
- General Path Comments
  - o Malignant tumors of SMG include ACCa, MECa and 3 types of BMT malignant transformations listed below
  - o ACCa specific comments
    - Pronounced tendency for perineural spread
  - o MECa specific comments
    - Tends to have associated malignant lymph nodes
  - o 3 types of malignancies are due to BMT transformation
    - Carcinoma-ex-pleomorphic adenoma (malignant mixed tumor)
    - Carcinosarcoma
    - Metastasizing benign mixed tumor

Submandibular Gland Carcinoma

- Carcinosarcoma
- Metastasizing benign mixed tumor
- Epidemiology
  - 45% of tumors of the SMG are malignant; 55% benign
  - Most common SMG carcinoma is ACCa (40%)

Gross Pathologic, Surgical Features
- Tan-white, infiltrating mass in SMS

Microscopic Features
- ACCa
  - Unencapsulated neoplasm with varied growth patterns consisting of cribriform, tubular and solid; individual tumors most commonly are composed of multiple growth patterns
- MECa
  - Malignant epithelial salivary gland tumor composed of a variable admixture of epidermoid, intermediate and mucous-secreting cells

Staging Criteria
- **T1**: Tumor $\leq$ 2 cm without extraparenchymal extension
- **T2**: Tumor 2-4 cm without extraparenchymal extension
- **T3**: Tumor 4-6 cm with extraparenchymal extension
- **T4**: Tumor > 6 cm and/or invades adjacent structures (mandible)

Clinical Issues

Presentation
- Painless submandibular swelling (same as BMT of SMG)

Treatment
- Surgical extirpation of tumor plus regional nodal dissection
- Post-operative radiotherapy routine

Prognosis
- 50% 5 year survival for all comers
- Metastatic disease accounts for 30% of deaths

Selected References
1. Camilleri IG et al: Malignant tumours of the submandibular salivary gland: a 15-year review. Br J Plast Surg 51:181-5, 1998
2. Weissman JL et al: Anterior facial vein and submandibular gland together: predicting the histology of submandibular masses with CT or MR imaging. Radiology 208:441-6, 1998
3. Kaneda T et al: MR of the submandibular gland: normal and pathologic states. AJNR 17:1575-81, 1996

Ameloblastoma

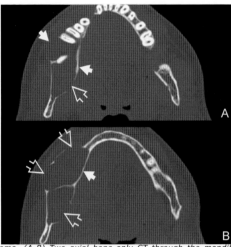

Ameloblastoma. (A-B) Two axial bone-only CT through the mandible reveal a multilocular, sharply-marginated, right-sided mass (arrows). Multiple areas of cortical dehiscence are evident (open arrows).

Key Facts
- Synonyms: Adamantoblastoma; adamantinoma
- Definition: Locally invasive, benign neoplasm, arising from the central mandibular or maxillary odontogenic epithelium
- Classic imaging appearance: Bubbly, multilocular, mixed cystic-solid mass in the posterior mandible-ramus associated with unerupted 3rd molar
- Unilocular and smaller multilocular ameloblastoma look very similar to dentigerous cysts and odontogenic keratocysts
  - Enhanced MR demonstration of **enhancing mural nodules** may differentiate ameloblastoma from these other lesions

Imaging Findings
General Features
- Mandible: Tumor tends to be confined by the thick cortex
  - Usually centered in the 3rd molar-ramus region
- Maxilla: Tumor more readily extends beyond bone into the maxillary sinus and nose because of the thin cortex of the maxilla
  - Usually centered in the premolar-1st molar region
  - Affects the maxillary sinus before the nose
CT Findings
- Uni- (20%) or **multilocular** (80%) with **scalloped borders**
- Bubbly pattern is typical but not pathognomonic
- Unerupted molar tooth association common
- Thinning of mandible or maxilla cortex is usually extensive
- Low-density, "osteolytic" lesion, such as ameloblastoma does not mineralize its matrix
- Enhanced CT
  - Smaller lesions with marginal enhancement only
  - Larger lesions with extraosseous extension show extensive soft tissue enhancement mixed with cystic low-density areas

Ameloblastoma

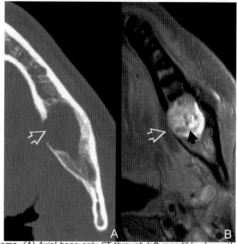

Ameloblastoma. (A) Axial bone-only CT through left mandible shows the tumor has dehisced the medial cortex (open arrow). (B) T1 C+ MR with fat sat reveals the tumor parenchyma enhances avidly. Open arrow: Mandibular cortical dehiscence.

MR Findings
- Smaller tumors show enhancing mural nodule
  - May represent "**tumor growth center**" which must be completely resected to achieve surgical cure
- High T2 signal helps differentiate from malignant tumors in larger lesions with extensive extraosseous components

Dental X-ray or Panorex
- Unilocular or multilocular radiolucent mass with scalloped borders

Imaging Recommendations
- Smaller lesions on Panorex: Enhanced thin-section CT best delineates both focal enhancing mural nodules as well as the tumor-bone relationships
- Larger lesions on Panorex: Enhanced MR imaging best defines the extraosseous components associations with critical neurovascular structures (especially true in maxillary tumors vs. sinus-nose-orbit)
  - Unenhanced, bone-only axial and coronal CT important adjunct

Differential Diagnosis: Mandibular Cystic Lesions

Dentigerous Cyst
- Unilocular cystic lesion surrounding the crown of a tooth
- No enhancing mural nodule

Odontogenic Keratocyst
- Unilocular or multilocular cystic lesion usually of the mandible associated with an unerupted tooth; no enhancing mural nodule
- Smaller, unilocular lesions indistinguishable from dentigerous cyst

Aneurysmal Bone Cyst
- Children more common than adults
- Large, round, multilocular mass with fluid-fluid levels
- No enhancing mural nodule

Ameloblastoma

Pathology
General
- General Path Comments
  - **Mandible to maxilla** ratio, **5:1**
    - Molar & ramus area > premolar area > symphysis
    - Unerupted 3rd molar tooth often a concurrent finding
  - Malignant transformation is rare (1%); referred to as **ameloblastic carcinoma**
- Etiology-Pathogenesis
  - Benign epithelial odontogenic tumor thought to arise from the ameloblast (epithelial cell in innermost layer of enamel organ)
- Epidemiology
  - Most common odontogenic tumor (35%)
  - 1% of all lesions of the mandible and maxilla

Gross Pathologic, Surgical Features
- Expansile, multilobular mass emanating from mandible or maxilla

Microscopic Features
- Unencapsulated
- Proliferating sheets or islands of odontogenic epithelium
- Odontogenic epithelium is made up of
  - Marginal, palisading, columnar cells with hyperchromatic, small nuclei arranged away from the basement membrane
  - Central, loosely-oriented cells confined by the columnar cells

Clinical Issues
Presentation
- Principal presenting symptom: Hard mandibular mass
- Other symptoms: Loose teeth, painless swelling
- Most commonly presents in 30-50 year olds

Natural History
- Slow growing, even indolent, benign neoplasm that takes years to become symptomatic in most cases

Treatment
- Conservative complete surgical excision when small
  - Curettement no longer acceptable therapy
- En bloc removal for larger lesions
- Chemotherapy and radiotherapy are contraindicated

Prognosis
- Tumor recurrence is common (33%) and may require a more aggressive second en bloc resection
  - Unilocular tumor occurs in a younger age group and recurs much less frequently (15%) than the multilocular group

Selected References
1. Reichart PA et al: Ameloblastoma: biological profile of 3677 cases. Eur J Cancer B Oral Oncol 31:86-99, 1995
2. Weissman JL et al: Ameloblastoma of the maxilla: CT and MR appearance. AJNR 14:223-6, 1993
3. Minami M et al: Ameloblastoma in the maxillomandibular region: MR imaging. Radiology 184:389-93, 1992

MASTICATOR SPACE

Masticator Space Abscess

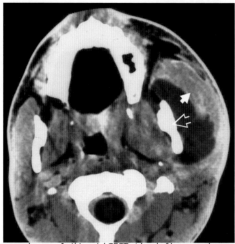

Masticator space abscess. In this axial CECT at level of low nasopharynx the abscess cavity can be seen widening the space between the more superficial masseter muscle (arrow) and the deeper ramus of the mandible (open arrow).

Key Facts

- Synonym: Odontogenous abscess in the masticator space (MS)
- Definition: Odontogenous infection= Originating in the teeth
- Classic imaging appearance = Walled-off fluid within the MS with associated molar root abscess & posterior mandibular osteomyelitis

Imaging Findings

<u>General Features</u>

- Anatomic considerations
  - Superficial layer of deep cervical fascia circumscribes the tissues of the MS
  - The MS contains the muscles of mastication, posterior body, ramus and condyle of the mandible, V3 as it passes into mandibular foramen
  - 2nd & 3rd molar abut the anterior surface of the MS
  - The **temporal fossa** is actually the **suprazygomatic MS**
  - The **infratemporal fossa** is the **nasopharyngeal MS**

<u>CT Findings</u>

- CECT shows focal fluid density within muscles of mastication with thick enhancing rim = MS abscess
  - Adjacent muscles are swollen, enhancing without fluid = myositis
  - Adjacent fatty planes are "dirty" = cellulitis
  - Linear markings in subcutaneous fat and thickening of skin when associated both help differentiate infection from malignant tumor
- Bone-only CT images show 2nd or 3rd molar root abscess with associated posterior mandibular body destructive change = **mandibular osteomyelitis**

<u>MR Findings</u>

- T1 low signal, T2 high signal in areas of abscess
- T1 C+ MR images show rim enhancing fluid collection
- Less sensitive to dental infection and osteomyelitis

Masticator Space Abscess

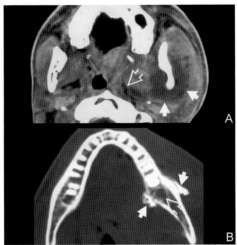

Masticator space abscess with mandibular osteomyelitis. (A) Axial CECT at level of nasopharynx shows masticator space abscess surrounding posterior mandibular ramus (arrows). Parapharyngeal space (open arrow). (B) Bone CT shows osteomyelitis of mandible (arrows). Open arrow: Empty molar socket.

Dental X-ray or Panorex
- Moth-eaten posterior mandibular body in vicinity of decaying molar tooth with associated root abscess

Imaging Recommendations
- In the setting of the acutely infected patient with trismus, limited jaw movement, CECT viewed in soft tissue and bone algorithm-window is best imaging approach
  - ○ Happens quickly, important for sick patient
  - ○ Shows extent of soft tissue abscess cavity
  - ○ Identifies offending tooth and extent of osteomyelitis if not blocked by dental amalgam artifact
- Questions for radiologist to answer while viewing scans
  - ○ Is mandibular osteomyelitis present? If so, requires more extensive surgical intervention and protracted antibiotic therapy
  - ○ Is the MS the only space with abscess? In general, surgeon needs one drain in per space or break through adjacent fascia
  - ○ Is the suprazygomatic MS involved? Infection tends to spread upward because the fascia is firmly attached to the under-surface of the mandible below

Differential Diagnosis: MS Mass

Masticator Muscle Hypertrophy
- The masticator muscles on one side are enlarged but lack focal rim-enhancing fluid or other cellulitis, myositis or fasciitis

Cellulitis-Phlegmon of MS
- The MS is swollen with cellulitis, myositis and/or fasciitis without focal rim-enhancing fluid

Masticator Space Abscess

Sarcoma of MS
- Infiltrating tissue density/intensity mass within MS with significant enhancement and minimal adjacent skin or soft tissue changes (lacks cellulitis, myositis or fasciitis) to suggest infection

Pathology
General
- Etiology-Pathogenesis
  - Dental infection (molar) or dental manipulation results in osteomyelitis of posterior body of mandible with cortical dehiscence placing pus within masticator space
- Epidemiology
  - Much less frequent infectious complication of dental decay in countries where antibiotics and dental care is readily available

Gross Pathologic, Surgical Features
- Irregular cystic lesion filled with green and white thick fluid surrounded by a thick wall made up of fibrous connective tissue
- Surrounding tissues are edematous

Microscopic Features
- Pus within the abscess cavity is made up of necrotic debris, polymorphonuclear leukocytes, lymphocytes and macrophages
- The abscess wall contains granulation tissue (capillaries, fibroblasts) and fibrous connective tissue (fibroblasts, collagen fibers)

Clinical Issues
Presentation
- Principal presenting symptoms: **Trismus**
- Fever, high white blood cell count
- Tender, swollen cheek
- History of bad dentition or dental manipulation common
- Physical exam: Tenderness and limited mouth opening makes PE difficult; CT becomes critical to assess pathology

Natural History
- Previous oral antibiotic treatment has inadequately treated simmering MS infection
- After termination of oral antibiotic, clinical recrudescence occurs

Treatment
- Surgical drainage combined with intravenous antibiotics
- Mandibular osteomyelitis may require subperiosteal drain and prolonged intravenous antibiotics

Prognosis
- Adequate drainage of pus loculi leads to rapid cure

Selected References
1. Yonetsu K et al: Deep facial infections of odontogenic origin: CT assessment of pathways of space involvement. AJNR 19:123-8, 1998
2. Curtin HD: Separation of the masticator space from the parapharyngeal space. Radiology 163:195-204, 1987
3. Hardin CW et al: Infection and tumor of the masticator space: CT evaluation. Radiology 157:413-7, 1986

Sarcoma of Masticator Space

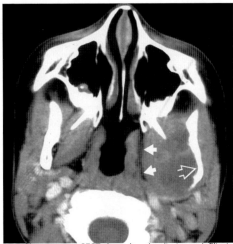

Masticator space fibrosarcoma. CECT shows low-density tumor infiltrates left medial masticator space, pushing the parapharyngeal space (arrows) posteromedially and eroding the inner table of the mandibular ramus (open arrow).

Key Facts
- Most common primary tumor of masticator space (MS) is sarcoma
- Sarcoma (MS) types: Osteosa, chondrosa, fibrosa, rhabdomyosa and Ewing's sarcoma
- Classic imaging appearance: Infiltrating mass in tissues of MS with associated mandibular destruction
  - Osteosa: Osseous matrix
  - Chondrosa: Chondroid calcifications

Imaging Findings
General Features
- Best imaging clue: Invasive mass in MS with mandibular destruction associated
- Osteosa & Ewing's Sarcoma: Arises from posterior mandible and ramus
- Chondrosa: Arises from TMJ, emanates inferiorly into MS
- Rhabdomyosa: Arises from muscles of mastication in children

CT Findings
- Osteosa: Tumor new bone in matrix (75%)
- Chondrosa: Cartilaginous calcifications in tumor matrix (50%)
- Fibrosa, rhabdomyosa, Ewing's: No osseous or calcified matrix

MR Findings
- Invasive mass of the muscles of mastication and posterior body-ramus of mandible
- Perineural tumor climbing V3 through foramen ovale may be seen
- Ossific or calcific matrix usually poorly seen with MR

Imaging Recommendations
- Enhanced MR imaging best delineates deep tissue extent and perineural tumor
- Bone-only unenhanced CT may be important to define bony destruction-involvement and type of tumor matrix if present

Sarcoma of Masticator Space

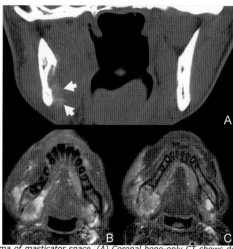

Osteosarcoma of masticator space. (A) Coronal bone-only CT shows destruction of mandible by a mass with tumor new bone in its matrix (arrows). (B & C) Osteosarcoma is seen arising from the mandibular ramus and body, spreading centrifugally into masticator space on these T1 C+ fat sat MR images.

Differential Diagnosis: Destructive Mass in MS

General Comment
- In the absence of tumor matrix ossification or calcification, sarcoma of the MS cannot be differentiated from NHL or metastatic tumor

Abscess of MS
- Septic patient with focal fluid in MS and wall enhancement
- Extensive associated inflammatory changes of skin, subcutaneous tissues; myositis, fasciitis and cellulitis

SCCa of Tonsil or Retromolar Trigone, Invasive
- Known mucosal tumor invades MS from mucosal surface

Non-Hodgkin Lymphoma
- If not associated with NHL of Waldeyer's ring and/or nodes, a primary focus of extranodal, extralymphatic NHL in MS is indistinguishable from non-matrix forming MS sarcoma

Metastatic Tumor
- If singular with clinically occult primary tumor, indistinguishable from non-matrix forming MS sarcoma

Pathology

General
- Etiology-Pathogenesis
  - Sarcoma arising from mandibular bone (osteosa or Ewing's), cartilage of TMJ (chondrosa), muscles of mastication (rhabdomyosa, fibrosa)
- Epidemiology
  - Osteosarcoma most common followed by chondrosarcoma
  - Rhabdomyosarcoma most common in children
  - Fibrosarcoma and Ewing's sarcoma very rare in MS

Microscopic Features
- Osteosa: Sarcoma stroma admixed with osteoid

Sarcoma of Masticator Space

- Chondrosa: Chondrocyte infiltrate with hyperchromatic, pleomorphic nuclei, prominent nucleoli, multinucleated cells
- Rhabdomyosa: Rhabdomyoblasts with wide range of appearances
- Fibrosa: Spindle-shaped cellular infiltrate with scanty cytoplasm

Staging Criteria: Sarcoma of Bone (Osteosa, Chondrosa, Ewing's)
- Stage **IA**: Low-grade, confined within cortex
- Stage **IB**: Low-grade, invades beyond cortex
- Stage **IIA**: High-grade, confined within cortex
- Stage **IIB**: High-grade, invades beyond cortex
- Stage **III**: Not defined
- Stage **IVA**: Regional lymph nodes positive
- Stage **IVB**: Distant metastasis

Staging Criteria: Soft Tissue Sarcoma (Fibrosa, Rhabdomyosa)
- Stage **IA**: Low-grade, small (< 5 cm), superficial and deep lesion
- Stage **IB**: Low-grade, large (> 5 cm), superficial lesion
- Stage **IIA**: Low-grade, large (>5 cm), deep lesion
- Stage **IIB**: High-grade, small, superficial and deep lesion
- Stage **IIC**: High-grade, large, superficial lesion
- Stage **III**: High-grade, large, deep lesion
- Stage **IV**: Any of above with any metastasis

Clinical Issues

Presentation
- Principal presenting symptom: Painless swelling of the jaw and cheek
- Other symptoms: Loss of molar teeth; chin numbness

Natural History
- Depends on sarcoma grade; high grade = undifferentiated sarcoma grows rapidly and results in patient demise within months

Treatment
- Wide surgical excision + postoperative radiotherapy

Prognosis
- Osteosarcoma: 33% 5 year survival
- Chondrosarcoma: 45% 5 year survival

Selected References
1. Patel SC et al: Sarcomas of the head and neck. Top Magn Reson Imaging 10:362-75, 1999
2. Wanebo HJ et al: Head and neck sarcoma: report of the Head and Neck Sarcoma Registry. Society of Head and Neck Surgeons Committee on Research. Head Neck 14:1-7, 1992
3. Hardin CW et al: Infection and tumor of the masticator space: CT evaluation. Radiology 157:413-7, 1986

PAROTID SPACE

Benign Lymphoepithelial Lesions

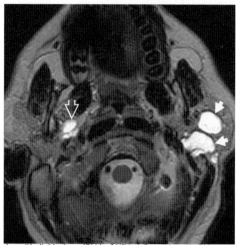

Benign lymphoepithelial lesions (BLL) of HIV. A Parotid cystic BLL are seen as high-signal intraparotid foci (arrows) on the left. Right parotid BLL are in deep lobe (open arrow) projecting into subjacent parapharyngeal space.

Key Facts
- Synonym: AIDS-related parotid cysts (ARPCs)
  - Since the patient need only be HIV+ to manifest this finding, this synonym probably should be avoided
- Definition: BLL-HIV = Mixed cystic-solid and cystic lesions found bilaterally in parotid glands in HIV+ patients
- Classic imaging appearance: Multiple mixed and cystic masses enlarging both parotid glands associated with tonsillar hyperplasia and cervical reactive-appearing adenopathy
- Treatment: Current antiretroviral drug therapy regimens are effective in diminishing this uncomfortable, cosmetic problem in > 80% of cases

Imaging Findings
General Features
- Best imaging clue: Bilateral parotid masses of cystic and mixed cystic-solid appearance
- Other complementary imaging findings include **cervical adenopathy, adenoidal, faucial** and **lingual tonsillar hypertrophy**
CT Findings
- CECT shows bilateral parotid enlargement secondary to a mixture of cystic and mixed cystic-solid lesions
- Non-necrotic cervical adenopathy with tonsillar hypertrophy can be an important clue to the BLL-HIV diagnosis with CT
MR Findings
- Cystic lesions: Low T1, high T2 with rim enhancement on T1 C+
- Mixed lesions: Mixed low, intermediate and high T1 may be seen in the same lesion; T2 signal may be intermediate or high
US Findings
- Wide spectrum of sonographic findings ranging from simple cysts to mixed masses with predominantly solid components

Benign Lymphoepithelial Lesions

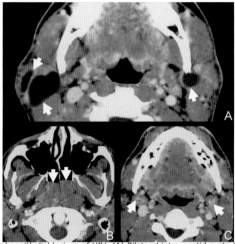

Benign lymphoepithelial lesions of HIV. (A) Bilateral intraparotid cysts (arrows) are identified on axial CECT. (B) Adenoid hyperplasia (arrows). (C) Reactive-appearing adenopathy (arrows). The triad of parotid cysts, adenoid hyperplasia and reactive adenopathy should suggest BLL-HIV to the imager.

- o Cystic lesions were not purely anechoic, often containing thin septa supplied by vessel pedicles; 40% had mural nodules
- o Mixed nodules may resemble parotid neoplasm

Imaging Recommendations
- CECT or CEMR from skull base to clavicles both will give the signature findings of bilateral parotid masses, tonsillar hyperplasia and cervical adenopathy

Differential Diagnosis: Bilateral Parotid Space Masses

Sjögren's Syndrome
- Clinical setting is compelling: Older women with Sicca syndrome (dry eyes, dry mouth, dry skin) and a connective tissue disorder (rheumatoid arthritis); antinuclear antibodies present
- Imaging picture may be identical to BLL-HIV

Sarcoidosis
- Extremely rare manifestation of sarcoidosis
- Cervical and mediastinal lymph nodes
- Imaging picture may be identical to BLL-HIV

Warthin's Tumor
- 20% are multiple, solid or mixed cystic-solid parotid masses
- Nodular walls; maximum of 2 lesions, unilateral or bilateral
- Lacks associated tonsillar hyperplasia and cervical adenopathy

NHL in Parotid Nodes
- Bilateral solid nodal-appearing masses in parotid
- Chronic systemic NHL is already apparent

Metastatic Disease to Parotid Glands
- Bilateral single or multiple parotid masses with invasive margins
- Primary malignancy and other nodal deposits already apparent

Benign Lymphoepithelial Lesions

Pathology
General
- Etiology-Pathogenesis
  - Hypothesis 1: Periductal lymphoid aggregates cause ductal radicular obstruction, periductal atrophy and distal cyst formation
  - Hypothesis 2: Cyst formation occurs in the included glandular epithelium within intraparotid nodes, so called "cystification"
- Epidemiology
  - 5% of HIV + patients develop BLL of parotids

Gross Pathologic, Surgical Features
- Diffusely enlarged parotid glands with multiple well-delineated nodules with a rubbery consistency and a smooth, tan-white, fleshy appearance

Microscopic Features
- Thin, smooth-walled cysts measuring a few mm to 3-4 cm
- Aspiration of cyst fluid reveals foamy macrophages, lymphoid and epithelial cells and multinucleated giant cells
  - Intense immunoexpression of S-100 and p24 (HIV-1) protein is present in the multinucleated giant cells

Clinical Issues
Presentation
- Principal presenting symptom: Bilateral parotid masses in HIV+ patient
- Other symptoms: Tonsillar hypertrophy + cervical reactive adenopathy
- Initially seen in HIV+ patients prior to AIDS onset

Natural History
- Left untreated, will grow to reach a chronic, mumps-like state with significant bilateral parotid enlargement
- Rarely may transform into B-cell lymphoma

Treatment
- Combination antiretroviral therapy for HIV tends to also completely or partially treat BLL-HIV of the parotid glands
- Radiotherapy has yielded mixed, non-lasting regression

Prognosis
- Patients' prognosis is dependent on their other HIV and AIDS-related diseases, not on BLL-HIV

Selected References
1. Holliday RA et al: Benign lymphoepithelial parotid cysts and hyperplastic cervical adenopathy in AIDS-risk patients: a new CT appearance. Radiology 168:439-41, 1998
2. Som PM et al: Nodal inclusion cysts of the parotid gland and parapharyngeal space: a discussion of lymphoepithelial, AIDS-related parotid, and branchial cysts, cystic Warthin's tumors, and cysts in Sjögren's syndrome. Laryngoscope 105:1122-8, 1995
3. Kirshenbaum KJ et al: Benign lymphoepithelial parotid tumors in AIDS patients: CT and MR findings in nine cases. AJNR 12:271-4, 1991

Sjogren's Syndrome

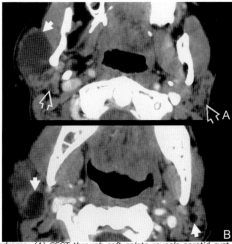

Sjogren syndrome. (A) CECT through soft palate reveals parotid cyst (arrow) and solid lesions (open arrows). (B) Bilateral cysts (arrows) are seen on this lower CECT image. Large cysts and lymphoid aggregates seen in a smaller, scarred parotid signals the process is chronic and severe.

Key Facts
- Synonym: Sicca syndrome
- Definition: Chronic systemic autoimmune exocrinopathy that causes salivary and lacrimal glands tissue destruction
  - Primary Sjogren's Syndrome (SjS) = Dry eyes and mouth; no collagen vascular disease (CVD)
  - Secondary SjS = Dry eyes and mouth with CVD
- Classic imaging appearance
  - Early: Diffuse bilateral small cysts (dilated distal ducts)
  - Late: Larger cystic (parenchymal destruction) and solid masses (lymphocyte aggregates) in both parotids

Imaging Findings
General Features
- Imaging appearance depends on the stage of disease and the presence or absence of lymphocyte aggregates within the parotid
  - Any stage may have solid pseudotumorous masses within the parotid glands secondary to lymphocytic accumulation
- Stage I SjS shows **punctate** cystic foci throughout enlarged parotid glands ≤ 1 mm
- Stage II SjS reveals diffuse **globular** cystic foci 1-2 mm
- Stage III SjS shows > 2 mm cystic lesions
- Stage IV SjS demonstrates **destructive areas** within the parotid gland parenchyma
- Invasive parotid mass and/or cervical adenopathy may signal malignant transformation of SjS
CT Findings
- CECT ranges from characteristic early diffuse 1 mm fluid density cystic lesions through late macrocystic change that may mimic BLL-HIV
- Punctate calcification may be diffusely present in both parotids

Sjogren's Syndrome

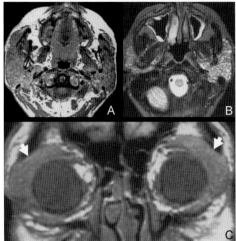

Sjogren syndrome with NHL. (A) T1 MR image shows many small, low-signal cysts within both enlarged parotids. (B) On T2 image cysts become high signal. (C) Coronal T1 image in same patient's orbit reveals both lacrimal glands to be enlarged (arrows) and infiltrated by NHL.

MR Findings
- Diffuse, bilateral low T1, high T2 1-2 mm foci (Stage I & II)
- Multiple high T2 signal > 2 mm foci (Stage III & IV)

Ultrasound Findings
- 1 mm or less punctate cystic changes (Stage I) may be missed
- Stage II-IV changes readily apparent on parotid ultrasound

Conventional Sialography & MR Sialography
- Equally sensitive to diagnosis of SjS
- Both will stage the severity of SjS
- Display punctate, globular, cavitary or destructive parotid distal ductal changes of SjS as contrast collections or focal high T2 signal

Imaging Recommendations
- MR with MR sialography single best imaging test if SjS is suspected
- Allows both cross-sectional analysis and MR sialography staging

Differential Diagnosis: Bilateral Parotid Cystic Masses

Benign Lymphoepithelial Lesions-HIV
- Mixed cystic-solid and cystic masses enlarging both parotids
- Tonsillar hyperplasia and cervical reactive-appearing adenopathy

Sarcoidosis
- Extremely rare manifestation of sarcoidosis
- Cervical and mediastinal lymph nodes
- Mixed cystic-solid and cystic masses enlarging both parotids with associated reactive-appearing cervical adenopathy

Warthin's Tumor
- 20% are multiple, solid or mixed cystic-solid parotid masses
- Nodular walls; maximum of 2 lesions, unilateral or bilateral
- Lacks associated tonsillar hyperplasia and cervical adenopathy

NHL in Parotid Nodes
- Bilateral, solid, nodal-appearing masses in parotid

Sjogren's Syndrome

- Chronic systemic NHL may already be apparent

Metastatic Disease to Parotid Glands
- Bilateral single or multiple parotid masses with invasive margins
- Primary malignancy and other nodal deposits already apparent

Pathology
General
- Etiology-Pathogenesis
  - ○ Autoimmune dysregulation leads to destruction of the acinar cells and ductal epithelia of the lacrimal and salivary glands
  - ○ Activated lymphocytes selectively home in on the lacrimal and salivary glands leading to tissue damage
- Epidemiology
  - ○ Incidence of SjS is about 0.5%

Gross Pathologic, Surgical Features
- Enlarged parotid glands with multiple small to large cysts

Microscopic Features
- Labial biopsy: CD4 positive T-cell lymphocytes
- Periductal lymphocytic infiltration and epimyoepithelial islands
  - ○ Lymphocytic infiltration obstructs intercalated ducts

Staging Criteria (Based on Conventional or MR Sialography)
- Stage **I**: **Punctate** contrast material/high signal ≤ 1 mm
- Stage **II**: **Globular** contrast material/high signal 1-2 mm
- Stage **III**: **Cavitary** contrast material/high signal > 2 mm
- Stage **IV**: Complete **destruction** of parotid gland parenchyma

Clinical Issues
Presentation
- Middle-aged to older women with firm swelling of both parotids
- Dry eyes, dry mouth, dry skin; connective tissue disorder
  - ○ Rheumatoid arthritis >> systemic lupus erythematosus > progressive systemic sclerosis
  - ○ Requires positive labial biopsy or autoantibody against Sjogren's associated A or B antigen for diagnosis to be assigned
- Schirmer's test is positive (decreased tear production)

Natural History
- Slowly progressive syndrome that evolves over years

Treatment
- Symptomatic unless bacterial superinfection requires parotidectomy

Prognosis
- **NHL** may complicate this otherwise chronic illness
- Intraparotid or GI locations most common sites of NHL

Selected References
1. Ohbayashi N et al: Sjogren syndrome: comparison of assessments with MR sialography and conventional sialography. Radiology 209:683-8, 1998
2. Izumi M et al: MR imaging of the parotid gland in Sjogren's syndrome: a proposal for new diagnostic criteria. AJR 166:1483-7, 1996
3. Takashima S et al: Sjorgren syndrome: comparison of sialography and ultrasonography. J Clin Ultrasound 20:99-109, 1992

Benign Mixed Tumor, PS

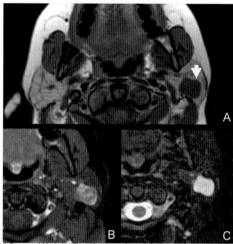

BMT, Parotid Space. (A) Axial T1 MR through oropharynx shows sharply marginated left intraparotid mass (arrow) with signal similar to muscle. (B) Magnified T1 C+ with fat saturation of BMT reveals inhomogeneous enhancement. (C) Magnified T2 images demonstrates uniform high signal.

Key Facts
- Synonym: Pleomorphic adenoma
- Definition: Benign heterogeneous tumor of parotid gland origin made up of an admixture of epithelial, myoepithelial and stromal components
- Classic imaging appearance
  - Small benign mixed tumor (BMT): Sharply-marginated, ovoid mass with uniform parenchymal enhancement
  - Large BMT: Lobulated mass with inhomogeneous enhancement
- BMT is the **most common parotid space (PS) mass** (80%)

Imaging Findings
General Features
- Best imaging clue: Ovoid, well-circumscribed, intraparotid mass
- May be found in parotid tail, superficial or deep lobe
- Small BMT: Appears as a sharply-circumscribed mass surrounded on all sides by parotid gland with homogeneous parenchyma
- Large BMT of the deep lobe: Multilobular, inhomogeneous mass that widens the stylomandibular notch as it pushes the parapharyngeal space medially; characteristic pear shape
  - May grow quite large before being discovered clinically
- Multicentric BMT very rare (cf. 20% Warthin's multicentricity)
CT Findings
- Small BMT: Smoothly marginated, homogenous, spherical mass that is higher density than the gland pre-contrast with mild to moderate contrast enhancement
- Larger BMT: Inhomogeneous, lobulated, mixed-density mass with areas of lower attenuation representing foci of degenerative necrosis and old hemorrhage
- Dystrophic calcification is rare

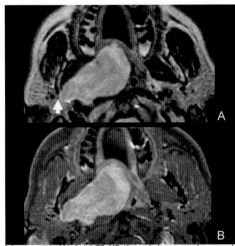

BMT, deep lobe parotid. (A) Axial T2 MR through low nasopharynx shows a pear-shaped well-delineated mass projecting from deep lobe of parotid gland medially. No fat separates the mass from deep lobe tissue (arrow). (B) T1 C+ with fat saturation MR images shows avid BMT enhancement with mild inhomogeneity.

MR Findings
- Small BMT: Sharply-marginated mass with low T1, high T2 signal
- Large BMT: Inhomogeneous mixed T1 and T2 signal; multilobular
- Enhancement pattern: Variable; homogeneous enhancement

Imaging Recommendations
- CECT or CEMR both can answer all imaging questions
- The facial nerve plane can be projected from the stylomastoid foramen, anteroinferiorly to just lateral to the retromandibular vein, from there out over the surface of the masseter muscle
  - This projected plane represents an imaging estimation of the line dividing the superficial and deep lobes of the parotid gland
- Is the mass superficial to the facial nerve plane? If so, mass is in superficial lobe
- Is the mass deep to the facial nerve plane? If so, mass is in deep lobe of parotid gland
- Does the mass widen the stylomandibular notch and push the parapharyngeal fat anteromedially? If so, you have further verification that the mass is centered in the deep lobe

Differential Diagnosis: Parotid Space Mass

Warthin's Tumor
- Multicentric 20%
- Mixed-intensity, well-circumscribed mass on T1 C+ MR

Adenoid Cystic Carcinoma
- Facial nerve paralysis may be present
- Enhancing infiltrating mass on T1 C+ MR

Mucoepidermoid Carcinoma
- Facial nerve paralysis may be present
- Mixed-intensity discrete mass with irregular margins on T1 C+ MR

SCCa or Melanoma Nodal Metastasis
- Primary lesion on or around skin of ear
- Multiple intraparotid masses, often with central necrosis

Pathology

General
- Etiology-Pathogenesis
  - Benign tumor arising from distal portions of the parotid ductal system, including the intercalated ducts and acini
- Epidemiology
  - **80%** of parotid tumors are BMT
  - 80% of head and neck BMT arise in parotid glands
  - 6.5% in submandibular glands
  - 6.5% arise from minor salivary glands
  - .5% in sublingual glands

Gross Pathologic, Surgical Features
- Tan-white mass encased in a fibrous capsule

Microscopic Features
- Interspersed epithelial, myoepithelial and stromal cellular components must be identified to diagnose BMT
- BMT of major salivary glands are encased in a fibrous capsule

Clinical Issues

Presentation
- Principal presenting symptom: Painless cheek mass
- Location dependent symptoms and signs
  - Superficial lobe: Cheek mass
  - Parotid tail: Angle of mandible mass
  - Deep lobe: "Parapharyngeal space" mass pushing tonsil into pharyngeal airway
- Facial nerve paralysis is rare
- Clinical epidemiology
  - 2:1, female:male ratio
  - Most common age of presentation: 30-60 years

Natural History
- Slowly-growing, painless, benign tumor

Treatment
- Complete surgical resection of encapsulated mass within an "adequate margin" of surrounding parotid gland tissue to avoid any **spillage** of tumor cells

Prognosis
- Recurrent tumor tends to be **multifocal**

Selected References
1. Ikeda K et al: The usefulness of MR in establishing the diagnosis of parotid pleomorphic adenoma. AJNR 17:555-9, 1996
2. Phillips PP et al: Recurrent pleomorphic adenoma of the parotid gland: report of 126 cases and a review of the literature. Ann Otol Rhinol Laryngol 104:100-41, 1995
3. Joe VQ et al: Tumors of the parotid gland: MR imaging characteristics of various histologic types. AJR 163:433-8, 1994

Warthin's Tumor, Parotid Space

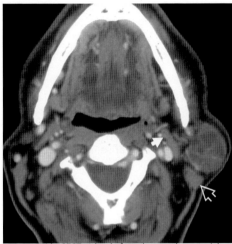

Warthin's tumor, parotid. CECT at level of oropharynx shows an inhomogeneously-enhancing mass in left parotid tail. Parotid tail location can be identified by its position lateral to posterior belly of digastric muscle (arrow) and anterolateral to sternomastoid muscle (open arrow).

Key Facts
- Synonyms: Papillary cystadenoma lymphomatosum; adenolymphoma; lymphomatous adenoma
- Definition: Benign parotid gland tumor with a characteristic histopathologic appearance composed of papillary structures, mature lymphocytic infiltrate and cystic changes
- Classic imaging appearance: Sharply-marginated tail of parotid mass with striking parenchymal inhomogeneity
- Second most common parotid space benign tumor behind BMT

Imaging Findings
General Features
- Well-marginated intraparotid or periparotid mass
- **Parenchymal inhomogeneity** is the rule
- 30% have cystic areas within the tumor parenchyma
CT Findings
- Mixed-density mass with mild contrast enhancement
- Focal low-density areas may be seen in 30%
MR Findings
- T1 shows multiple high-signal areas within tumor parenchyma secondary to proteinaceous debris and/or hemorrhage
- T2 signal is intermediate unless cystic areas are present, in which case these cystic foci are high T2 signal
- No or minimal enhancement on T1 C+ MR is characteristic
Nuclear Medicine Findings
- Increased and prolonged uptake of technetium-99m that does not "wash out" after sialogue administration
- Increased uptake of FDG-PET
  - PET may incidentally diagnose while looking for malignancy

Warthin's Tumor, Parotid Space

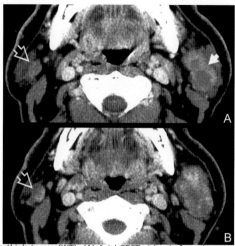

Bilateral Warthin's tumor (WT). (A) Axial CECT at level of oropharynx shows large, left, mixed-density WT in parotid tail. Open arrow: smaller right WT (open arrow) is better seen on this image. (B) CT below (A) reveals both WTs extend inferiorly.

Imaging Recommendations
- Parotid mass lesions best evaluated with enhanced MR
- MR best delineates their intra- vs. extraparotid location, relationship to facial nerve plane, deep tissue extent and perineural tumor spread

Differential Diagnosis: Unilateral Parotid Space (PS) Mass

Benign Lymphoepithelial Lesion-HIV
- When unilateral and singular, may strongly mimic Warthin's
- Tonsillar hyperplasia and cervical adenopathy help differentiate

BMT-PS
- Well-circumscribed, homogenous, intraparotid mass when small
- Larger lesions may be inhomogeneous and mimic Warthin's

Malignant Tumor-PS (ACCa/MECa)
- Low-grade parotid malignancy may be well demarcated
- Higher grade, more advanced parotid malignancy easily differentiated given invasive appearance on imaging

Pathology

General
- Embryology
  - The parotid gland undergoes "late encapsulation," incorporating lymphoid tissue-nodes within the superficial layer of deep cervical fascia
  - Warthin's tumor is thought to arise within this lymphoid tissue
- Etiology-Pathogenesis
  - Smoking-induced, benign tumor arising from salivary-lymphoid tissue in intraparotid and periparotid lymph nodes
- Epidemiology
  - 5% all salivary gland tumors
  - 12% of benign parotid gland tumors

Warthin's Tumor, Parotid Space

- o **20% multicentric**, unilateral or bilateral, synchronous or metachronous

Gross Pathologic, Surgical Features
- Encapsulated, soft, ovoid mass with a smooth but lobulated surface
- Tan tissue with cystic spaces which contain a tenacious, mucoid, brown fluid or a thin, yellow fluid with cholesterol crystals
  - o Papillary projections can also be seen within these cystic areas

Microscopic Features
- Epithelial and lymphoid components dominate histopath picture
- The papillary projections are lined with a double epithelial layer
  - o Inner-luminal layer: Tall columnar cells with their nuclei oriented toward the lumen
  - o Outer-basal layer: Cuboidal or polygonal cells with vesicular nuclei
- The inner lymphoid component of the papillary projection is composed of mature lymphoid aggregates with germinal centers

Clinical Issues

Presentation
- Principal presenting symptom: angle of mandible (tail of parotid) mass
- Other symptoms: Mass is painless; multiple masses ≤ 20%
- Mean age at presentation is 60 years
- Male:female ratio 3:1
- 90% of patients with this tumor **smoke**

Natural History
- Slowly-growing, benign tumor with very low malignant transformation potential

Treatment
- Resection of mass within a collar of normal parotid tissue without injury to the intraparotid facial nerve is treatment goal

Prognosis
- "Recurrent" Warthin's tumor may be from inadequate resection or from metachronous second lesion

Selected References
1. Yoo GH et al: Warthin's tumor: a 40-year experience at The Johns Hopkins Hospital. Laryngoscope 104:799-803, 1994
2. Joe VQ et al: Tumors of the parotid gland: MR imaging characteristics of various histologic types. AJR 163:433-8, 1994
3. Minami M et al: Warthin tumor of the parotid gland: MR-pathologic correlation. AJNR 14:209-14, 1993

MECa & ACCa, Parotid Space

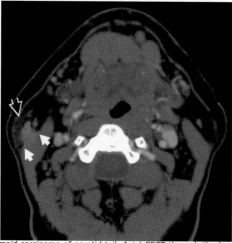

Mucoepidermoid carcinoma of parotid tail. Axial CECT through the low oropharynx shows an invasive mass projecting posteriorly from the right parotid tail (open arrow). The enhancing MECa invades along the surface of the deeper sternomastoid muscle (arrows).

Key Facts
- The two major carcinomas of the parotid space are mucoepidermoid carcinoma (MECa) and adenoid cystic carcinoma (ACCa)
- Classic imaging appearance: Poorly-circumscribed, invasive mass arising within the parotid gland is carcinoma until proven otherwise

Imaging Findings
General Features
- Best imaging clue: **Invasive** mass in parotid gland
- Imaging appearance based on histologic grade of tumor
  - Low-grade malignancy: Well-circumscribed mass mimicking BMT
  - High-grade malignancy: Invasive margins
- Adjacent malignant adenopathy may be present (esp. with MECa)
  - 1st order nodes = jugulodigastric group

CT Findings
- Low grade: Enhancing homogenous mass with sharp margins
- High grade: Enhancing invasive mass with shaggy margins

MR Findings
- High grade: Mass with inhomogeneous signal intensity on T1 and T2 sequences with invasive margins
- If in high, deep PS look for **perineural spread**
  - Stylomastoid foramen up mastoid segment of facial nerve

Imaging Recommendations
- MR imaging is recommended to evaluate a parotid mass since deep tissue spread and perineural tumor are better defined by MR
  - Surprisingly, **T1 unenhanced** images best delineates the mass
- Long term (5-10 year) imaging follow-up recommended given the tendency of these tumors to recur late

MECa & ACCa, Parotid Space

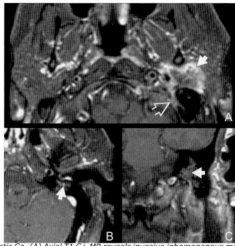

Adenoid cystic Ca. (A) Axial T1 C+ MR reveals invasive inhomogenous mass involving deep posterior parotid (arrow) & stylomastoid foramen (open arrow). (B) Magnified axial T1 C+ image shows perineural tumor on mastoid VII (arrow) and surrounding air cells. (C) Arrow in coronal T1 C+ image: Perineural tumor (VII).

- The radiologist and invasive parotid space (PS) masses
  - In masses of the cheek area, first decide if the mass is **intraparotid** (BMT, Warthin's, MECa, ACCa, etc.) or **extraparotid** (in the CS, MS, PPS or PMS)
  - If intrinsic to the parotid gland, is the mass in the superficial lobe or deep lobe?
    - Determined by relationship to projected facial nerve plane just lateral to retromandibular vein
  - If in high, deep PS, check for **perineural tumor** on mastoid VII
  - Beyond this localization, a prediction of benign vs. malignant can be made based on sharp or invasive margins respectively
    - Beware! Benign tumors can incite focal obstructive sialadenitis and low-grade malignancy may have sharp margins

Differential Diagnosis: Parotid Space Mass
Benign Mixed Tumor
- Well-demarcated, solid intraparotid mass that is homogeneous and ovoid when small but inhomogeneous & lobulated when large
Warthin's Tumor
- Multicentric 20%
- Mixed-intensity, well-circumscribed mass on T1 C+ MR
Non-Hodgkin Lymphoma
- Parenchymal: Invasive tumor of parotid tissue indistinguishable from high-grade MECa or ACCa
- Nodal: Multiple intraparotid nodal-appearing masses
Nodal Metastasis from EAC Skin SCCa or Melanoma
- Primary lesion on or around skin of ear
- Multiple intraparotid masses, often with central necrosis

MECa & ACCa, Parotid Space

Pathology

General

- General Path Comments
  - The two most common malignant tumors = MECa and ACCa
    - MECa: Tends to have associated malignant lymph nodes
    - ACCa: Tendency for perineural spread; mets to lungs & bones
- Epidemiology
  - The larger the salivary gland, the fewer the malignancies found
    - **Parotid** gland: **20%** are malignant
    - Submandibular gland: 50% malignant
    - Sublingual gland: 70% malignant
  - MECa is most common carcinoma of PS (60%)

Gross Pathologic, Surgical Features

- Tan-white, infiltrating mass

Microscopic Features

- MECa
  - Malignant, epithelial, salivary gland tumor composed of a variable admixture of epidermoid, intermediate and mucous-secreting cells
  - Arises in glandular ductal epithelium
- ACCa
  - Unencapsulated neoplasm with varied growth patterns consisting of cribriform, tubular and solid; individual tumors most commonly are composed of multiple growth patterns
  - Arises in peripheral parotid ducts

Staging Criteria

- **T1**: Tumor 2 cm or less without extraparenchymal extension
- **T2**: Tumor 2-4 cm without extraparenchymal extension
- **T3**: Tumor 4-6 cm with extraparenchymal extension
- **T4**: Tumor > 6 cm and/or invades adjacent structures (mandible, skull base, deep spaces of suprahyoid neck)

Clinical Issues

Presentation

- Principal presenting symptom: Painful parotid mass
- Other symptoms: Rock-hard mass; facial nerve paralysis

Treatment

- Surgical removal of tumor with surrounding normal parotid tissue
  - Superficial parotidectomy if possible
  - Total parotidectomy may be necessary if involves deep lobe
- Post operative radiotherapy routine

Prognosis

- MECa: Recurrence and survival rates depend on tumor grade
  - 6% for low-grade tumors with 90% 10-year survival rate
  - 50% for high-grade tumors with 40% 10-year survival rate
- ACCa: Recurrence and survival rates depend on tumor grade
  - 65% overall 10-year survival rate

Selected References

1. Schlakman BN et al: MR of intraparotid masses. AJNR 14:1173-80, 1993
2. Freling NJM A et al: Malignant parotid tumors: clinical use of MR imaging and histologic correlation. Radiology 185:691-6, 1992
3. Som PM et al: High-grade malignancies of the parotid glands: identification with MR imaging. Radiology 173:823-6, 1989

Parotid Nodal Malignancy

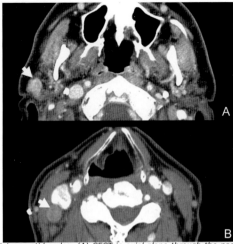

Metastatic intraparotid nodes. (A) CECT in axial plane through the nasopharynx in patient with known SCCa of the periauricular skin shows right parotid metastatic node (arrow). (B) Inferior CT image shows the nodal metastasis has also spread to the deep cervical nodes (arrow).

Key Facts
- Definition: Skin SCCa and melanoma from the scalp, auricle and face spread to their 1st order intra- and periparotid nodal station
- Classic imaging appearance: One or more focal masses in the superficial or deep lobe of the parotid gland, often with associated pre-auricular and/or cervical nodal masses
- The primary skin lesion may not be clinically apparent at the time of parotid nodal involvement as it may be hidden above the hairline
- Remember that the parotid space is the **first order nodal station** for skin malignancy from the upper face, scalp and auricle-EAC

Imaging Findings
General Features
- One or more intraparotid masses with sharp margins (early) or invasive margins (late, extranodal spread)
- Preauricular and/or cervical nodal masses may also be present
- Skin thickening (primary skin malignancy) in area of auricle
CT Findings
- Single or multiple masses with or without central nodal necrosis
- Intraparotid, preauricular and cervical nodes may all be seen
MR Findings
- No distinctive features
- Single or multiple intraparotid masses with or without central nodal inhomogeneity of signal
Imaging Recommendations
- MR imaging is recommended to evaluate parotid masses since deep tissue spread and perineural tumor are better defined by MR
  - Surprisingly, **T1 unenhanced** images best delineate the mass

Parotid Nodal Malignancy

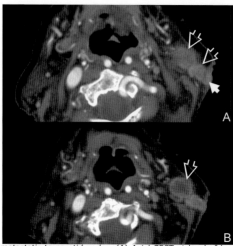

Skin SCCa metastatic to parotid nodes. (A) Axial CECT at level of low oropharynx shows the primary skin SCCa (arrow) with deep spread to parotid tail lymph nodes (open arrows). (B) Just inferior to (A) the nodal necrosis is better delineated (open arrow).

- All patients with invasive skin SCCa or melanoma on the skin of the face, scalp and auricle should be considered for staging MR searching for intraparotid nodes and/or nodes in the cervical neck
  - As PET staging is common in metastatic melanoma, the PET and MR findings should be cross correlated

Differential Diagnosis: Multiple Unilateral Parotid Masses
Early Benign Lymphoepithelial Lesions-HIV
- Mixed cystic and cystic-solid masses
- Tonsillar hyperplasia and cervical adenopathy associated
Sjogren's Syndrome
- Multiple small cysts mixed with cystic-solid masses
- No tonsillar hyperplasia and cervical adenopathy associated
Multicentric Warthin's Tumor
- Two mixed-intensity, well-circumscribed masses on T1 C+ MR
NHL in Parotid Nodes
- Multiple intraparotid nodal-appearing masses

Pathology
General
- Embryology-Anatomy
  - The parotid gland undergoes "late encapsulation," incorporating lymph nodes within its capsule
  - Consequently, the parotid gland is a commonly forgotten nodal station above the deep cervical and spinal accessory chains
  - Skin malignancy from the face, scalp and auricle-EAC have as their first order drainage station the parotid nodal group
- Etiology-Pathogenesis
  - Face, scalp and auricular-EAC skin SCCa or melanoma primary seeds 1st order intraparotid nodes

Parotid Nodal Malignancy

- Epidemiology
  - Intraparotid nodal spread seen more common in regions of increased sun exposure (eg. Arizona) where skin malignancy is more prevalent

Gross Pathologic, Surgical Features
- SCCa node: Tan-yellow, firm nodules within normal parotid
- Melanoma node: Black, brown, pink or white rubbery mass

Microscopic Features
- **SCCa**: Lymph node is partially or entirely replaced by an epithelial-lined structure with central cystic change
  - The epithelium lining of the cystic spaces is composed of a hypercellular and pleomorphic cell population, with loss of polarity and increased mitotic activity
- **Melanoma**: Diffuse proliferation of epithelioid and/or spindle cells with abundant eosinophilic cytoplasm and prominent nucleoli
  - Immunohistochemistry: S-100 protein and HMB-45 present

Clinical Issues

Presentation
- Non-healing sore (skin SCCa or melanoma) on the skin of the face, scalp or auricle-EAC associated with cheek mass (parotid nodes)
- Needle biopsy reveals parotid mass to be SCCa or melanoma with skin lesion then found above the hairline in suprazygomatic area

Treatment
- SCCa: Superficial or total parotidectomy and neck dissection dictated imaging and physical exam; postoperative radiotherapy
- Melanoma: Superficial or total parotidectomy and neck dissection dictated by lymphatic mapping and sentinel nodal identification; adjuvant radiotherapy and/or chemotherapy depends on context

Prognosis
- SCCa: 70% 5 year survival for all comers
- Melanoma: Poor prognosis although rare patients may survive a long period of time following surgery

Selected References
1. Prayson RA et al: Parotid gland malignant melanoma. Arch Pathol Lab Med 124:1780-84, 2000
2. Schroeder WA et al: Malignant neoplastic disease of the parotid lymph nodes. Laryngoscope 108:1514-9, 1998
3. delCharco JO et al: Carcinoma of the skin metastatic to the parotid area lymph nodes. Head Neck 20:369-73, 1998

CAROTID SPACE

Jugular Vein Thrombosis

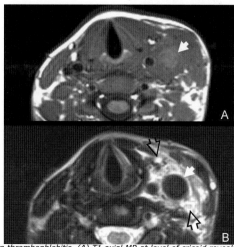

Jugular vein thrombophlebitis. (A) T1 axial MR at level of cricoid reveals high signal (methemoglobin) clot in thrombosed internal jugular vein (arrow). (B) T2 MR shows clot to be very low signal (arrow). The inflammatory edema surrounding the vein is seen as high signal in adjacent soft tissues (open arrow).

Key Facts

- Definitions
  - **Jugular vein thrombophlebitis (JVT)**: Acute to subacute thrombosis of internal jugular vein (IJV) with associated adjacent tissue inflammation (myositis and fasciitis)
  - **Jugular vein thrombosis**: Chronic IJV thrombosis (> 7 days) where clot persists within lumen but soft-tissue inflammation gone
- JVT presents to radiologists in its acute phase as "rule out abscess"; in its chronic phase, as "evaluate tumor extent"
- Classic imaging appearance: Luminal clot is present in most or all of IJV with soft-tissue inflammatory changes when acute-subacute

Imaging Findings

General Features
- Best imaging clue: Clot seen in IJV lumen
- Findings depend on the stage of the disease
- **Acute-subacute thrombophlebitic phases** (< 7 days): Imaging shows inflammation-induced loss of soft-tissue planes surrounding the enlarged, thrombus-filled IJV with vein wall rim enhancement
- **Chronic thrombotic phase** (> 7 days): Imaging shows a well-marginated, tubular mass without adjacent inflammation
  - Multiple venous collaterals are seen bypassing the thrombosis
- Edema fluid may be present in RPS as a secondary sign of JVT

CT Findings
- Acute-subacute thrombophlebitic phase: CECT shows increased density in fat surrounding carotid space (CS) secondary to cellulitis
  - IJV is enlarged and filled with a low-density thrombus
  - Vasa vasorum of IJV wall enhances as a thin, hyperdense rim
- Chronic thrombotic phase: Enhanced CT shows a tubular mass where the IJV should live without increased density in adjacent fat

Jugular Vein Thrombosis

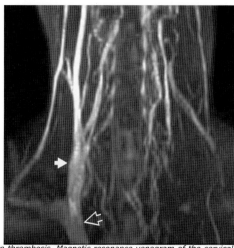

Jugular vein thrombosis. Magnetic resonance venogram of the cervical neck shows complete absence of the deep venous system secondary to venous thrombosis. Normal right internal jugular vein (arrow) and brachiocephalic vein (open arrow) are readily apparent in the low left neck.

MR Findings
- Acute-subacute phase: May have a bizarre tumorous appearance, especially on coronal plane; adjacent fat appears infiltrated
- Subacute to chronic phase: Tubular mass in the posterolateral CS with high signal on T1 images secondary to T1 shortening from the paramagnetic effect of methemoglobin
- MRV will show absent signal throughout most of the IJV

Imaging Recommendations
- CECT in these sick patients permits rapid diagnosis of JVT

Differential Diagnosis: Infrahyoid Neck CS Mass

Slow or Turbulent Flow in IJV
- High signal intensity on T1 MR images may be seen
- Look at all sequences, usually one will show flow
- If not, consider MRV to work this out

Reactive Adenopathy-Lymphadenitis
- Multiple focal masses along CS course of cervical neck

Cervical Neck Abscess
- Focal walled-off fluid collection in any space of infrahyoid neck

SCCa Malignant Adenopathy
- Multiple focal, necrotic, and non-necrotic masses along the course of the cervical CS and posterior cervical space

Pathology

General
- General Path Comments
  - JVT is different from intraparenchymal hematoma
  - In JVT there is lamination of thrombus, no hemosiderin deposition, and a delay in evolution of blood products (especially methemoglobin)

Jugular Vein Thrombosis

- o **Lemierre's syndrome**
  - ▪ Septic thrombophlebitis of IJV associated with disseminated metastatic abscesses in wake of an acute oropharyngeal infection in a young patient
  - ▪ Fusobacterium necrophorum, an obligate anaerobic, pleomorphic, gram-negative rod is grown from the blood or pus of these patients
- Pathogenesis: 3 mechanisms for thrombosis
  - o Endothelial damage from an indwelling line or infection, altered blood flow and a hypercoagulable state
  - o Venous stasis from compression of the IJV in the neck (nodes) or mediastinum (SVC syndrome) can also incite thrombosis
  - o Migratory IJV thrombophlebitis (Trousseau's syndrome) associated with malignancy (pancreas, lung and ovary)
    - ▪ Elevated factor VIII and accelerated generation of thromboplastin cause the hypercoagulable state

Clinical Issues
Presentation
- Principal presenting symptom: Swollen lateral infrahyoid neck
- Clinical diagnosis is unreliable
- Patient's history
  - o Previous neck surgery, central venous catheterization, drug abuse, hypercoagulable state or malignancy
  - o May be spontaneous clinical event
- **Acute thrombophlebitic phase**: Tender, red mass with low-grade fever; radiology requisition often reads "rule-out abscess"
- **Chronic thrombotic phase**: Hard, nontender mass; requisition reads "evaluate tumor extent"
Natural History
- IJV thrombophlebitis gives way to thrombosis over a 7-14 period with decreased soft-tissue swelling
Treatment
- Aggressive antibiotics are given to treat any underlying infection; surgical drainage of focal pus is completed if seen on CT
- As clinically significant thromboembolism to the lungs is relatively rare in IJV thrombosis, anticoagulant therapy is usually not used
Prognosis
- Prognosis is related to the underlying cause of the IJV thrombosis
- IJV thrombosis itself is self-limited, with venous collaterals forming to circumvent the occluded vein

Selected References
1. Poe LB et al: Acute internal jugular vein thrombosis associated with pseudoabscess of the retropharyngeal space. AJNR 16:892-6, 1995
2. Albertyn LE et al: Diagnosis of internal jugular vein thrombosis. Radiology 162:505-8, 1987
3. Erdman WA et al: Venous thrombosis: clinical and experimental MR imaging. Radiology 161:233-8, 1986

Glomus Vagale Paraganglioma

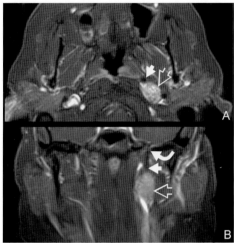

Glomus vagale paraganglioma (GVP). (A) Axial T1 C+ MR with fat sat shows the enhancing GVP (open arrow) displacing the ICA anteromedially (arrow). (B) Coronal images reveals the ovoid GVP (open arrow) with its cephalad margin (arrow) distinct from the skull base (curved arrow).

Key Facts
- Synonym: Vagal body tumors
- Definition: Benign vascular tumor derived from primitive neural crest that begins in the ganglia of the vagus nerve
- Classic imaging appearance: **Nasopharyngeal carotid space mass** displacing the parapharyngeal fat anteriorly, the ICA anteromedial; avid enhancement with CT, high-velocity flow voids on T1 MR

Imaging Findings
General Features
- Mass is centered 1-2 cm below floor of jugular foramen in nasopharyngeal carotid space(s)
- CS mass displaces parapharyngeal space anteriorly
- Internal carotid artery is displaced anteriorly or medially
- Both CT and MR are diagnostic
CT Findings
- Avidly-enhancing mass in nasopharyngeal CS
MR Findings
- **T1 MR** images show "salt and pepper"
- "Salt" or high-signal areas within the tumor parenchyma rarely seen; secondary to subacute hemorrhage
- "Pepper" is low-signal foci from the high-velocity flow voids of feeding arteries commonly seen; punctate or curvilinear
Angiographic Findings
- Enlarged feeding vessels with prolonged, intense vascular blush with early draining veins seen secondary to arteriovenous shunting
- Ascending pharyngeal artery is principal tumor feeder
Imaging Recommendations
- In familial patient group, screening MR beginning at 20 years old
- MR and angiography done before surgery

Glomus Vagale Paraganglioma

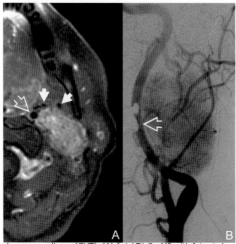

Glomus vagale paraganglioma (GVT). (A) Axial T1 C+ MR with fat sat shows enhancing GVT in left carotid space, displacing ICA anteromedially (open arrow). Arrows: high-velocity flow voids = "pepper." (B) Carotid angio: Tumor blush above bifurcation. Arrow: ICA anteromedial displacement.

- Angiographic challenges
  - To provide a vascular road map for the surgeon
  - Evaluates collateral arterial and venous circulation of the brain, should sacrifice of a major vessel become necessary
  - Searches for multicentric tumors
  - Preoperative embolization for prophylactic hemostasis

Differential Diagnosis: Nasopharyngeal Carotid Space Mass
Vagal Schwannoma
- MR shows fusiform enhancing mass in carotid space
- MRA shows ICA bowed over anterior surface of mass
- Absence of tumor blush or enlarged feeding arteries on angiography
Meningioma of Carotid Space
- Extends from jugular foramen above
- CT shows permeative sclerotic bony changes of the jugular foramen (JF) bony margins
- Dural thickening (tails) present along cephalad margin of JF
- Prolonged but mild tumor blush during angiography
Glomus Jugulare Paraganglioma
- Mass centered in JF with permeative bony margins (CT) and high velocity flow voids (T1 MR)
Carotid Body Paraganglioma
- Mass centered in crotch of ICA-ECA at the carotid bifurcation
- T1 MR images show high-velocity flow voids

Pathology
General
- Genetics
  - Paraganglioma occurs in a sporadic and a familial form
    - The familial form is autosomal dominant

Glomus Vagale Paraganglioma

- Etiology-Pathogenesis
  - Arise from **glomus bodies**, aka **paraganglia**
  - Glomus bodies are composed of chemoreceptor cells derived from the primitive neural crest
- Epidemiology
  - Rarest of paragangliomas; 2.5% of all paragangliomas
  - 5% multicentric in non-familial group
  - Familial incidence of multicentricity may reach 90%

Gross Pathologic, Surgical Features
- Lobulated, reddish-purple mass with fibrous pseudocapsule

Microscopic Features
- Chief cells and sustentacular cells are surrounded by a fibromuscular stroma
- Nests of chief cells are characteristic (zellballen)
- Electronmicroscopy shows neurosecretory granules

Clinical Issues
Presentation
- Principal presenting symptom: Vocal cord paralysis
  - 50% have vocal cord paralysis at presentation
- Pulsatile lateral retropharyngeal mass
- Rarely hormonally active

Treatment
- Surgical excision is treatment of choice
- Radiotherapy is used for lesion control in poor surgical candidates
- If bilateral GVP, surgery on one, radiotherapy on other to preserve unilateral vagus nerve function

Prognosis
- 100% have unilateral vagus nerve paralysis from surgery
- Teflon injection of ipsilateral vocal cord usually necessary
- Cricopharyngeal myotomy completed if dysphagia severe

Selected References
1. Rao AB et al: Paragangliomas of the head and neck: Radiologic-pathologic correlation. RadioGraphics 19: 1605-32, 1999
2. Urquhart AC et al: Glomus Vagale: paraganglioma of the vagus nerve. Laryngoscope 104:440-5, 1994
3. Olsen WL et al: MR imaging of paragangliomas. AJR 148: 201-4, 1987

Carotid Body Paraganglioma

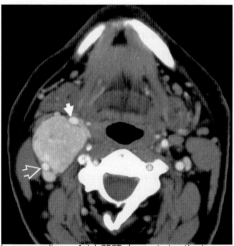

Carotid body paraganglioma. Axial CECT demonstrates the tumor as an avidly enhancing mass in the notch between the ECA (arrow) and the ICA (open arrow). Viewing the normal left ECA and ICA reveals the degree of splaying of these vessels on the affected right side.

Key Facts
- Synonyms: Carotid body tumor; chemodectoma; non-chromaffin paraganglioma
- Definition: Carotid body paraganglioma (CBP) is a benign vascular tumor derived from primitive neural crest that in the glomus bodies in the crotch of the ECA and ICA at the carotid bifurcation
- Classic imaging appearance: Oropharyngeal carotid space mass splaying the ECA and ICA at the carotid bifurcation; avid enhancement with CT, high velocity flow voids on T1 MR

Imaging Findings
General Features
- Best imaging clue: ECA and ICA are splayed
- Mass is centered in the crotch of the carotid bifurcation
- ICA is characteristically displaced posterolaterally
- Both CT and MR appearances are diagnostic
CT Findings
- Avidly-enhancing mass in the crotch between the ECA and ICA at the carotid bifurcation
MR Findings
- **T1 MR** images show "salt and pepper"
- "Salt" or high-signal areas within the tumor parenchyma seen only in larger tumors; secondary to subacute hemorrhage
- "Pepper" is low-signal foci from the high-velocity flow voids of feeding arteries commonly seen; punctate or curvilinear
- MRA will show splayed ECA-ICA but not the capillary bed of CBP
Angiographic Findings
- Enlarged feeding vessels with prolonged, intense vascular blush with early draining veins seen secondary to arteriovenous shunting
- Ascending pharyngeal artery branches are principal tumor feeder

Carotid Body Paraganglioma

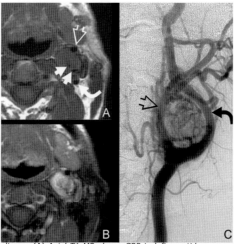

CB paraganglioma. (A) Axial T1 MR shows CBP in left carotid space, splaying ECA (open arrow) and ICA (curved arrow). Arrows: High-velocity flow voids. (B) T1 C+ MR with fat sat shows avid CBT enhancement. (C) Carotid angio shows tumor blush in bifurcation. Open arrow: ECA; Curved arrow: ICA.

<u>Imaging Recommendations</u>
- In familial patient group, screening MR beginning at 20 years old
- MR and angiography done before surgery
- Angiographic challenges
  - To provide a vascular road map for the surgeon
  - Evaluates collateral arterial and venous circulation of the brain, should sacrifice of a major vessel become necessary
  - Searches for multicentric tumors
  - Preoperative embolization for prophylactic hemostasis

Differential Diagnosis: Oropharyngeal Carotid Space Mass
<u>Carotid Bulb Ectasia</u>
- Enlarged, ectatic, calcified carotid bulb secondary to atherosclerosis
<u>Jugulodigastric (JD) Lymph Node Hyperplasia</u>
- Enlarged, non-necrotic JD node pulsates against carotid bulb
<u>Vagal Schwannoma</u>
- MR shows fusiform enhancing mass in carotid space
- MRA shows ICA bowed over anterior surface of mass
- Absence of tumor blush or enlarged feeding arteries on angiography
<u>Vagal Neurofibroma</u>
- CECT shows low-density, well-circumscribed mass in CS
- MR imaging cannot differentiate from vagal schwannoma
<u>Glomus Vagale Paraganglioma</u>
- Mass centered approximately 2 cm below the skull base
- High-velocity flow voids on T1 MR images

Pathology
<u>General</u>
- Genetics
  - All paraganglioma occurs in a sporadic and a familial form

Carotid Body Paraganglioma

- Familial paraganglioma is autosomal dominant
- Etiology-Pathogenesis
  - Arise from glomus bodies (paraganglia) in the carotid body
  - Glomus bodies are composed of chemoreceptor cells derived from the primitive neural crest
  - Glomus bodies are found in the temporal bone, jugular foramen and the upper carotid space to the level of the carotid bifurcation
- Epidemiology
  - CBP is the most common location for paraganglioma
  - 40% of all paragangliomas found are CBP
  - 5% of paragangliomas are multicentric in non-familial group
  - Familial incidence of multicentricity may reach 90%

Gross Pathologic, Surgical Features
- Lobulated, reddish-purple mass with fibrous pseudocapsule

Microscopic Features
- Chief cells and sustentacular cells are surrounded by a fibromuscular stroma
- Nests of chief cells are characteristic (zellballen)
- Electronmicroscopy shows neurosecretory granules

Clinical Issues

Presentation
- Principal presenting symptom: Pulsatile angle of mandible mass
- 20% have vagal and/or hypoglossal neuropathy
- Catecholamine-secreting CBP is rare

Treatment
- Surgical excision is treatment of choice
- Radiotherapy is used for lesion control in poor surgical candidates
- Malignant transformation is extremely rare

Prognosis
- Surgical cure without lasting post-operative cranial neuropathy is expected in CBP < 5 cm
- Complications of surgery, especially permanent vagal and/or hypoglossal neuropathy, increase in tumors > 5 cm

Selected References
1. Rao AB et al: Paragangliomas of the head and neck: Radiologic-pathologic correlation. RadioGraphics 19: 1605-32, 1999
2. Muhm M et al: Diagnostic and therapeutic approaches to carotid body tumors. Review of 24 patients. Arch Surg 132:279-84, 1997
3. Olsen WL et al: MR imaging of paragangliomas. AJR 148: 201-4, 1987

Vagal Schwannoma, Carotid Space

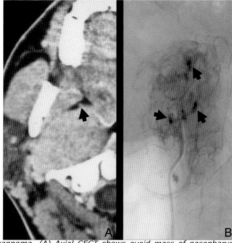

Vagal schwannoma. (A) Axial CECT shows ovoid mass of nasopharyngeal carotid space pushing parapharyngeal fat anteriorly (arrow). (B) Capillary phase of lateral view of carotid angio shows characteristic "puddling" of contrast in tumor parenchyma (arrows).

Key Facts
- Synonyms: Neuroma; neurilemmoma
- Definition: Benign tumor of Schwann cells that wrap the vagus nerve in the carotid space of the extracranial head and neck
- Classic imaging appearance: Fusiform mass in CS of neck that displaces the carotid artery anteromedially; enhancement is typical although T1 MR shows **no** high-velocity flow voids

Imaging Findings
General Features
- Best imaging clue: Fusiform mass in CS
- Smooth, sharply-circumscribed tumor
- Tumor may be solid, contain multiple small cysts or coalesce these cysts into a large, central cyst
- In **suprahyoid neck**, mass has characteristic displacement pattern
  - Displaces parapharyngeal space fat anteriorly and posterior belly of digastric muscle laterally
  - Internal carotid artery (ICA) is bowed over anteromedial surface
- In **infrahyoid neck**, mass displaces thyroid and trachea to contralateral neck, common carotid artery anteromedial and posterior cervical space posterolaterally

CT Findings
- In axial plane CECT shows mass to be round, sharply marginated and avidly enhancing

MR Findings
- Coronal and sagittal MR reveals the fusiform shape of tumor best
- T1 C+ MR images shows bright, uniform enhancement
  - Intramural cysts may be present in larger tumors
  - MRA will show carotid artery displacement only

Vagal Schwannoma, Carotid Space

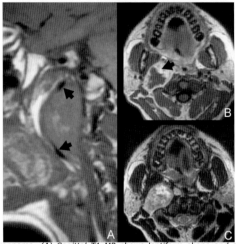

Vagal schwannoma. (A) Sagittal T1 MR shows lentiform shape and anterior ICA displacement (arrows) characteristic of schwannoma of carotid space. (B) Axial T1 C+: Tumor cystic change (arrow). (C) T2 shows well-circumscribed tumor with inhomogeneous signal.

Angiographic Findings
- Tumor is moderately vascular, with tortuous but not enlarged feeding vessels feeding the tumor
- Scattered contrast "**puddles**" without arteriovenous shunting or vascular encasement is characteristic

Imaging Recommendations
- CECT or MR can be used to make this diagnosis
- The displacement patterns described above allow diagnosis of a CS mass
  - Lack of high-velocity flow voids within the tumor allows correct identification of a solitary nerve sheath tumor

Differential Diagnosis: Carotid Space Mass
Vagal Neurofibroma
- CECT shows low-density, well-circumscribed mass in CS
- MR imaging cannot differentiate from vagal schwannoma

Sympathetic Plexus Schwannoma
- Centered in lateral wall of RPS
- Otherwise indistinguishable from vagal schwannoma

Glomus Vagale Paraganglioma
- Mass centered 2 cm below the skull base
- High-velocity flow voids on T1 MR images

Carotid Body Paraganglioma
- Mass centered in common carotid bifurcation
- High velocity flow voids on T1 MR images

Pathology
General
- Etiology-Pathogenesis

Vagal Schwannoma, Carotid Space

- o   Arises from Schwann cells wrapping the vagus nerve in the neck
- Epidemiology
- o   Rare tumor of the extracranial head and neck

Gross Pathologic, Surgical Features
- White-tan, smooth, encapsulated, sausage-shaped mass

Microscopic Features
- Differentiated neoplastic Schwann cells
- Spindle cells with elongated nuclei and alternating areas of organized, compact cells (Antoni A) and loosely arranged, relatively acellular tissue (Antoni B) present in all cases
- Immunochemistry: Strong, diffuse, immuno-staining for S-100 protein = Neural-crest marker antigen present in the supporting cell of the nervous system

Clinical Issues

Presentation
- Principal presenting symptom
- o   Lateral retropharyngeal mass (suprahyoid vagal schwannoma)
- o   Anterolateral cervical neck (infrahyoid vagal schwannoma)
- Rarely Horner's syndrome

Natural History
- Slow but persistent growth until airway compromise or cosmetic issues supervene

Treatment
- Surgical removal in total is treatment of choice
- Severe transient bradycardia may occur during removal

Prognosis
- Vagus nerve preservation is not possible at surgery
- o   End-to-end anastomosis or interposition of nerve graft is done

Selected References
1.   Colreavy PM et al: Head and neck schwannoma: a 10 year review. J Laryngol Otol 114:119-24, 2000
2.   Gilmer-Hill HS et al: Neurogenic tumors of the cervical vagus nerve: report of four cases and review of the literature. Neurosurgery 46:1498-503, 2000
3.   Abramowitz J et al: Angiographic diagnosis and management of head and neck schwannomas. AJNR 12:97-84, 1991

MIDLINE SPACES

Retropharyngeal Space Abscess

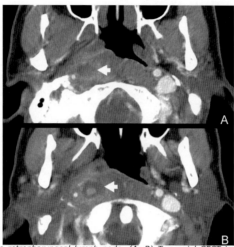

*Suppurative retropharyngeal lymph node. (A, B) Two axial CECT images of the nasopharynx depict a right suppurative retropharyngeal node (arrows). Initial reaction of a lymph node to seeding by a pathogen is to react, then suppurate. Another term for a suppurative node is **intranodal abscess**.*

Key Facts
- Definition: Abscess within the retropharyngeal space
- Classic imaging appearance: Unilateral suppurative node, early; rectangular to ovoid fluid collection filling the RPS with thick, enhancing wall, late
- Progression of inflammatory disease is usually a primary suppurative unilateral node, which ruptures into RPS
- RPS infection is now often diagnosed before RPS abscess has fully formed; RPS suppurative node with cellulitis more commonly found
- Antibiotics alone may suffice in the early stages of infection

Imaging Findings
General Features
- Best imaging clue: Focal RPS fluid
- Imaging appearance depends on stage of infection
- Early: Unilateral, suppurative RPS node is seen with RPS cellulitis
- Late: Walled-off fluid fills the entire RPS, extending inferiorly toward the mediastinum
CT Findings
- Early: Lateral RPS cystic mass (suppurative node) with low density in the adjacent RPS (cellulitis); no enhancing wall, asymmetric airway effacement
  - Narrowing of ipsilateral ICA may be seen in children
- Late: Shows fluid filling the RPS from side to side
  - Thick, enhancing wall is seen identifying mature RPS abscess
  - Anterior bowing of pharyngeal wall by RPS abscess
  - Posterior flattening of prevertebral muscles
  - If large, fluid may extend into mediastinum
Plain Films of Cervical Neck Soft Tissues
- Prevertebral soft-tissue swelling

Retropharyngeal Space Abscess

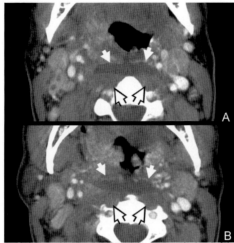

Retropharyngeal abscess. (A, B) Two CECT axial images at the level of the oropharynx reveal an abscess (arrows) situated between the anterior pharyngeal mucosal space and the posterior prevertebral muscles (open arrows).

- Loss of normal cervical lordosis
- Air in prevertebral soft tissues (uncommon)

<u>Imaging Recommendations</u>
- CECT of neck from skull base to carina best exam when RPS abscess is suspected
- CT permits differentiation between suppurative RPS node with edema and RPS abscess
- Be careful of early arterial phase scanning as abscess wall may enhance late

Differential Diagnosis: Retropharyngeal Space Lesion
<u>Retropharyngeal Space Edema</u>
- Secondary to jugular vein thrombosis or post-radical neck dissection with IJV resection
- Fluid seen in RPS with associated JV thrombosis or IJV resection

<u>RPS Suppurative Node with RPS Edema</u>
- Cystic node seen in lateral RPS
- Fluid within adjacent RPS has no enhancing wall

<u>RPS Malignant Adenopathy</u>
- Enlarged RPS node ± central nodal necrosis
- H & N SCCa, melanoma or other metastatic disease

Pathology
<u>General</u>
- Embryology-Anatomy
  - Only the suprahyoid RPS contains nodes
  - All RPS abscesses begin in suprahyoid neck RPS
  - RPS extends from skull base above to T4 below
  - Inferior continuity between RPS and **danger space** provides conduit for RPS abscess to mediastinum

Retropharyngeal Space Abscess

- Etiology-Pathogenesis
  - Pharyngitis or tooth infection seeds RPS lymph nodes
  - RPS nodes react, then suppurate, forming **intranodal abscess**
  - Pus ruptures from suppurative node into adjacent RPS
  - When walled off, an RPS abscess is formed
- Epidemiology
  - Increasingly rare to see full-blown RPS abscess
  - 25% RPS abscess
  - 75% RPS suppurative node with cellulitis

Gross Pathologic, Surgical Features
- Yellow-green fluid drains from distended RPS
- Thick abscess wall is fibrous connective tissue

Microscopic Features
- Pus = necrotic debris, polymorphonuclear leukocytes, lymphocytes and macrophages
- Abscess wall = granulation tissue (capillaries, fibroblasts) and fibrous connective tissue (fibroblasts, collagen fibers)

Clinical Issues

Presentation
- Most patients < 10 years old unless immunocompromised
- 2:1 males
- Very sick, septic-appearing patient
- Fever, chills, sore throat & elevated white blood cell count
- Infants present with stridor or airway obstruction
- Physical exam: Posterior wall of pharynx bulges inward

Natural History
- Untreated abscess may spread either inferiorly via danger space into mediastinum or locally into adjacent spaces

Treatment
- When infection is found at early stages (reactive or suppurative node, and/or cellulitis), antibiotic therapy & airway support, and follow-up imaging considered treatment of choice
- When suppurative node has ruptured and retropharyngeal space has filled with pus, surgical intervention is warranted

Prognosis
- Surgical drainage with aggressive intravenous antibiotics creates excellent prognosis in vast majority of cases

Selected References
1. Boucher C et al: Retropharyngeal abscesses: a clinical and radiologic correlation. J Otolaryngol 28:134-7, 1999
2. Huag RH et al: Diagnosis and treatment of the retropharyngeal abscess in adults. Br J Maxillofac Surg 28:34-8, 1990
3. Davis WL et al: Retropharyngeal space: evaluation of normal anatomy and diseases with CT and MR imaging. Radiology 174:59-64, 1990

RPS Nodal Malignancy

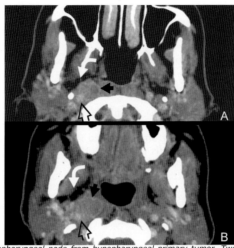

SCCa retropharyngeal node from hypopharyngeal primary tumor. Two axial CECT through nasopharynx (A) and high oropharynx (B) reveal a large right necrotic retropharyngeal node (arrow) that displaces the internal carotid artery laterally (open arrow) and elevates the medial parapharyngeal space (curved arrow).

Key Facts
- Multiple head and neck malignancies can spread to the RPS nodes
- Pharyngeal SCCa, especially nasopharyngeal carcinoma (NPCa), is the most common malignancy that spreads to retropharyngeal space (RPS) nodes
- Since there are no RPS nodes below the hyoid bone, RPS malignant adenopathy (RPS-MA) is a suprahyoid neck phenomenon
- Classic imaging appearance: Cystic-necrotic oval to round mass > 1cm in the RPS just medial to the ICA

Imaging Findings
General Features
- Lateral RPS-MA displaces the PPS fat anteromedially
  - Care must be taken not to mistake this lesion for carotid space (CS) mass
  - CS masses are centered more lateral in the midst of the carotid artery and internal jugular vein
- RPS malignant nodes are identified by
  - Any size node with central nodal necrosis
  - > 1 cm RPS node in an adult
CT Findings
- Often difficult to identify on CT, especially if the patient is thin
- SCCa RPS node: Oval to round mass just medial to the ICA associated with NPCa, posterior wall oropharynx (OP) or hypopharynx primary SCCa
- Thyroid Ca RPS node: May have Ca++ or prominent cystic change
- Other RPS-MA: Adult with known malignancy with RPS node > 1cm
  - Especially melanoma & non-Hodgkin lymphoma (NHL)

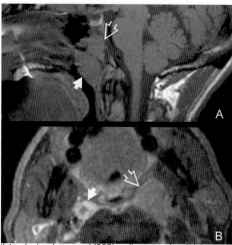

NPCa with bilateral retropharyngeal (RPS) malignant nodes. (A) Sagittal T1 MR shows a nasopharyngeal mass (arrow) invading clivus (open arrow). (B) Axial T1 C+ MR through oropharynx shows bilateral malignant RPS nodes. Right RPS node (arrow), central nodal necrosis; left RPS node (open arrow) malignant by size.

MR Findings
- MR clearly distinguishes NPCa, OPCa and hypopharyngeal Ca primary tumor from more posterior RPS malignant node
- Thyroid Ca nodes may have high T1 signal (thyroglobulin)

Nuclear Medicine Findings
- PET: Valuable complementary information in nodal SCCa staging
- I-131: May first identify high lateral RPS nodal involvement

Imaging Recommendations
- If RPS-MA is incidentally observed on brain MR, follow-up MR imaging of the nasopharynx (NPCa), oropharynx (OPCa), thyroid (Ca) and neck nodes (NHL) should be undertaken
- MR is more sensitive to the presence of RPS-MA than CT
- If a primary pharyngeal SCCa is clinically overt, MR imaging should both stage the primary and nodal extent simultaneously

Differential Diagnosis: RPS Masses

Reactive RPS Adenopathy
- Homogeneous RPS mass less than 1 cm
- Usually in < 30 year old with multiple other reactive-appearing nodes and tonsillar hyperplasia

Suppurative RPS Adenopathy
- Clinical pharyngitis is present in a septic patient
- Usually in < 30 year old with tonsillar hyperplasia
- RPS edema or early abscess may be associated

Direct Invasion, Posterior Pharyngeal Wall SCCa
- Clinically overt posterior pharyngeal wall SCCa (OP or hypopharynx)
- Imaging shows contiguous, invasive mass in the PMS and RPS

RPS Nodal Malignancy

Pathology
General
- General Path Comments
  - H & N and systemic malignancies can spread to RPS nodes
  - Pharyngeal SCCa > NHL > Thyroid Ca > Melanoma
  - Pharyngeal SCCa breakdown: NP >> OP & HP primary sites
  - If OP or NP, primary on posterior wall
- Embryology
  - During formation of the RPS, medial and lateral (nodes of Rouviere) lymph **nodes** are **in** the **suprahyoid RPS**
  - The RPS nodes are primary drainage for the posterior nasal cavity, ethmoid and sphenoid sinus, hard and soft palate, the **nasopharynx** and the posterior wall of oro- and **hypopharynx**
    - The postcricoid hypopharynx, cervical esophagus and posterior capsule of the **thyroid** gland may also drain into RPS nodes
  - No lymph nodes are incorporated in the infrahyoid RPS
- Etiology-Pathogenesis
  - Primary tumors of head and neck seed RPS lymph nodes
- Epidemiology
  - 75% of NPCa have RPS malignant adenopathy at presentation
  - 20% of posterior OP and HP wall SCCa have RPS-MA
  - < 5% of thyroid carcinoma have RPS-MA

Microscopic Features
- SCCa: Lymph node is replaced by epithelial-lined structures with central cystic change
  - Epithelial lining of the cystic spaces is composed of hypercellular pleomorphic cells with increased mitotic activity
- Thyroid Ca: Papillary and/or follicular cells seen with thyroglobulin
- Melanoma: Epithelioid and/or spindle cells with melanin deposition

Staging Criteria
- RPS-MA not specifically mentioned in nodal staging criteria
- Considered a negative prognostic indicator

Clinical Issues
Presentation
- RPS malignant adenopathy is often clinically occult
- If large, bulging of the posterolateral wall of the NP or OP

Treatment
- For NPCa, included in XRT boost field
- For OP and HP SCCa RPS-MA, surgical nodal dissection
- For thyroid carcinoma, surgical removal prior to I-131 therapy
- For melanoma, if isolated, aggressive surgical excision

Prognosis
- RPS-MA in SCCa and melanoma is a strong predictor of poor prognosis
- For thyroid carcinoma, RPS-MA does not affect prognosis

Selected References
1. King AD et al: Neck node metastases from nasopharyngeal carcinoma: MR imaging of patterns of disease. Head Neck 22:275-81, 2000
2. McLaughlin MP et al: Retropharyngeal adenopathy as a predictor of outcome in squamous cell carcinoma of the head and neck. Head Neck 190-8, 1995
3. Davis WL et al: Retropharyngeal space: evaluation of normal anatomy and diseases with CT and MR imaging. Radiology 174:59-64, 1990

Prevertebral Abscess

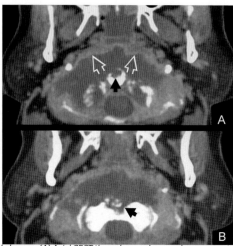

Prevertebral abscess. (A) Axial CECT through nasopharynx shows prevertebral abscess elevating prevertebral muscles (open arrows). Odontoid process of C2 & associated vertebral body are eroded by osteomyelitis (arrow). (B) CECT below (A) again shows prevertebral abscess. Arrow: C2 body osteomyelitis erosion.

Key Facts
- Synonym: Vertebral osteomyelitis with perivertebral space abscess
- Definition: Osteomyelitis of a cervical vertebral body (VB) spreads to become a prevertebral abscess (PVA) or phlegmon
- Classic imaging appearance: Cervical VB destruction associated with prevertebral area and epidural enhancement (plegmon) or fluid (abscess)
- Worldwide primary offending organism is M. tuberculosis; in USA primary offending organism is staphylococcus aureus (S. aureus)

Imaging Findings
General Features
- Pyogenic osteomyelitis
  - Cervical VB and disc space destruction
  - Edema-cellulitis extensive in adjacent soft tissues
  - Prevertebral muscles are lifted and/or engulfed by infection
  - Posterior elements not involved (cf. VB metastases)
- Tuberculous osteomyelitis
  - Cervical VB destruction involving 2 consecutive levels
  - **Sparing of the intervertebral disc** characteristic
  - VB **fragments** characteristic
  - Disc herniation into the VB, epidural involvement and PVA
CT Findings
- Pyogenic osteomyelitis
  - Disc space narrowing is earliest imaging sign
  - Superior and inferior VB endplate erosion, then loss next
- Tuberculous osteomyelitis
  - Disc and endplate sparing common
  - VB **fragments** with bony debris seen in epidural area (70%)

Prevertebral Abscess

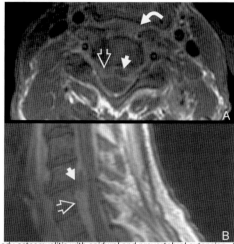

Vertebral body osteomyelitis with epidural and prevertebral extension. Axial (A) and sagittal (B) T1 C+ MR images show epidural abscess (arrow) and phlegmon (open arrow) from disk space infection. Curved arrow marks phlegmon extending into prevertebral soft tissues.

MR Findings
- Pyogenic osteomyelitis
  - Decreased T1 signal, increased T2 signal in cervical VB and disc
  - T1 C+ enhancement of disc and VB
- Tuberculous osteomyelitis
  - 2 consecutive cervical vertebrae are involved
  - Disc sparing common
  - Prevertebral soft tissue infection (phlegmon or abscess) common

Plain Films Findings
- Early (< 6 wks) cervical subluxation may be only finding
  - Disc space narrowing and/or endplate erosion can be early clues
- Late (> 6 wks) VB destruction (osteomyelitis) ± abnormal thickness to prevertebral soft tissues (PVA)

Imaging Recommendations
- Plain films with flexion and extension
- CECT looking at cervical soft tissues and vertebrae
- MR is used if any clinical or CT suspicion of epidural infection

Differential Diagnosis: Vertebral Body Destructive Lesion

Vertebral Body Metastatic Tumor
- VB destruction with disc sparing on CT & MR
- Posterior elements involved (75%)
- Adjacent soft tissue planes intact; do not show edema
- MR, bone scan or PET shows multiple other metastases

Pathology

General
- Anatomy-Embryology
  - The deep layer of deep cervical fascia surrounds the **perivertebral space** (PVS) completely

Prevertebral Abscess

- o   A fascial slip that reaches to the transverse process divides the PVS into anterior **prevertebral** and posterior **paraspinal** spaces
- o   PVA is confined by this fascia, forcing the infection into the epidural space within the spinal canal
- • Etiology-Pathogenesis
  - o   PVA caused by hematogenous spread of infection, penetrating spine or neck trauma or cervical surgical procedures
  - o   Hematogenous spread = most common inoculation mechanism
    - ▪ Genitourinary infection, IV drug use, respiratory infection and spinal trauma may all initiate the hematogenous process
- • Epidemiology
  - o   Worldwide the most common cause of **cervical osteomyelitis** is **tuberculous spondylitis**
  - o   In US, S. aureus is most common pathogen

Gross Pathologic, Surgical Features
- • In advance-cases, the vertebral body is soft and fragmented

Microscopic Features: Microbiology
- • 60% of pyogenic vertebral osteomyelitis secondary to S. aureus
- • Gram-negative osteomyelitis (Pseudomonas) seen with IV drug use
- • M. tuberculosis most commonly seen among the destitute

Clinical Issues

Presentation
- • Cervical osteomyelitis
  - o   Most common: Fever, localized neck pain and stiffness
  - o   Less common: Malaise, weight loss and torticollis
  - o   20% present with myelopathy associated with epidural mass
- • Prevertebral abscess
  - o   Dysphagia, odynophagia and shortness of breath
- • History of urinary tract infection, neck surgery, instrumentation or IV drug abuse may be present

Natural History
- • Left untreated, cervical osteomyelitis with PVA will spread deep to create epidural abscess and anteriorly to form retropharyngeal abscess

Treatment
- • Intravenous antibiotics
- • Identification of offending organism + abscess drainage if present
- • Surgical intervention to debride dead bone and create supportive bony fusion if collapse or kyphosis has resulted

Prognosis
- • Neurologic deficits may not recover after treatment

Selected References
1.   Dagirmanjian A et al: MR imaging of vertebral osteomyelitis revisited. AJR 167:1539-43, 1996
2.   Davis WL et al: CT and MRI of the normal and diseased perivertebral space. Neuroradiology 37:388-94, 1995
3.   Battista RA et al: Prevertebral space infections associated with cervical osteomyelitis. Otolaryngol Head Neck Surg 108:160-6, 1993

Prevertebral Metastases

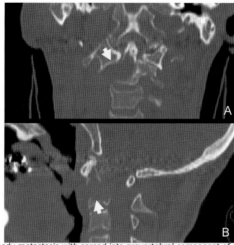

Vertebral body metastasis with spread into prevertebral component of perivertebral space. Coronal (A) and sagittal (B) CT reformations of upper cervical spine delineate a C2 vertebral body metastasis (arrows) as a focal bony destructive process.

Key Facts
- Definition: Any metastatic tumor involving the cervical vertebral body (VB) with invasion of the adjacent prevertebral area
- Classic imaging appearance: Cervical VB and posterior element destruction associated with prevertebral and epidural tumor

Imaging Findings
General Features
- Best imaging clue: Cervical VB destruction with disc space sparing
- 75% have **posterior elements** involved by tumor
- Soft tissue mass in prevertebral and epidural spaces
- Prevertebral muscles are lifted and/or engulfed by tumor
- Multiple bony lesions possible
CT Findings
- Fragmentary VB destruction with bony debris
- Epidural spread may be hard to see
MR Findings
- Prevertebral soft tissue commonly associated
- Epidural mass ± cord compression
Plain Films Findings
- VB destruction **without** significant prevertebral swelling
Bone Scintigraphy
- Positive when VB cortical involvement is present
- Often negative when metastasis is small and located within the VB medullary cavity
- MR may be + when bone scintigraphy is negative
Imaging Recommendations
- Bone scintigraphy may show multiple metastatic foci in other parts of spine or other distant bones

Prevertebral Metastases

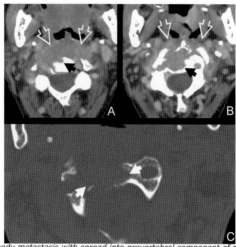

Vertebral body metastasis with spread into prevertebral component of perivertebral space. (A, B) Axial CECT of C2 vertebral body reveals destructive metastasis (arrows) with prevertebral spread confined by deep layer of deep cervical fascia. (C) Bone-only axial image shows destructive metastasis (arrows).

- Bone-only CT with multiplanar reconstruction best defines degree of spine instability; delineates surgical stabilization challenges
- MR excellent in delineating epidural foci; if found, consider also screening the T- and L-spines
  - Cord compression best detected by MR
  - Early, non-cortical VB metastases may only be seen with MR

Differential Diagnosis: Vertebral Body Destructive Mass
VB Osteomyelitis: Aerobic or Anaerobic
- VB destruction; + endplate and disc
- Posterior elements uninvolved
VB Osteomyelitis: Tuberculous
- May be precise mimic of metastatic tumor
- VB destruction with disc sparing on CT & MR
- VB bone fragments are distinctive
- Adjacent soft tissue planes show edema or abscess
Non-Hodgkin Lymphoma
- Arises in PVS, secondarily affects VB
Cervical Chordoma
- Very rare lesion
- Indistinguishable from VB metastasis

Pathology
General
- Anatomy-Embryology
  - The deep layer of deep cervical fascia surrounds the **perivertebral space** (PVS)
  - A fascial slip that reaches to the transverse process divides the PVS into the anterior **prevertebral** and posterior **paraspinal spaces**

Prevertebral Metastases

- o Vertebral metastases are confined by this fascia, forcing the tumor into the epidural space within the spinal canal
- Etiology-Pathogenesis
  - o Vertebral body metastases caused by hematogenous spread of malignancy or penetration of posterior pharyngeal wall SCCa
  - o Hematogenous spread = most common mechanism
- Epidemiology
  - o Most common lesion of the VB and PVS is metastases (30%)

Microscopic Features
- Histology often obtained by needle biopsy
- No predominant histopathology

Clinical Issues
Presentation
- Principal presenting symptom: Neck pain
- Other symptoms: Myeloradiculopathy
- Known primary tumor of lung, breast, kidney, soft tissues

Natural History
- Left untreated, VB metastatic disease will invade epidural space, compress the spinal cord and cause myelopathy

Treatment
- External XRT with steroid therapy
- Surgical resection with spine stabilization when no response to XRT
  - o Laminectomy vs. anterior vertebral body resection

Prognosis
- Neurologic deficits will not recover after treatment
- Poor prognosis with some dependence on tumor histology

Selected References
1. Taoka T et al: Factors influencing visualization of vertebral metastases on MR imaging versus bone scintigraphy. AJR 176:1525-30, 2001
2. Gupta RK et al: Problems in distinguishing spinal tuberculosis from neoplasia on MRI. Neuroradiology 38:97-104, 1996
3. Davis WL et al: CT and MRI of the normal and diseased perivertebral space. Neuroradiology 37:388-94, 1995

VISCERAL SPACE

Multinodular Goiter

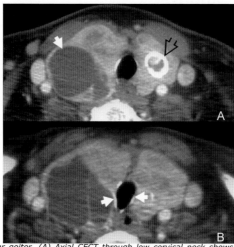

Multinodular goiter. (A) Axial CECT through low cervical neck shows holothyroid enlargement with intrathyroidal cysts (arrow) and calcifications (open arrow). (B) Just inferior to (A) the trachea is narrowed by compression on both sides (arrows) from the thyromegaly.

Key Facts

- Synonyms: Nodular goiter, nontoxic goiter or simple goiter
- Definitions
  - **Multinodular goiter** (MNG) = Enlargement of thyroid gland in response to inadequate endogenous thyroid hormone production
    - Diffuse hyperplasia mixed with degenerative nodules gives gland its multinodular appearance
  - Plunging or substernal goiter = MNG that has grown into mediastinum from inferior thyroid gland poles
- Classic imaging appearance: Holothyroid enlargement with sharp margins and multiple cystic, calcified, intraglandular nodules causing inhomogeneous enhancement

Imaging Findings

General Features

- Best imaging clue: Bizarre inhomogeneous thyromegaly
  - When first encountered, MNG bizarre imaging appearance suggests malignancy to the uninitiated
- Sharply-marginated **holothyroid enlargement** within visceral space of infrahyoid neck
  - Displaces carotid spaces away from midline
  - Pinches trachea between swollen thyroid lobes
- Multiple complex masses within the enlarged thyroid
- Calcifications, degenerative cysts and hemorrhage make for wild densities/intensities on CT/MR respectively
- No normal thyroid identified; no associated lymph nodes

CT Findings

- CECT shows large, inhomogeneously-enhancing thyroid
- 90% have focal calcifications (amorphous, ring-like, curvilinear)
- Low-density areas of degenerative and colloidal cysts

Multinodular Goiter

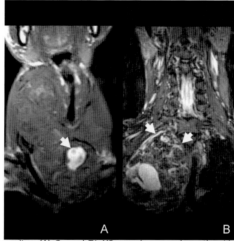

Multinodular goiter. (A) Coronal T1 MR reveals a very large thyroid mass in the cervical neck with a central area of high protein colloid (arrow). (B) On coronal T2 MR more posterior than (A) the inferior lobule of the multinodular goiter (MNG) (arrows) is seen. Bizarre mixed intensity is highly suggestive of MNG.

- Mixed-density areas of old and new hemorrhage

MR Findings
- Nodules within enlarged thyroid gland have **bizarre inhomogeneous signals** from protein and hemorrhage effects
- On coronal sequences, enlarged thyroid has **chevron shape**
- Coronal images show **"cradling"** of inferior extent of substernal MNG by brachiocephalic vessels

Chest X-ray Findings
- If suprasternal, may be normal or show mild tracheal deviation
- If substernal, tracheal deviation with superior mediastinal mass

Radioiodine Scintigraphy
- Effective in recognizing a mediastinal mass as thyroid in nature

Imaging Recommendations
- CECT is exam of choice for routine questions related to MNG
  - Imaging questions include
    - Extent and severity of airway compression
    - Presence and extent of substernal MNG
    - Unusual extensions of MNG (e.g. retroesophageal)
- If FNA suggests malignancy, MR imaging is used to stage nodal extent, without compromising subsequent I-131 therapy

Differential Diagnosis: Large Visceral Space Mass
Hemorrhagic Colloid Cyst
- Large, cystic mass within thyroid
- Unilateral with normal thyroid tissue seen

Follicular Adenoma
- Solitary intrathyroidal mass without local invasion or adenopathy
- No imaging modality reliably differentiates from early carcinoma

Papillary Thyroid Carcinoma
- Tumor may occupy all or part of the thyroid gland

- Thyroid gland margins may be invasive
- 50% have cervical or upper mediastinal malignant nodes

Anaplastic Thyroid Carcinoma
- Rapidly enlarging, invasive tumor originating from the thyroid
- Esophagus, trachea, carotid space may be invaded

Non-Hodgkin Lymphoma
- Large, invasive tumor originating from the thyroid
- May be indistinguishable from anaplastic carcinoma

Pathology
General
- Etiology-Pathogenesis
  o Thyroid gland in its basal state cannot supply the body with adequate thyroid hormone in MNG cases
  o Thyroid hyperplasia results with gradual glandular enlargement
  o Thyroid follicles degenerate within the enlarged gland giving it a multinodular imaging appearance
- Epidemiology
  o In US, incidence = 1.5% per year; 250,000 new cases annually
  o 95% MNG benign; 5% malignant

Microscopic Features
- Distended follicles with colloid and hyperplasia of thyroid tissue
- Follicle degeneration leads to hemorrhage, infarction, fibrosis, cyst formation and calcification

Clinical Issues
Presentation
- Principal presenting symptom: Large lower neck mass
- Bilateral lobular masses in lower cervical neck
- Airway compression (55%); hoarseness (15%); dysphagia (10%); superior vena cava syndrome (10%)
- Most are nontoxic (normal TSH levels)
- 2:1 female; older patients
- At risk: History of exposure to external irradiation

Treatment
- No treatment for asymptomatic, non-palpable MNG identified on U/S, CT or MR of neck done for other reasons
- Patients with prominent, growing, hard nodule may have FNA for cytology to exclude malignancy
- Large, non-toxic MNG with compressive symptoms: Surgical removal
- Toxic MNG: Surgery or radioiodine therapy
- Substernal MNG: Suprasternal collar incision alone usually adequate
  o Median sternotomy rarely necessary (< 2%)

Prognosis
- Thyroid gland removal accompanied by thyroid hormone replacement provides excellent relief from MNG

Selected References
1. Hurley DL et al: Evaluation and management of multinodular goiter. Otolaryngol Clin North Am 29:527-40, 1996
2. Singh B et al: Substernal goiter: a clinical review. Am J Otolaryngol 15:409-16, 1994
3. Bashist B et al: Computed tomography of intrathoracic goiters. AJR 140:455-60, 1983

Differentiated Thyroid Carcinoma

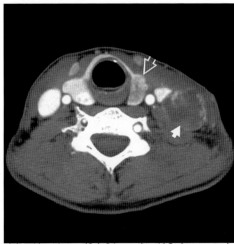

Differentiated thyroid carcinoma (Ca). Primary thyroid Ca (open arrow) and adjacent node (arrow) with mixed cystic, solid-enhancing regions is seen on axial CECT through the thyroid bed. Although MR is preferred in staging differentiated thyroid carcinoma, CT is often done when thyroid nature is unsuspected.

Key Facts
- Synonyms: Papillary, papillary-follicular or follicular carcinoma
- Definitions: Differentiated thyroid carcinoma (DTCa) = thyroid malignancies with well-defined histologies; includes **papillary** (90%) and **follicular** (10%) groups
- Classic imaging appearance: Focal, unilateral, intrathyroidal mass with irregular margins; may have extracapsular invasion and/or regional lymph node metastases
- Useful adage = **"Weird looking" nodes** in the cervical neck of a young female, think DTCa

Imaging Findings
General Features
- Primary tumor appearance: 10% bilateral; irregular or ill-defined borders of tumor mass with associated soft tissue invasion
- Lymph node appearance: May be small, hyperplastic appearing, cystic, hemorrhagic or contain calcification

CT Findings
- Cystic change (hypodensity), calcifications (hyperdensity) or well-defined borders to a thyroid mass does not exclude malignancy
- Metastatic adenopathy may appear "reactive" and small or contain areas of cystic change, calcification or nodular enhancement

MR Findings
- Mixed low- and high-signal intrathyroidal mass with heterogeneous enhancement; invasive margins help make malignant diagnosis
- Metastatic adenopathy may have areas of high signal on T1 pre-contrast images caused by hemorrhage and/or thyroglobulin

Ultrasound Findings
- Solid hypoechoic or isoechoic mass with or without calcification
- Calcification seen as hyperechoic acoustic shadowing

Differentiated Thyroid Carcinoma

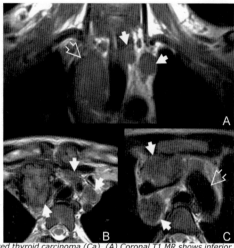

Differentiated thyroid carcinoma (Ca). (A) Coronal T1 MR shows inferior extension of thyroid Ca nodal disease (arrows) into superior mediastinum. Open arrow: Large right paratracheal nodal tumor. (B-C) Axial T2 MR through upper mediastinum reveals multiple metastatic nodes (arrows). Open arrow: Aortic arch.

- Echopenic halo around mass is incomplete
- Used to guide FNA in suspicious solitary nodules

Nuclear Medicine Findings
- Tc99m pertechnetate: Cold nodule most likely malignant (25%)
- I-131: Used for substernal thyroid glands or to perform whole body imaging after thyroidectomy to detect metastatic foci

Imaging Recommendations
- Radiologist must determine
  - Whether thyroid gland capsule is violated = extracapsular spread
  - Specific areas of extraglandular invasion (trachea, CS, RPS, PVS)
  - Presence and location of metastatic adenopathy
- Staging of DTCa best accomplished with **MR**
  - Extent of exam: Oropharynx to **carina**
- **Iodinated contrast** used in CECT **may postpone I-131 therapy**

Differential Diagnosis: Intrathyroidal Mass

Hemorrhagic Colloid Cyst
- Large, cystic mass within thyroid
- Unilateral with normal thyroid tissue seen

Follicular Adenoma
- Solitary intrathyroidal mass without local invasion or adenopathy
- No imaging modality reliably differentiates from early DTCa

Multinodular Goiter
- Multiple nodules in an enlarged thyroid gland

Medullary Carcinoma
- May exactly mimic DTCa when imaged

Anaplastic Carcinoma
- Rapidly enlarging, invasive tumor originating from the thyroid
- Esophagus, trachea, carotid space may be invaded

Differentiated Thyroid Carcinoma

Non-Hodgkin Lymphoma
- Also seen as a rapidly enlarging, invasive thyroid mass
- Rarely calcified or necrotic
- When lymph nodes associated, rarely necrotic

Pathology
General
- General Path Comments
  - Papillary (50%) >> follicular (10%) nodal spread at presentation
  - 5% have distant metastases at presentation (lungs, bone, CNS)
- Embryology-Anatomy
  - Nodal drainage from thyroid includes deep cervical, spinal accessory, retropharyngeal and **paratracheal** chains
  - The **paratracheal chain** takes DTCa into the mediastinum
- Etiology-Pathogenesis
  - Sporadic or radiation-induced malignant thyroid tumor
- Epidemiology
  - 80% of all thyroid malignancy is DTCa
  - DTCa is most frequent endocrine malignant neoplasm
    - 1% of all human malignant tumors
Microscopic Features
- Psammoma bodies = laminated calcific spherules (40%)
- Ground-glass nuclei; branching pattern within fibrovacular stroma
Staging Criteria: Primary Tumor (T)
- **T1**: Intrathyroidal tumor, ≤ 1 cm
- **T2**: Intrathyroidal tumor, 1-4 cm
- **T3**: Intrathyroidal tumor, > 4 cm
- **T4**: Tumor extends beyond the thyroid capsule
Staging Criteria: Regional Lymph Nodes (N)
- **N0**: No regional metastasis
- **N1**: Regional nodal metastasis
  - **N1a**: Nodal metastasis in ipsilateral cervical neck
  - **N1b**: Bilateral, midline or contralateral cervical or mediastinal

Clinical Issues
Presentation
- Principal presenting symptom: Paramedian lower cervical neck mass
- Risk factors: Previous radiation exposure (Chernobyl syndrome)
Treatment
- Total thyroidectomy and regional lymphadenectomy (if nodes present clinically or on imaging)
- Therapeutic I-131 follows surgical debulking to "mop up"
Prognosis
- 20-year survival rate = 90% (papillary), 75% (follicular)
- Rising serum thyroglobulin indicates recurrence (< 10%); I-131 then identifies the site of recurrence

Selected References
1. Takashima S et al: Differentiated thyroid carcinomas: prediction of tumor invasion with MR imaging. Acta Radiologica 41:377-83, 2000
2. Toubert ME et al: Cervicomediastinal MRI in persistent or recurrent papillary thyroid carcinoma: clinical use and limits. Thyroid 9:591-7, 1999
3. Mazzaferri EL: An overview of the management of papillary and follicular thyroid carcinoma. Thyroid 9:421-7, 1999

Anaplastic Thyroid Carcinoma

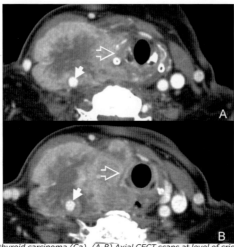

Anaplastic thyroid carcinoma (Ca). (A-B) Axial CECT scans at level of cricoid cartilage reveal invasive right thyroid mass. The larynx is being invaded (open arrow) through its protective cartilage. Engulfed common carotid artery is seen in the posterolateral margin of the anaplastic Ca (arrow).

Key Facts
- Synonym: Undifferentiated thyroid carcinoma
- Definition: Anaplastic thyroid carcinoma (ATCa) = lethal, uncommon, thyroid malignancy that affects older patients and is poorly responsive to multimodality therapy
- Classic imaging appearance: Rapidly growing, poorly-marginated thyroid mass that invades multiple adjacent infrahyoid neck spaces
- ATCa does not concentrate iodine or express thyroglobulin
- Multimodality therapy is palliative with life expectancy measured in months, not years

Imaging Findings
General Features
- Best imaging clue: Large (> 5 cm), very invasive thyroid mass
- Invades adjacent structures of visceral space including larynx, trachea, recurrent laryngeal nerve and esophagus
- Invades adjacent IHN spaces including the CS, RPS, PVS and PCS
- If ATCa arises out of multinodular goiter (MNG), thyromegaly is present
- Nodal metastasis present 40%
- Distant metastasis present 25%
CT Findings
- Dense, amorphous calcifications seen within mass (60%)
- Necrosis within tumor mass (75%)
- Necrotic metastatic adenopathy seen 50%
MR Findings
- Invasive mass with complex signal characteristics
Ultrasound Findings
- Hypoechoic mass that invades structures of the neck
Imaging Recommendations
- MR of cervical neck and mediastinum is exam of choice

Anaplastic Thyroid Carcinoma

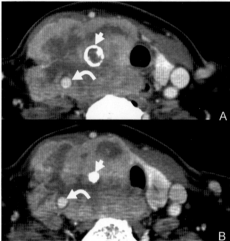

Anaplastic thyroid carcinoma (Ca). (A-B) An invasive tumor is seen centered in the right thyroid gland on axial CECT images. Benign-appearing calcifications (arrows) suggest that this anaplastic Ca arose from multinodular goiter. Curved arrow: Common carotid artery fixation by anaplastic Ca.

- o Iodinated contrast used in CECT may postpone I-131 therapy if tumor turns out to be differentiated thyroid carcinoma
- If diagnosis known before imaging, CECT faster and cheaper (cf. MR)

Differential Diagnosis: Intrathyroidal Mass
Hemorrhagic Colloid Cyst
- Large, cystic mass within thyroid
- Unilateral with normal thyroid tissue seen
Follicular Adenoma
- Solitary intrathyroidal mass without local invasion or adenopathy
- No imaging modality reliably differentiates from early DTCa
Multinodular Goiter
- Multiple nodules in an enlarged thyroid gland
Differentiated Thyroid Carcinoma
- Unilateral poorly-marginated thyroid mass with adenopathy
Medullary Carcinoma
- May exactly mimic differentiated thyroid Ca when imaged
Non-Hodgkin Lymphoma
- Also seen as a rapidly enlarging, invasive thyroid mass
- Rarely calcified or necrotic
- When lymph nodes associated, rarely necrotic

Pathology
General
- General Path Comments
  - o In up to 33% of cases, ATCa arises out of MNG
  - o May coexist with other forms of thyroid Ca, especially papillary
- Etiology-Pathogenesis

Anaplastic Thyroid Carcinoma

- o Best hypothesis = Prolonged stimulation of MNG or differentiated carcinoma by thyroid-stimulating hormone transforms these conditions into the highly malignant ATCa
- Epidemiology
  - o 5-10% of thyroid carcinoma group

Microscopic Features
- Tumors classified according to predominant cell type
- Small cell, giant cell, spindle cell or mixed spindle-giant cell Ca
- 25% have concomitant follicular or papillary thyroid Ca

Clinical Issues
Presentation
- Principal presenting symptom: Rapidly growing, large, (> 5 cm) painful mass in thyroid area
- Elderly patient group with mean age at presentation = 65 years
- Other symptoms if invasion of
  - o Larynx or trachea: Dyspnea
  - o Recurrent laryngeal nerve: Hoarseness
  - o Esophagus: Dysphagia
- Medical history: History of radiation to neck (15%); previous MNG

Natural History
- ATCa is one of the most aggressive neoplasms seen in humans
- Rapid growth and lack of response to therapy lead to quick demise

Treatment
- Multimodality with surgery, and/or radiotherapy and chemotherapy
- Biopsy with tracheostomy followed by combined radio-chemotherapy most commonly employed
- Aggressive surgery probably only warranted when tumor is caught early and has not invaded widely into adjacent spaces

Prognosis
- Poor prognosis is universally accepted
- Rapidly fatal with mean survival of 6 months after diagnosis

Selected References
1. Giuffrida D et al: Anaplastic thyroid carcinoma: current diagnosis and treatment. Ann Oncol 11:1083-9, 2000
2. Takashima S et al: CT evaluation of anaplastic thyroid carcinoma. AJNR 11:361-7, 1990
3. Nel CJ et al: Anaplastic carcinoma of thyroid: a clinicopathologic study of 82 cases. Mayo Clin Proc 60:51-8, 1985

PEDIATRIC LESIONS

First Branchial Cleft Cyst

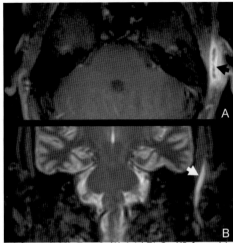

1st branchial cleft cyst (BCC), Type I. (A) Axial T1 C+ MR focused just above left auricle shows rim-enhancing 1st BCC (arrow). (B) Coronal T2 MR image through the posterior temporal bone reveals the high signal 1st BCC (arrow) following a course projecting inferiorly to just below the left auricle (open arrow).

Key Facts

- Synonyms: Cervicoaural cyst, branchial cleft remnant, branchial cleft sinus, fistula, or cyst
- Definition: First branchial cleft cyst (1st BCC) = benign, congenital cyst that occurs either in parotid or submandibular space or preauricular region
  - Remnant of the 1st branchial cleft
- Classic imaging appearance: Well-circumscribed, non-enhancing cyst
  - **Type I 1st BCC**
    - Presents either below or posterior to the pinna
    - Runs parallel to the EAC
  - **Type II 1st BCC**
    - Presents in parotid space and periparotid area
    - If sinus exists, found at angle of mandible
    - Deep projection to bony-cartilaginous junction of EAC
- Clinical presentation: Soft, painless EAC or parotid space mass in a child; recurrent swelling is typical

Imaging Findings

General Features

- Best imaging clue: Ovoid cystic mass in the area around the EAC (Type I) or in the area of the parotid space (Type II)
- Type I 1st BCC: Ovoid cystic mass below or posterior to pinna
- Type II 1st BCC: Ovoid well-marginated cystic mass found in parotid space or periparotid area
  - Periparotid area includes
    - Parapharyngeal space
    - Superficial space over the surface of the parotid gland

First Branchial Cleft Cyst

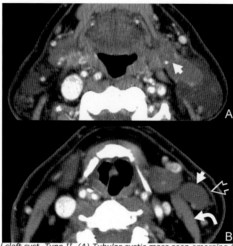

1st branchial cleft cyst, Type II. (A) Tubular cystic mass seen emerging (arrow) from inferior margin of parotid tail (open arrow) on axial CECT. (B) At level of hyoid bone the 1st BCC is seen as an oval low-density lesion (arrow) hanging from the parotid tail. Open arrow: Platysma; Curved arrow: Sternomastoid.

CT Findings
- CECT shows well-circumscribed, non-enhancing or rim-enhancing, low-density mass
- Thick, enhancing rim suggests superinfection

MR Findings
- Low signal on T1; high signal on T2
- No wall enhancement on T1 C+ MR images is typical

Ultrasound Findings
- Anechoic mass in the area of the EAC or parotid space

Imaging Recommendations
- CECT is recommended imaging procedure
- Both soft tissues and bony EAC can be assessed

Differential Diagnosis: Cystic Parotid Space Mass in a Child
Cystic Hygroma
- Imaging: Most commonly multilocular, insinuating lesion
  - If unilocular, may be difficult to differentiate from 1st BCC
- Clinical: Rarely involves area of parotid space

Neck Abscess
- Imaging: Thick-walled, lobulated mass most commonly seen in node-bearing space (retropharyngeal or submandibular space)
  - Associated cellulitis expected
- Clinical: Presents with marked tenderness and fever

Suppurative Parotid Lymph Node
- Imaging: Thick-walled, ovoid, cystic mass within parotid; if single, may look like infected 1st BCC
- Clinical: Presents with marked tenderness and fever

First Branchial Cleft Cyst

Pathology

<u>General</u>
- Embryology-Anatomy
  - Remnant of 1st branchial apparatus
  - 1st branchial apparatus composed of dorsal and ventral portions
    - Dorsal gives rise to the incus body, malleus head, pinna, EAC, eustachian tube, middle ear cavity and mastoid air cells
    - Ventral gives rise to the remainder of the malleus
- Etiology-Pathogenesis
  - Persistence of the first branchial apparatus
- Epidemiology
- Very rare lesions
- 1st BCC accounts for only 8% of branchial cleft remnants
- 2nd BCC most common

<u>Gross Pathologic, Surgical Features</u>
- Cystic neck mass, easily dissected at surgery unless there has been repeated infection
- Facial nerve may be medial or lateral to 1st BCC
  - Cystic remnant may split the facial nerve trunk

<u>Microscopic Features</u>
- Thin outer layer of fibrous tissue
- Inner layer of flat squamoid epithelium
- Germinal centers may be present in cyst wall

Clinical Issues

<u>Presentation</u>
- Principal presenting symptom: Compressible neck mass in the EAC, parotid or periparotid area
- Other symptoms
  - Persistent otorrhea without middle ear disease
    - Seen when connects to bony-cartilaginous junction of EAC
  - Rarely associated facial nerve palsy
- Age of presentation: Majority present < 10 years old

<u>Natural History</u>
- May enlarge with upper respiratory track infection
- Often incised and drained as an "abscess," only to recur

<u>Treatment</u>
- Complete surgical resection
- Proximity to the facial nerve puts the nerve at risk during surgery

<u>Prognosis</u>
- Depends on surgical resection
- May recur if residual cyst wall remains

Selected References
1. Benson MT et al: Congenital anomalies of the branchial apparatus: embryology and pathologic anatomy. RadioGraphics 12:943-60, 1992
2. Finn DG et al: First branchial cleft cysts: clinical update. Laryngoscope 97:136-40, 1987
3. Belenky WM et al: First branchial cleft anomalies. Laryngoscope 90:28-39, 1980

Second Branchial Cleft Cyst

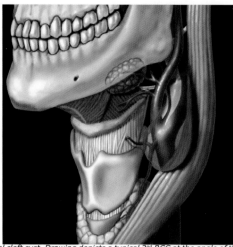

2nd branchial cleft cyst. Drawing depicts a typical 2nd BCC at the angle of the mandible. The sternomastoid muscle is pushed posterolaterally while the carotid is pushed medially. If the cyst has a deep sinus, it passes between the external and internal carotid arteries to surface in the faucial tonsillar crypts.

Key Facts
- Synonyms: Branchial apparatus remnant, branchial cleft anomaly
- Definition: Second branchial cleft cyst (2nd BCC) = cystic remnant cleft related to developmental alterations of the second branchial apparatus
- Classic imaging appearance: Non-enhancing well-circumscribed mass at anterior margin of sternomastoid muscle, just posterior to the submandibular gland and lateral to the internal jugular vein
  - If infected, wall may be thicker and enhance
- Most common branchial anomaly, accounting for 95% of lesions
- Branchial cleft anomalies may be cysts, fistulae or sinuses

Imaging Findings
General Features
- Best imaging clue: **Cystic mass** displaces submandibular gland anteromedially, carotid space medially and sternomastoid muscle posterolaterally
- Ovoid cystic mass at angle of mandible
- Other locations 2nd BCC may be found
  - Superiorly into parapharyngeal space (PPS) or carotid space (CS)
  - Inferior along anterior surface of infrahyoid carotid space
CT Findings
- Well-circumscribed, non-enhancing, ovoid cystic mass
- If infected, wall is thicker and enhances with surrounding soft tissues appearing "dirty" (cellulitis)
MR Findings
- T1 signal depends on protein content
  - If low, hypointense; if high, may become hyperintense
- Hyperintense on T2 images
- T1 C+ MR shows no enhancement if uninfected

Second Branchial Cleft Cyst

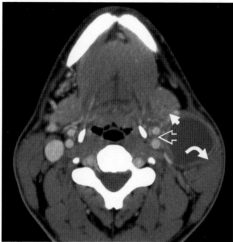

2nd branchial cleft cyst (BCC). CECT shows a round, low-density mass with a thick, enhancing wall. This 2nd BCC manifests the classic displacement pattern by pushing submandibular gland anteromedially (arrow), carotid space medially (open arrow) and sternomastoid muscle posterolaterally (curved arrow).

Imaging Recommendations
- Either CT or MR can easily suggest this diagnosis
- Contrast is used to aid in differentiation from a solid mass

Differential Diagnosis: Cystic Neck Mass
Cystic Hygroma
- **Multilocularity** is common
- If unilocular, may be difficult to differentiate from 2nd BCC if it occurs in location typical for 2nd BCC
Thymic Cyst
- Cyst is inferior in cervical neck
- Centered in lateral visceral space
Benign Reactive Lymph Node
- Solid lesion with central enhancement; often multiple
Cystic Vagal Schwannoma
- Tumor centered behind carotid space with displacement of IJV an ICA expected
- Cystic schwannoma has thick, enhancing wall
Necrotic Malignant Adenopathy
- Solid lesion, or necrotic with thick, enhancing wall
- Occasionally necrotic adenopathy may have cystic appearance similar to 2nd BCC
  - Papillary carcinoma of the thyroid malignant nodes may be cystic

Pathology
General
- General Path Comments
  - Squamous epithelial-lined cyst often with lymphoid tissue in wall
  - Presence of lymphoid tissue suggests epithelial rests may be entrapped within cervical lymph nodes during embryogenesis

Second Branchial Cleft Cyst

- Embryology
  - Branchial apparatus is anlagen of many structures of H & N
  - 2nd branchial arch overgrows the second, third, and fourth clefts, forming a cavity called the cervical sinus
  - Completed by 6-7 weeks gestation
  - Failure of obliteration of cervical sinus results in 2nd branchial cleft remnants, either a cyst, sinus or fistulae
  - 2nd branchial cleft fistula extends from the SCM muscle, through the carotid artery bifurcation and terminates in tonsillar fossa
- Etiology-Pathogenesis
  - Failure of obliteration of cervical sinus, leading to a 2nd BCC
- Epidemiology
  - **2nd BCC** account for **> 90%** of all branchial cleft anomalies

Gross Path-Surgical Features
- Well-defined cyst, lateral to the carotid sheath
- Filled with cheesy material or serous, mucoid or purulent fluid

Microscopic Features
- Squamous epithelial-lined cyst
- Lymphoid infiltrate in wall, often in form of germinal centers

Clinical Issues
Presentation
- Principal presenting symptom: Mass at angle of mandible
- Other symptoms
  - Intermittent, soft, painless, compressible lateral neck mass
  - 1-10 cm in diameter
  - May get larger with upper respiratory infection
  - If infected, mass becomes painful
- Age of presentation: Teenage years to young adult

Natural History
- If untreated, may become repeatedly infected and inflamed, making surgical resection more difficult

Treatment
- Complete surgical resection is treatment of choice
- Surgeon must dissect around the cyst bed to exclude the possibility of an associated fistula or tract
- If a tract goes superomedially, it passes through carotid bifurcation into the crypts of the facial (palatine) tonsil
- If a tract goes inferiorly, it passes along the anterior carotid space, reaching the skin in the supraclavicular area
  - If fistula present, it is seen at birth
  - Mucoid secretions are emitted from the skin opening

Prognosis
- Excellent if lesion is completely resected

Selected References
1. Nakagawa T et al: Differential diagnosis of a lateral cervical cyst and solitary cystic lymph node metastases of occult thyroid papillary carcinoma. J Laryngol Otol 115:240-2, 2001
2. Lev S et al: Imaging of cystic lesions: Radiol Clin North Am 38:1013-27, 2000
3. Harnsberger HR et al: Branchial cleft anomalies and their mimics: Computed tomographic evaluation. Radiology 152:739-48, 1984

Thyroglossal Duct Cyst

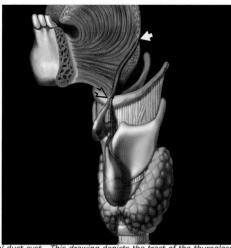

Thyroglossal duct cyst. This drawing depicts the tract of the thyroglossal duct as it passes from the cephalad foramen cecum (arrow) to the distal thyroid bed. The tract passes close to the mid-hyoid bone (open arrow). In the infrahyoid neck, the TGDC fades off midline to a paramedian location.

Key Facts
- Definition: Thyroglossal duct cyst (TGDC) = remnant of the thyroglossal duct found between foramen cecum of tongue base and thyroid bed of infrahyoid neck
- Classic imaging appearance: Cystic neck mass with thin rim of peripheral enhancement, located in midline
  - Can occur in tongue base, at hyoid bone, or embedded in infrahyoid strap muscles
  - The more inferior the TGDC, the more paramedian
- Most common congenital neck lesion
- Presents as asymptomatic **midline** or paramedian neck mass

Imaging Findings
General Features
- Best imaging clue: Midline cystic neck mass embedded in infrahyoid strap muscles
- Benign-appearing, cystic neck mass
- Wall may enhance if infected
- Location is important key to diagnosis
  - Above the hyoid bone, occurs at base of tongue or within posterior floor of mouth
  - At level of hyoid bone, found in midline abutting hyoid
    - May project into **pre-epiglottic space**
  - In the infrahyoid neck, **embedded in strap muscles**
- Carcinoma is associated with TGDC (< 1%)
- Differentiated thyroid Ca (85% papillary carcinoma)
CT Findings
- Low-density mass, occasionally septated
- If associated thyroid carcinoma, solid eccentric mass, often with calcifications, associated with the cyst

Thyroglossal Duct Cyst

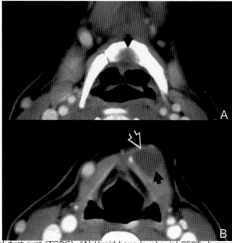

Thyroglossal duct cyst (TGDC). (A) Hyoid bone level axial CECT shows a bony notch in the mid-portion of the tripartite hyoid bone associated with small cystic mass. (B) CECT inferior to (A) reveals a TGDC nestled in the infrahyoid strap muscles (arrow). Beaking of the muscles over the cyst (open arrow) is common.

MR Findings
- Low signal on T1, hyperintense on T2
- No enhancement with T1 C+

Ultrasound Findings
- Anechoic midline neck mass

Imaging Recommendations
- TGDC in children have a classic clinical presentation
- May not require pre-operative imaging
- CT or MR more than adequate to task of defining nature and extent
- Imaging is recommended in most adults if the cyst is suprahyoid in location, if there is question about the diagnosis, if the mass is infected, or when there is a suspicion of associated carcinoma

Differential Diagnosis: Anterior Neck Mass

Lingual or Sublingual Thyroid
- Ectopic thyroidal tissue will enhance and appear solid on CT/MR

Lymphadenopathy
- Usually multiple, paramedian, non-cystic unless necrotic

Dermoid of the Tongue
- Dermoid will be fat density on CT, hyperintense on T1 MR

Mixed Laryngocele
- Laryngocele can be traced back to laryngeal origin
- Laryngocele will not be embedded within strap muscles

Malignant Necrotic Node, Anterior Neck (Delphian Chain)
- May be difficult to differentiate necrotic node from infected TGDC

Pathology

General
- Embryology-Anatomy
  - Thyroglossal duct originates near the foramen cecum

Thyroglossal Duct Cyst

- - Descends through the base of the tongue, the floor of the mouth, around or through the hyoid bone area, anterior to the strap muscles, to the final position in the thyroid bed anterior to thyroid or cricoid cartilage
- Etiology-Pathogenesis
  - Failure of involution of the thyroglossal duct and persistent secretion of the epithelial cells lining the duct result in TGDC
  - TGDC can occur anywhere along the route of descent
  - Ectopic thyroid tissue can also occur anywhere along this course
- Epidemiology
  - TGDC is most common congenital neck mass

Gross Pathologic, Surgical Features
- Smooth, benign-appearing cyst, usually with a tract to the hyoid bone ± the foramen cecum

Microscopic Features
- Cyst lined by respiratory or squamous epithelium
- Small deposits of thyroid tissue commonly associated

Clinical Issues

Presentation
- Principal presenting symptom: Midline neck mass
- Other presenting symptoms: Recurrent, soft, mobile, asymptomatic, midline or slightly paramedian neck mass
- Often has a history of recurrent, intermittent neck swelling, or multiple prior incision and drainage procedures
- Age of presentation: < 10 years (90%); 10% are 20-35 year olds
- Physical examination: When the TGDC surrounds the hyoid bone, it moves with tongue movement

Natural History
- Recurrent, intermittent swelling of the mass, usually following a minor upper respiratory infection

Treatment
- Complete surgical resection, termed a **Sistrunk procedure**
  - Entire cyst and midline portion of hyoid bone is resected and tract to foramen cecum dissected free, to prevent recurrence

Prognosis
- Excellent with complete surgical resection

Selected References
1. Glastonbury CM et al: The CT and MR imaging features of carcinoma arising in thyroglossal duct remnants. AJNR 4:770-4, 2000
2. Radkowski D et al: Thyroglossal duct remnants. Arch Otolaryngol Head Neck Surg 117:1378-81, 1991
3. Reede DL et al: CT of thyroglossal duct cysts. Radiology 157:121-5, 1985

Cystic Hygroma

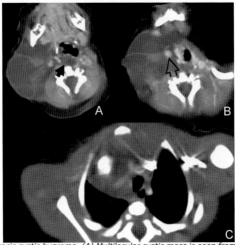

Cervicothoracic cystic hygroma. (A) Multilocular cystic mass is seen from the level of the hyoid bone (A) to the upper mediastinum (C) on these 3 axial CECT images. A thumb of cystic hygroma projects into the retropharyngeal space (arrow, A). Common carotid artery is surrounded by the lesion (open arrow, B).

Key Facts
- Synonyms: Lymphangioma, vasculolymphatic malformation
- Definition: Cystic Hygroma (CH) is a non-encapsulated **lymphatic rest**
  - CH is most common of the lymphangiomas (there are 4 types)
  - Transpatial (multiple contiguous spaces) congenital neck mass
- Classic imaging appearance: Uni- or multiloculated, non-enhancing, cystic neck mass that invaginates and insinuates between vessels and other normal structures
- Other key facts
  - Lymphangiomas are a spectrum of lesions, differentiated by size of lymphatic channels within lesion
  - 80% of CH occur in neck or lower face
  - Etiology is abnormal development of lymphatic sacs
  - Composed of dilated lymphatic spaces

Imaging Findings
General Features
- Best imaging clue: **Insinuating, multilocular** cystic mass
- Usually found in multiple contiguous spaces, i.e., is **transpatial**
- Common in the posterior cervical space of infrahyoid neck, masticator and submandibular spaces of suprahyoid neck
- Tends to invaginate between normal structures without mass effect
- May be unilocular or multilocular
CT Findings
- Hypodense, poorly-circumscribed, non-enhancing cystic mass
MR Findings
- Low T1 signal, high T2 signal
  - May be hyperintense on T1 suggesting prior hemorrhage
- T1 C+ images show no enhancement or subtle rim enhancement

Cystic Hygroma

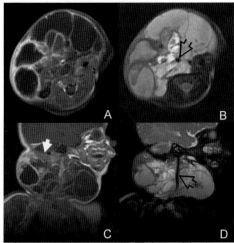

Cervical cystic hygroma. Axial T1 C+ (A) & T2 (B) show multilocular cystic transpatial mass in this infant. Open arrow: carotid artery. Sagittal T1 C+ (C) & T2 (D) images again reveal cystic hygroma surrounding carotid (open arrow). Arrow in (C) shows enhancing tissue due to mixed venous vascular components in rest.

 o If areas of enhancement seen, most likely a mixed rest with venous vascular or hemangiomatous components

Ultrasound Findings
- Primarily hypo- or anechoic transpatial mass
- May be septated and multilocular
- May be detected on prenatal U/S
- Fluid-fluid levels suggest prior hemorrhage

Imaging Recommendations
- MR, especially T2 images, is most helpful
- High signal on T2 makes definition of local extension, proximity to normal structures, including vessels, straightforward

Differential Diagnosis: Cystic Neck Mass

2nd Branchial Cleft Cyst
- Ovoid unilocular mass at angle of mandible with characteristic displacement pattern (see "2nd BCC")

Thyroglossal Duct Cyst
- Ovoid unilocular cystic mass in midline in vicinity of hyoid bone
- Engulfed by infrahyoid strap muscles

Neck Abscess
- Thick, enhancing wall surrounds fluid collection
- Adjacent soft tissues have cellulitis, myositis and fasciitis

Pathology

General
- Genetics
  - o Frequently seen in Turner's syndrome, Noonan's syndrome, fetal alcohol syndrome and other less common syndromes
- Embryology

Cystic Hygroma

- o   Failure of embryologic fusion between primordial lymph sac and central venous system
- o   Arise from **sequestrations** of embryonic lymph sacs
- Etiology-Pathogenesis
  - o   CH comes from rests of embryonic lymph sacs left behind during embryogenesis
- Epidemiology
  - o   May be sporadic or part of congenital syndromes, most notably Turner's syndrome

Gross Pathologic, Surgical Features
- Smooth, gray, glistening, non-encapsulated mass

Microscopic Features
- Dilated lymphatic spaces, with septations that vary in thickness
- May have dilated, thin-walled vessels within the mass
- 4 types of lymphangioma
  - o   **Cystic hygroma**, cavernous lymphangioma, capillary lymphangioma, and vasculolymphatic malformation
  - o   Both lymphatic and venous vascular malformation may occur in same lesion = **vasculolymphatic malformation**
  - o   Size of the lymphatic spaces within the lesion differentiates one from another
  - o   Imaging cannot differentiate the subtypes of lymphangioma

Clinical Issues

Presentation
- Principal presenting symptom: Neck mass
- Age of presentation: Most commonly present at birth or within first two years of life; small early adult group
- Physical exam: Soft, compressible, painless neck mass, usually in the posterior cervical space or submandibular space
- May involve mucosal surface of oral cavity, tongue or airway
- Respiratory compromise is present for large airway mucosal lesions

Treatment
- Surgical resection if the lesion is isolated, unilocular and not associated with major vessels or nerves
- Sclerosing agents may be used with extensive, transpatial lesions with significant vascular component

Prognosis
- High local recurrence rate due to incomplete surgical resection

Selected References
1.   Koeller KK et al: congenital cystic masses of the neck: Radiologic-pathologic correlation. RadioGraphics 19:121-46, 1999
2.   Zadvinskis DP et al: congenital malformations of the cervico-thoracic lymphatic system: Embryology and pathogenesis. RadioGraphics 12:1175-89, 1992
3.   Bill AA et al: A unified concept of lymphangioma and cystic hygroma. Surg Gynecol Obstet 120:79-86, 1965

Cervical Thymic Cyst

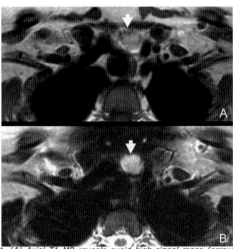

Thymic cyst. (A) Axial T1 MR reveals ovoid high-signal mass (arrow) in inferior visceral space. High signal is due to the high protein content of the thymic cyst. (B) On T2 MR the thymic cyst (arrow) is seen as a high-signal, well-circumscribed mass nestled among the great vessels (arrow) of the low visceral space.

Key Facts
- Synonym: Persistent **thymopharyngeal duct**
- Definition: Cervical thymic cyst (CTC) = cystic neck mass found along course of embryologic tract from pyriform sinus to mediastinum which results from failure of complete involution of thymopharyngeal duct
- Classic imaging appearance: Non-enhancing cyst, found near the carotid sheath from the angle of the mandible to the thoracic inlet
  - Solid components along cyst wall contain aberrant thymic tissue, lymphoid aggregates or parathyroid tissue
- Larger CTC may present as a dumbbell cervicothoracic mass
- **Hassall's corpuscles** in cyst wall confirm diagnosis of CTC

Imaging Findings
General Features
- Best imaging clue: Cystic mass in the lateral infrahyoid neck
- Remnants of the thymopharyngeal duct can occur from the angle of the mandible to the chest, so location is variable
- Usually lateral in location, paralleling sternocleidomastoid muscle and close to carotid sheath
- Primarily cystic, but nodules of aberrant thymic tissue, lymphoid aggregates or parathyroid glands may be seen as solid components
CT Findings
- Low-density, non-enhancing, unilocular, lateral neck mass
MR Findings
- Low signal on T1, high-signal T2
- No enhancement T1 C+ images
U/S Findings
- Anechoic lateral neck mass

Cervical Thymic Cyst

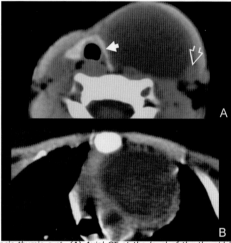

Cervicothoracic thymic cyst. (A) Axial CT at the level of the thyroid bed shows a unilocular cyst centered in the lateral neck between the thyroid lobe (arrow) and the carotid space (open arrow). (B) The thymic cyst is seen to dumbbell into the anterior upper mediastinum on this CT through upper chest.

Imaging Recommendations
- CT or MR are preferable to U/S, as long length of lesion and intrathoracic component may not be detected with U/S alone
- CTC may enlarge with Valsalva maneuver

Differential Diagnosis: Lateral Cystic Neck Mass
Branchial Cleft Remnants
- 2nd, 3rd and 4th branchial cleft cysts (BCC)
- 2nd BCC usually at angle of mandible, when lower may mimic CTC
- 3rd BCC in posterior cervical space
- 4th BCC communicates with inferior pyriform sinus

Unilocular Cystic Hygroma
- Usually in posterior cervical space, not related to carotid sheath
- Insinuates spaces available to it; often with complex shape
- Giant infantile cervicothoracic cystic hygroma may closely mimic large, infantile, cervicothoracic thymic cyst

Suppurative Lymph Nodes
- Nodal wall enhances; usually thick
- Usually multiple, bilateral

Pathology
General
- Embryology
  - Thymus and parathyroid glands arise from the third and fourth pharyngeal pouches, respectively
  - Embryologic migration follows a caudal course along the thymopharyngeal duct during first trimester
  - **Thymopharyngeal duct** arises from pyriform sinus and descends into mediastinum

Cervical Thymic Cyst

- Etiology-Pathogenesis
  - Remnants of thymopharyngeal duct or thymic rests result in CTC
- Epidemiology
  - Only 1/3 present after first decade
  - Slightly more common in boys
  - Rare lesion as compared with other congenital neck masses

Gross Pathologic, Surgical Features
- Smooth, thin-walled, < 1 cm in diameter cervical cyst, often with cephalad fibrous strand
- Filled with brownish fluid
- Cyst wall may be nodular, with foci of lymphoid tissue, parathyroid or thymic remnants

Microscopic Features
- **Hassall's corpuscles** in cyst wall confirm diagnosis
- Lymphoid tissue, parathyroid or thymic tissue may be in cyst wall
- Cholesterol crystals and granulomas are frequently found in cyst wall, probably from prior hemorrhage

Clinical Issues

Presentation
- Principal presenting symptom: Asymptomatic lateral neck mass
- Age at presentation: 2/3 present in first decade
- Large, infantile, cervicothoracic thymic cyst: Respiratory compromise
- Rarely may be associated with disordered calcium metabolism, if parathyroid component is functioning

Treatment
- Complete surgical resection
- Recurrence rate is high if entire remnant is not resected

Prognosis
- Excellent, with complete surgical resection

Selected References
1. Koeller KK et al: Congenital cystic masses of the neck: radiologic-pathologic correlation. RadioGraphics 19:121-46, 1999
2. Burton EM et al: Cervical thymic cysts: CT appearance of two cases including a persistent thymopharyngeal duct cyst. Pediatric Radiology 25:363-5, 1994
3. Tovi F et al: The aberrant cervical thymus: embryology, pathology, and clinical implications. Am J Surg 136:631-7, 1978

Rhabdomyosarcoma

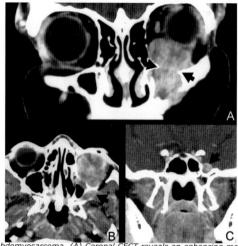

Orbital rhabdomyosarcoma. (A) Coronal CECT reveals an enhancing mass centered on inferior rectus muscle. Tumor has eroded through anterior orbital floor (arrows) into maxillary sinus. (B) Axial CECT shows perineural V2 tumor filling pterygopalatine fossa (arrow). (C) Perineural tumor (arrow) in foramen rotundum.

Key Facts
- Definition: Soft-tissue sarcoma of skeletal cells
- Classic imaging appearance: Heterogeneous mass with mild, diffuse enhancement and local bone destruction
- Most common childhood soft-tissue sarcoma
  - Head and neck most common location (40%)
- Three categories: Orbital, parameningeal & other H & N locations

Imaging Findings
General Features
- Best imaging clue: Invasive heterogeneous mass
- May have associated osseous destruction or intracranial extension
- Up to 30% have hemorrhage
- Orbit > nasopharynx > temporal bone > sinonasal cavity

CT Findings
- NCCT: Isodense with brain/muscle with indistinct margins
- CECT: Variable enhancement; usually mild, diffuse

MR Findings
- Poorly-defined, heterogeneous mass
- Isointense to muscle on T1
- Hyperintense to muscle on T2
- T1 C+ shows diffuse enhancement following contrast
- **Intracranial/perineural spread common**

Imaging Recommendations
- **MR** is imaging **tool of choice** in parameningeal rhabdomyosarcoma
- T1 C+ fat sat skull base/orbit to evaluate intracranial extension

Differential Diagnosis: H&N Tumors in Young Adults
Plexiform Neurofibroma
- Imaging: Heterogeneously hyperintense T2; strong enhancement

Rhabdomyosarcoma

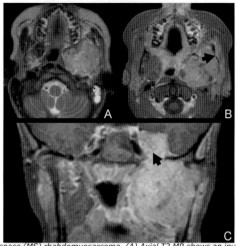

Masticator space (MS) rhabdomyosarcoma. (A) Axial T2 MR shows an invasive tumor filling the MS. (B) T1 C+ fat sat image reveals tumor destruction of mandible (arrow). (C) Coronal T1 C+ fat sat image shows perineural V3 tumor going through large foramen ovale (arrow).

- o   Well-circumscribed margins, no osseous destruction
- • Clinical: NF-2

Non-Hodgkin Lymphoma
- • Imaging: Homogeneous, enhancing skull base lesion
- • Clinical: Young adults

Nasopharyngeal Carcinoma
- • Imaging: Heterogeneous, enhancing PMS mass; skull base invasion
- • Clinical: Older age group but may affect the young

Synovial Sarcoma
- • Imaging: Well-defined mass with cysts, hemorrhage, Ca++
- • Loculation: Hypopharynx, masticator space and parapharyngeal space

Pathology
General
- • General Path Comments
  - o   Divided into three groups
    - ▪ Parameningeal (middle ear, nasopharynx, sinonasal)
    - ▪ Orbital
    - ▪ Other H & N locations
- • Genetics
  - o   PAX3-FKHR & variant PAX7-FKHR gene fusions observed
- • Etiology-Pathogenesis
  - o   Arise from primitive mesenchymal cells committed to skeletal muscle differentiation
  - o   Three types: Embryonal, differentiated & alveolar
- • Epidemiology
  - o   20% of all sarcomas; most common sarcoma of H & N
  - o   40% of rhabdomyosarcoma arise in H & N
  - o   Most common sarcoma in pediatric, adolescent and young adults

Rhabdomyosarcoma

Gross Pathologic, Surgical Features
- Pink/gray mass with frequent areas of hemorrhage and necrosis
- May be grape-like (sarcoma botryoides)

Microscopic Features
- Malignant tumor of skeletal cells = **rhabdomyoblasts** in varying stages of differentiation
- Three histologic forms of rhabdomyosarcoma
  - Embryonal, pleomorphic & alveolar
  - Embryonal - common in H & N
    - Primitive cellular structure corresponding to early stages of development of skeletal muscle cell
    - Round or elongated cells; hyperchromatic, irregular nuclei with numerous mitoses; cytoplasm with vacuolation (glycogen)
- Immunohistochemistry: positive for desmin & vimentin

Staging Criteria (Controversial)
- Intergroup Rhabdomyosarcoma Study Group (IRSG)
  - Group I: Complete resection
  - Group II: Gross resection with microscopic residual
  - Group III: Incomplete resection
  - Group IV: Distant metastasis
- TNM: Tumor site, size (5 cm), local invasiveness, lymph nodes, distant metastases
- Low risk, intermediate risk and high risk

Clinical Issues

Presentation
- Depends on location
  - Orbit: Proptosis, decreased vision (optic nerve compression)
  - T-bone: Bloody discharge, otitis media & otorrhea
  - Sinonasal: Nasal obstruction, epistaxis
  - Other: Pain, swelling, mass & neurologic deficits
- Up to 55% of parameningeal-intracranial extension at presentation
- Most common 1st and 2nd decades (rare in adults)

Natural History
- Depends on location & staging; parameningeal has worst prognosis
- Lymph node metastases in 30% cases
- Distant metastases: Lungs and bones

Treatment
- Treatment: Combined therapy—surgery, XRT & chemotherapy

Prognosis
- Prognosis determined by clinical group, stage, histology, age at diagnosis - more favorable in children & adolescents
- Orbital - best prognosis (80-90% disease-free survival)
- Parameningeal - worst prognosis (40-50% disease-free survival)

Selected References
1. Feldman BA: Rhabdomyosarcomas of the head and neck. Laryngoscope 92:424-40, 1992
2. Yousem DM et al: Rhabdomyosarcomas in the head and neck: MR imaging evaluation. Radiology 177:683-6, 1990
3. Latack JT et al: Imaging of rhabdomyosarcomas of the head and neck. AJNR 8:353-9, 1987

Index of Diagnoses

NOTES

NOTES

NOTES

NOTES